Pulmonary Manifestations of Primary Immunodeficiency Diseases

Seyed Alireza Mahdaviani • Nima Rezaei
Editors

Pulmonary Manifestations of Primary Immunodeficiency Diseases

Springer

Editors
Seyed Alireza Mahdaviani
Pediatric Respiratory Diseases
Research Center, National Research
Institute of Tuberculosis
and Lung Diseases (NRITLD)
Shahid Beheshti University
of Medical Sciences
Tehran
Iran

Nima Rezaei
Research Center for Immunodeficiencies
Children's Medical Center
Tehran University of Medical
Sciences (TUMS)
Tehran
Iran

Network of Immunity in Infection
Malignancy and Autoimmunity (NIIMA)
Universal Scientific Education
and Research Network (USERN)
Tehran
Iran

Department of Immunology
School of Medicine
Tehran University of Medical Sciences
Tehran
Iran

ISBN 978-3-030-00879-6 ISBN 978-3-030-00880-2 (eBook)
https://doi.org/10.1007/978-3-030-00880-2

Library of Congress Control Number: 2018963301

This Springer imprint is published by the registered company Springer Nature Switzerland AG
The registered company address is: Gewerbestrasse 11, 6330 Cham, Switzerland

Preface

Primary immunodeficiency diseases (PIDs) are a heterogeneous group of disorders, characterized by increased susceptibility of infections, mainly in respiratory system. More than 350 different PIDs have already been recognized and classified into 8 groups. Many patients with PIDs firstly present with upper and lower respiratory tract manifestations, while delay in diagnosis can lead to morbidity and even mortality of affected patients. Our understanding on PIDs is rapidly improving, which helps us in making definite diagnosis managing more efficiently.

This book is an attempt to gather the most recent advances in pulmonary problems of patients with PIDs, where diagnosis and management of pulmonary manifestations have also been discussed. The first chapter gives an overview on PIDs and pulmonary manifestations of PIDs, in general. In Chaps. 2, 3, 4, 5, 6, 7, 8, and 9, pulmonary manifestations of eight groups of PIDs are discussed in detail. Treatment of pulmonary manifestations of PIDs is also presented in Chap. 10.

We would like to acknowledge the expertise of all contributors for generously giving their time and considerable effort in preparing their respective chapters. We are also grateful to Springer for giving us the opportunity to publish this book, and we hope that this book will be comprehensible, cogent, and manageable for physicians and nurses, who wish to learn more about pulmonary manifestations of PIDs.

Tehran, Iran — Nima Rezaei
Tehran, Iran — Seyed Alireza Mahdaviani

Acknowledgment

We would like to express our gratitude to the technical editor of this book, Dr. Sara Hanaei.

Nima Rezaei
Seyed Alireza Mahdaviani

Contents

Chapter 1
General Considerations

Mikko Seppänen and Nima Rezaei

1.1 Lungs Are an Immunologic Battlefield

Focus on the most obvious function of our lungs, gas exchange, has greatly shaped the practice of respiratory medicine. However, blood contributes approximately 40–50% of the weight of human lungs [1]. Our lungs harbor a wide range of hematopoietic progenitors, with the capacity to repopulate the bone marrow after irradiation. The lung is also an especial primary site for platelet biogenesis from megakaryocytes, responsible for the origin of 50% of our platelets [2]. For blood to oxygenate, circulating blood cells and their products traverse through the respiratory zone of lungs. Daily, over 10,000 L of ambient air in our lungs constantly and effectively exposes our immune system to the outside environment through an alveolar surface that exceeds 100–150 m^2 in a human adult, which consists the largest epithelial surface in the body [3]. Consequently, our respiratory tract is equipped

M. Seppänen (✉)
Rare Disease Center, New Children's Hospital, University of Helsinki and Helsinki University Hospital, Helsinki, Finland

Adult Primary Immunodeficiency Clinic, Inflammation Center, University of Helsinki and Helsinki University Hospital, Helsinki, Finland
e-mail: mikko.seppanen@hus.fi

N. Rezaei
Research Center for Immunodeficiencies, Children's Medical Center, Tehran University of Medical Sciences, Tehran, Iran

Network of Immunity in Infection, Malignancy and Autoimmunity (NIIMA), Universal Scientific Education and Research Network (USERN), Tehran, Iran

Department of Immunology, School of Medicine, Tehran University of Medical Sciences, Tehran, Iran
e-mail: rezaei_nima@tums.ac.ir

S. A. Mahdaviani, N. Rezaei (eds.), *Pulmonary Manifestations of Primary Immunodeficiency Diseases*, https://doi.org/10.1007/978-3-030-00880-2_1

with a highly specialized localized immune system with an effective mucociliary clearance machinery and specialized type II alveolar cells which produce innate immunity surfactant proteins and cytokines. Type II cells in turn trigger resident immune cells like alveolar macrophages and dendritic cells as well as the highly complex adaptive immunity [4]. Any breaches in immunity, barrier, and clearance functions of the local or systemic immunity predispose our lungs to impaired, prolonged, and/or hyperactivated immune reactions [5]. Thus, it is no wonder that many genetic and acquired immune-mediated diseases affect the human respiratory system.

1.1.1 Introduction to Primary Immunodeficiency Diseases

Many primary immunodeficiency diseases (PIDs) firstly present with lung and upper airway manifestations and symptoms, giving the well-versed practicing pulmonologist a unique opportunity to suspect these often highly debilitating and potentially fatal diseases, with no delay or undue ensuing mortality. PIDs are inherited, mostly monogenic and systemic disorders of immunity. Systemic PIDs are essentially diseases of hematopoietic immune cells with genetically impaired or dysregulated function. An increasing number of PIDs are due to impaired immunity caused by genetic dysregulation of immune pathways by organ-specific tissues like the skin [6]. Tissue-specific pulmonary PIDs (e.g., surfactant protein deficiencies, cystic fibrosis, primary ciliary dyskinesia syndromes) could be envisaged but are presently not classified as such and are thus outside the scope of this book, except when differential diagnostic issues are discussed.

If suspecting PID, irrespective of a patient's age, one should always exclude human immunodeficiency virus (HIV) infection and obtain careful information on received immunosuppressive treatments. If the onset of matching symptoms or findings precedes any immunomodulatory therapy, especially if the ensuing depth of given immunosuppression exceeds that normally seen, one should consider whether a patient's immunodeficiency is truly secondary or indeed primary. In a rapidly growing number of PIDs and patients, the onset seems delayed well into adult life [7].

Currently, there are more than 350 known PIDs. In variable combinations, these diseases predispose individuals to infections, inflammatory complications, and malignancies, often hematologic or virally induced cancers. Dysregulated acquired immunity leads to autoimmunity and severe early-onset atopy, while dysregulated innate immunity may lead to autoinflammation and impaired barrier function. Similar to blood disorders, systemic PIDs often give rise to various hematologic findings like cytopenias; deficient, disorganized, or hypoplastic lymphatic system; lymphoproliferation; myelodysplasia; or bone marrow failure. Biopsies may further reveal aberrant immune reactions like granulomas or hemophagocytosis (Fig. 1.1).

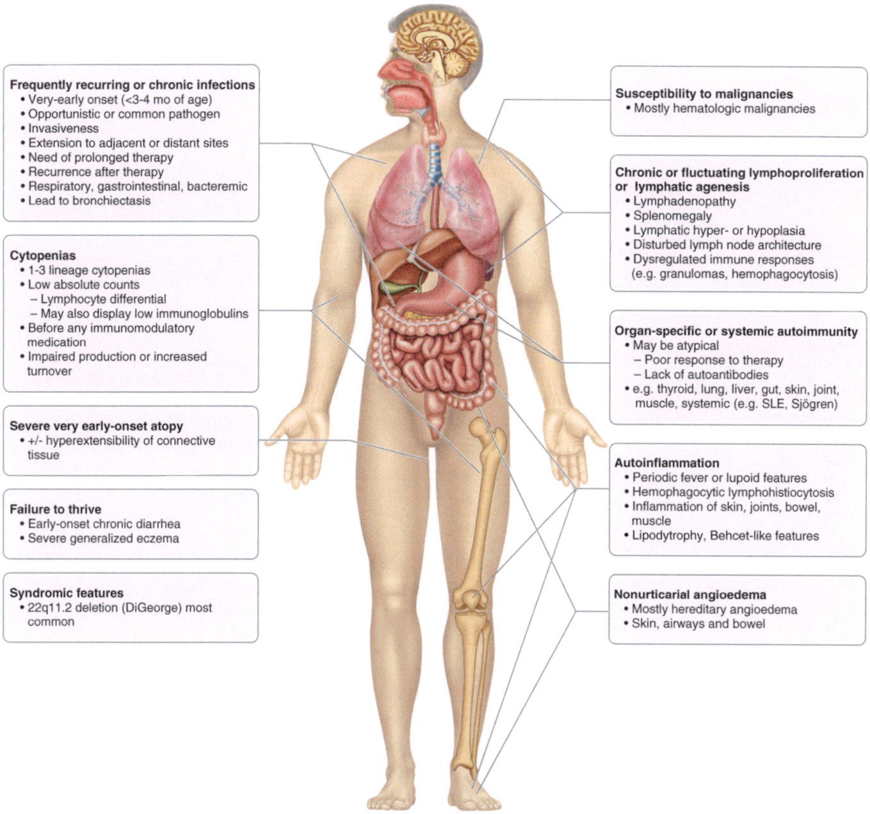

Fig. 1.1 Common features in primary immunodeficiency diseases. Usually ≥2 features present (except in hereditary angioedema). If SCID is suspected in an infant, PID doctor should be consulted urgently

1.1.2 Classification of Primary Immunodeficiency Diseases

Although there are no universally accepted classification systems for PIDs, the most commonly accepted one, endorsed by the International Union of Immunological Societies (IUIS), divides PIDs into eight different categories and further subcategories. IUIS classification is based on the affected cell types (e.g., B-cells, T-cells, and phagocytes), arms of immunity (e.g., antibodies, complement system, intrinsic and innate immunity), affected signaling pathways (e.g., type I interferons, IL-12-IFN-γ axis), or predominant clinical manifestations (e.g., immune dysregulation diseases, autoinflammatory diseases) [6, 8]. However, due to the complex nature of our immunity, a known genetic disease often has features from multiple disease groups. Helping clinical assessment, the defined PID categories commonly display pulmonary complications typical for either just one or a few categories (Tables 1.1, 1.2, and 1.3). IUIS maintains and updates regularly the list of known PIDs as well as

Table 1.1 Sentinel respiratory infections and their complications that most likely should result in screening for immunodeficiency

Infection	Setting	Note
Upper respiratory tract	Recurrent upper respiratory tract	In most PIDs with infection susceptibility
	Deep tissue infection	For example, mastoiditis after otitis media or tonsillar abscess in infant: MyD88/IRAK4, phagocyte, and antibody deficiencies
Severe viral infections	Interstitial pneumonitis	SCIDs, range of other CIDs (e.g., WAS, deficiencies of DOCK2, MALT1, CARD11, BCL10, TCRα, IL-21R, IKBKB, NIK, WIP) Innate and intrinsic immunity defects predisposing to severe viral infections (e.g., STAT1 AR-LOF, deficiencies of STAT2, IRF7, IFNAR2, CD16, MDA)
Pyogenic pneumonia	Failure to thrive	Susceptibility to a wide array of gram-positive and gram-negative microorganisms (also to viruses, fungi, parasites), interstitial pneumonitis: SCID and T-cell deficiencies
	Recurrent	Exclude a wide range of PIDs. Evaluate latest if >2–3 pneumonias during lifetime, earlier if warning signs: In various loci, leads to bronchiectasis or bronchial dilatation. In-between-episodes bronchial wall thickening, signs of cryptogenic organizing pneumonia, lymphoid interstitial pneumonitis, follicular bronchiolitis or granulomas atypical for sarcoidosis (i.e., low immunoglobulins/primary lymphopenia) Concurrent non-respiratory invasive infections, recurrent bacterial rhinosinusitis, very early-onset recurrent otitis media, adult-onset recurrent otitis media, slow systemic inflammatory response, or no demonstrable serum IgE
	Complicated	Pneumatocele formation: STAT3 deficiency Empyema or abscess: CGD, other phagocyte defects, STAT3 deficiency Bronchiectasis or interstitial pneumonitis: wide range of PIDs
	Early-onset (<3–4 mo)	Phagocyte deficiencies, MyD88/IRAK4 deficiency, SCID, T-cell deficiencies, congenital asplenia (*RPSA, NKX2–5*), FADD deficiency (functional hyposplenism)
Pyogenic sepsis +/– pneumonia/ meningitis	Recurrent	Antibody deficiencies, phagocyte deficiencies, complement deficiencies, SCID and various rather profound CIDs, MyD88/IRAK4 deficiency, CD40/CD40L deficiency, congenital asplenia (*RPSA, NKX2–5*), NEMO/*IKBKG*, GATA2 deficiency (+/-PAP), FADD deficiency
	Early-onset (<3–4 mo)	Like in pyogenic pneumonias above

(continued)

Table 1.1 (continued)

Infection	Setting	Note
Pneumocystis jirovecii	Pneumonia	SCIDs
		CID (e.g., DN *STAT3*; VODI; deficiencies of CD40, CD40L CARD 11, MALT1, BCL10, TCRα, MHC II, CD40/CD40L, IKBKB, IL-21R, NIK, MTHFD1, STAT5b; idiopathic CD4 deficiency)
		Syndromic CID (e.g., WAS, NEMO/*IKBKG*, *IKBA*, VODI, immune-osseous dysplasias, bone marrow failures like dyskeratosis congenita, Schaller sd)
		Reported rarely in XLA and CVID, also remember thymoma with hypogammaglobulinemia and anti-IFN-γ-autoantibodies
Aspergillus spp., other filamentous fungi	Invasive	Phagocyte defects: especially CGD (also mulch pneumonitis, *Nocardia, Paecilomyces, Trichosporon, S. aureus,* rare opportunistic bacteria, *Burkholderia cepacia, Serratia marcescens*), occasionally in SCN, LAD 1, Pearson sd
		Occasionally in SCID and CID; infections by other opportunistic and pyogenic pathogens predominate
		CID/T-cell def., e.g., *STAT3*-DN, *STAT1*-GOF GATA2 deficiency[a], WAS, 22q11.2 del, APLAID/*PLCG2*
		Also in idiopathic CD4 lymphopenia, thymoma with hypogammaglobulinemia (Good sd)
Dimorphic fungi[a]	Invasive	As part of MSMD: IL12Rβ1 and IFNγR1 deficiencies
		CID (e.g., *CARD9*, *STAT1*-GOF, *DOCK8*, *CD40LG*, GATA2 deficiency), idiopathic CD4 lymphopenia
Nontuberculous mycobacteria (NTM)	Mendelian Susceptibility to Mycobacterial Diseases (MSMD)	Affecting IL-12-IFN-γ -signaling (e.g., *IL12RB1*, *IL12*, *IFNGR1*, *IFNGR2*, AD *STAT1*-LOF): recurrent nontuberculous mycobacteriosis +/− salmonellosis, BCG-itis, osteomyelitis, *Klebsiella* spp., intracellular bacteria and viruses, invasive dimorphic fungi, leishmaniasis
		Dendritic cell deficiencies and GATA2 and AR/AD IRF8 def; AD *STAT1*-GOF, JAK1-LOF, deficiencies of Tyk2, ISG15, RORc
		Other: SCID, 22q11.2 del (especially BCGosis), CGD (especially BCGosis in *CYBB*), DN-*STAT3*, CD40L /CD40 def, anti-IFN-γ-autoantibodies

Always look also for sentinel nonpulmonary infections that alert to the possibility of PID in lung patient: cutaneous herpes simplex, chronic EBV viremia, EBV-associated lymphoproliferation, +/− hemophagocytic lymphohistiocytosis, chronic CMV, severe cutaneous papilloma virus or molluscum contagiosum, invasive or chronic mucocutaneous candidiasis, chronic *Cryptosporidium*, invasive *Neisseria*

[a]Histoplasmosis, coccidioidomycosis, paracoccidioidomycosis

Table 1.2 Typical infections in various impaired arms of immunity

	Specific (adaptive) immunity		Innate immunity		
Arm of immunity	B-cells	T-cell or combined	Phagocytic cells	Complement	Spleen[a]
Infectious complications	Upper respiratory Lung Gastrointestinal Skin, joint, meningeal Urinary tract	Systemic viral Gastrointestinal Pyogenic bacterial	Lymphadenitis Skin Gingivitis, aphtous Liver abscesses Lung abscesses Gastrointestinal Urinary tract	Bacteremic infections (encapsulated bacteria) Meningococcal and other pyogenic meningitides Disseminated *Neisseria gonorrhoeae*	Septic and meningeal by encapsulated pathogens, overwhelming postsplenectomy infection (OPSI)
Causative agents	**Pyogenic bacteria** Pneumococcus *Haemophilus influenzae* *Staphylococcus aureus* *Enterococcus* *Salmonella* *Campylobacter* *Mycoplasma* sp. **Parasites** *Giardia lamblia* **Viruses** Enteroviruses VZV, HSV	**Viruses** EBV,CMV, HPV,HSV, VZV Adenovirus, measles *Molluscum contagiosum.* **Pyogenic bacteria** *Pseudomonas* *Haemophilus* Pneumococcus *Campylobacter* Mycobacteria *Listeria* **Fungal:** *Candida,* *Aspergillus* *Pneumocystis jirovecii* **Parasites:** *Cryptosporidium*	**Bacterial** (often catalase+) *S. aureus* *Klebsiella* *Burkholderia cepacia Proteus* *Nocardia* *Serratia marcescens* **Fungal:** *Aspergillus* sp. Other filamentous fungi **Bacteria:** *Salmonella*	**Pyogenic bacteria** *Neisseriae* *S. pneumoniae* *H. influenzae*	*S. pneumoniae* *N. meningitidis* *H. influenzae* *E. coli* *S. aureus* Group B streptococci *P. aeruginosa* *C. canimorsus*

[a]Also asplenia and functional hyposplenism may be genetic or acquired

Table 1.3 Examples of noninfectious pulmonary complications in various primary immunodeficiency categories

PID category	Examples	Described noninfectious pulmonary complications besides bronchiectasis
1. Affect cellular and humoral immunity (combined immunodeficiencies, CID)	Severe combined immunodeficiencies (SCID) (T-B+ or T-B-)	ILD (exclude adenovirus, CMV, RSV, *P. jirovecii*)
	Somewhat less severe CID	ILD, LIP (*STAT5B*)
2. Combined immunodeficiencies with associated or syndromic features	Wiskott-Aldrich sd (WAS)	Pulmonary NHL
	Ataxia-telangiectasia (AT)	ILD, PF, aspiration
	Nijmegen breakage sd (NBS)	Pulmonary NHL
	22q11.2 sd (DiGeorge sd, velocardiofacial sd)	Structural defects, aspiration, tracheobronchomalacia
	Cartilage-hair hypoplasia (CHH)	PF, pulmonary NHL
	AD-HIES (DN-*STAT3*)	Pulmonary NHL
	Dyskeratosis congenita: AD-DKCs, AR-DKCs, XL-DKC	PF
	Anhidrotic ectodermodysplasia with immunodeficiency	ILD
	Hepatic veno-occlusive disease with immunodeficiency (VODI)	ILD
	CD40L and MST1 deficiencies	Pulmonary NHL
	Somech syndrome	PF
3. Predominantly antibody deficiencies	Agammaglobulinemias (B- or severely reduced)	ILD
	Hypogammaglobulinemias (usually B+)	ILD, GLILD, OP, LIP, PF, NSIP
4. Diseases of immune dysregulation	Familial hemophagocytic lymphohistiocytosis (FHL)	ILD and pulmonary NHL (*SH2D1A*)
	FHL with hypopigmentation: Hermansky-Pudlak type 2 (HPS2)	PF
	Regulatory T-cell defects (autoimmunity): IPEX, STAT3 GOF, LRBA def, CTLA-4 def	ILD, OP (*LRBA*), DIP, GLILD (*CTLA4*)
	Autoimmunity +/– lymphoproliferation: APECED, ITCH def	ILD, NSIP
	Autoimmune lymphoproliferative sds (ALPS)	Pulmonary NHL
	Susceptibility to EBV-associated lymphoproliferation	ILD (CD27 def)
5. Congenital phagocyte disorders Other nonlymphoid defects	Chronic granulomatous diseases (CGDs): XL-CGD, AR-CGDs	"Mulch pneumonitis" (hypersensitivity)
	GATA2 def	PAP, ILD, OP, GLILD
	Pulmonary alveolar proteinosis sds (PAP)	PAP, PF

(continued)

Table 1.3 (continued)

PID category	Examples	Described noninfectious pulmonary complications besides bronchiectasis
6. Defects of innate and intrinsic immunity	Predisposition to severe viral infections: AR STAT1 LOF	ILD
	Chronic mucocutaneous candidiasis	ILD and vascular aneurysms (*STAT1* GOF)
7. Autoinflammatory disorders	Type I interferonopathies: STING vasculopathy	ILD, NSIP
	Inflammasomopathies	ILD, NSIP (DIRA/*IL1RN*, APLAID/*PLCG2*)
	Non-inflammasome-related	ILD, alveolar hemorrhage (Copa defect)
	ADA2 deficiency	ILD, pulmonary vasculitis
8. Complement deficiencies	Deficiencies of circulating and membrane-associated factors	ILD (SLE), pulmonary embolism

DIP desquamative interstitial pneumonia, *GLILD* granulomatous-lymphocytic interstitial lung disease, *ILD* interstitial lung disease (not specified), *LIP* lymphocytic interstitial pneumonia, *NSIP* nonspecific interstitial pneumonia, *OP* organizing pneumonia, *PF* pulmonary fibrosis. *Bronchiectasis* seen in all groups at least occasionally, though rare in autoinflammatory disorders without antibody deficiency and severe congenital neutropenias, not listed separately

helpful flowcharts to ease their identification based on clinical and immunologic phenotype [8].

1.1.3 Epidemiology of Primary Immunodeficiency Diseases

Many erroneously believe that PIDs would be extremely rare, present exclusively in children, and incurable. The first two notions are true for the most severe PIDs, e.g., severe combined immunodeficiencies (SCIDs), early diagnosis of SCID and hematopoietic stem cell transplantation before 3.5 months of age lead to long-term survival in over 94% of SCID [9]. Currently, many countries screen newborns for SCIDs and note a rising prevalence in concurrently found milder PID cases. Even before SCID screening, the overall incidence rate of PIDs in national or regional registries exceeded 1 in 10,000 person years, while PID prevalence was close to 2:10,000 [10, 11].

Available worldwide data come from physician-confirmed regional registry data and large patient surveys covering up to 140,000 patients [12–16]. Due to pronounced geographic variability in their incidence, it is important to know the local epidemiology of autosomal recessive PIDs [13, 17]. While in highly consanguineous areas and genetic isolates, the combined prevalence of all PIDs may exceed 3:10,000; the prevalence of common variable immunodeficiency (CVID) exceeds 0.7:10,000 [13, 18]. Due to the relative commonness of X-linked PIDs, approximately 58% of PID patients are males [16]. Proportions of different PIDs thus considerably differ according to the geographical area. Higher proportions of various categories other than primarily antibody deficiencies are usually seen in consanguineous populations. In general, approximately 50% (ranging 20–75%) of PID patients have had predominantly antibody deficiencies, 14% (ranging 5–30%) other well-defined immunodeficiency syndromes, 8% (ranging 1–15%) autoinflammatory disorders, 8% (ranging 5–60%) combined immune deficiencies, 6% (ranging 4–35%) phagocytic disorders, 6% (ranging 2–15%) complement deficiencies, 4% (ranging 1–13%) disorders of immune dysregulation, and 1% (ranging 0–3%) innate immunity defects, while 1–5% have remained unclassified [12–16].

1.1.4 Primary Immunodeficiency Diseases Need to Be Diagnosed Early

Numerous studies have indicated that early diagnosis of PID reduces mortality and morbidity [9, 19]. As reported by various surveys, up to 60–75% of people affected with PID have survived to adulthood with improved diagnosis and therapy [12, 14, 16, 20], especially in CVID and some milder combined immunodeficiencies resembling that, which may present at any age [7, 18, 21]. In a European study on 2212 CVID patients, disease onset in two-thirds of the patients took place after 10 years of age [21]. In the majority, CVID was diagnosed in adulthood, and surprisingly in approximately 20% of patients, the diagnosis has been made at 50 years of age or later. In antibody deficiencies, a timely diagnosis and substitution therapy with IgG seem to improve the patient's prognosis in average by over 30 years [22]. Fascinatingly, even the innate immunity may be trained during an individual's life in order to provide a better protection [23]. Consequently, susceptibility to infections and complications due to dysregulated immunity from almost all genetic defects seems to be aggravated and accumulated with aging, emphasizing the need for timely diagnosis of PID. This may further save the patient from severe iatrogenic complications like disseminated infections caused by live attenuated vaccines and excessive immunosuppressive medication.

1.1.5 How to Recognize Primary Immunodeficiency Diseases

Early clinical recognition of a potential PID patient is largely based on "general impression, shape, and size" or "jizz" (Fig. 1.1) [24]. Most PID patients present with no immediately obvious clinical findings of an underlying disease. Typical "sentinel" (e.g., warning sign) airway infections are listed in Table 1.1, and extrapulmonary infections are listed as footnotes. It is noteworthy that such *sentinel infections* either present themselves in highly exposed surface niches of the body (lungs, skin, gut) or involve cunning pathogens which due to effective immune evasion establish chronic carrier state even in individuals with "normal" immunity. The nature of associated infections often reveals which so-called arms of immunity may be affected and thus how the patient should be screened for PID (Tables 1.1 and 1.2).

Examples of typical noninfectious pulmonary complications are listed in Table 1.3 and involve immune dysregulation. This, due to chronic ensuing inflammation, may further impair normal barrier function, like in bronchiectasis. When carefully analyzed, most PID patients commonly have general *sentinel immune dysregulatory features* in variable combinations. These general sentinel features in PIDs are depicted in Fig. 1.1. The presence of two or more of such features suggests a potential underlying PID. Furthermore, one can list numerous rare *sentinel clinical findings* that suggest more specifically some rare monogenic defects. Denoting these would more efficiently help in targeted testing. If found and necessary, it is recommended to consult further standard PID textbooks, local pediatric PID specialist, and clinical geneticist (Table 1.4). Moreover, if a monogenic disease is found, genetic counseling is needed [13, 25]. Due to its relative commonness, all pulmonologists should be able to discern CVID – almost invariably affecting the respiratory system – and screen for it (Fig. 1.2) [26].

Collectively, the most common complication in PIDs is susceptibility to recurrent, chronic, or opportunistic infections, most commonly in upper or lower airways. If the offending pathogen is opportunistic, e.g., of nature normally seen only in immunocompromised individuals, and the patient has no known secondary immunodeficiency, suspicion of PID may be straightforward. In SCID infants who almost totally lack T+/-B lymphocytes, often multiple opportunistic infections are found at presentation. Frequently, however, a single episode of respiratory infection like pneumonia and even inflammatory complications like those resembling sarcoidosis does not differ from those seen in individuals without immune compromise (Tables 1.1 and 1.3) [27, 28]. Therefore, keys to finding PIDs include remembering their existence and realizing their chronic, often systemic, and complex nature, all necessitating a carefully conducted review of lifelong patient and careful family history and findings from all organ systems (Fig. 1.1).

In childhood, atopy and PIDs may be present superficially rather similarly and display recurrent viral infections. Particularly in respiratory and skin infections, there is considerable overlap between recurrent infections in antibody deficient patients and in those with Th2-dominant immune response (Table 1.1) [29, 30]. Actually, if other members of a large family are perfectly healthy, this argues against common polygenic traits like chronic asthma or severe atopy that predispose to recurrent rhinosinusitis, skin infections, and – to an extent – to recurrent pneumonias. Early-onset severe atopy and life-threatening opportunistic infections are seen in Omenn syndrome (OS). OS is caused by various hypomorphic or "leaky" SCIDs, most often RAG1 and RAG2 deficiencies. In OS, expansion of oligoclonal T-cells and defective AIRE expression in thymus lead to autoreactivity, lymphadenopathy, hepatosplenomegaly, alopecia, exudative erythroderma, hypereosinophilia, and increased serum levels of IgE despite the absence of B-cells. The term leaky SCID

Table 1.4 Examples of sentinel early-onset clinical findings not directly related to immune dysfunction, which point toward rare monogenic primary immunodeficiency diseases

Hematologic	Lack of or dysmorphic lymphatic tissue (e.g., thymus, tonsils, lymphnodes, lymphangiectasia, primary lymphedema), congenital thrombopenia, thrombasthenia, small platelets, bleeding diathesis, bone marrow hypo-/dysplasia or failure, hepatomegaly, splenomegaly, asplenia
Nervous system	Microcephaly, macrocephaly, progressive neurologic deficits, psychomotor/ mental retardation, ataxia, porencephalic cysts, cerebral infarction, optic atrophy, retinal dystrophy and abnormalities, cataracts, strabismus, ptosis, coloboma, cranial nerve dysfunction, autism, sensorineural hearing loss, cerebellar hypoplasia, agenesis of corpus callosum, cerebral calcifications, cerebral palsy, focal cortical heterotopy, hydrocephalus, cerebral cysts, cerebral atrophy
Skin and appendages	Severe erythrodermia or eczema, congenital ichthyosis, ectodermal dysplasia, hypo-/anhidrosis, absent or disfigured teeth, enamel defects, delayed or incomplete eruption of teeth, microdontia, absent hair, hypotrichosis/fine and course or sparse hair, trichorrhexis (bamboo hair), congenital alopecia, premature graying of the hair, partial albinism/oculocutaneous hypopigmentation, skin hypo-/hyperpigmentation, poikiloderma, incontinentia pigmenti, telangiectasia, poor wound healing, ulcerative/vesicular skin lesions, nail dystrophy, photosensitivity, multiple pigmented nevi, lipodystrophy, reduced facial fat, palmar hyperkeratosis
Skeletal	Scapular spurring, anterior rib cupping, flared costochondral junctions, cartilage hypoplasia, joint hypermobility, osteopenia, high palate, kyphomelic dysplasia, metaphyseal dysplasia, spondylo- or multiple epiphyseal dysplasia, spondyloenchondrodysplasia, short limb dwarfism, scoliosis, craniosynostosis, osteopetrosis, vertebral anomalies, butterfly vertebrae, cervical spine instability, myopathy, hypotonia
Kidneys	Kidney and ureter anomalies (e.g., single/horseshoe kidney, duplication of the renal pelvis and ureter), nephrotic syndrome, abnormalities, kidney cysts, renal mesangial sclerosis, hypouricemia, reduced urinary uric acid excretion, kidney amyloidosis
Endocrine	Hypogonadism, ovarian dysgenesis, bifid uterus, testicular atrophy, genital hypoplasia, impaired fertility, growth hormone deficiency/insensitivity, hyperprolactinemia, neonatal diabetes, hypocalcemia, hypoparathyroidism, hypopituitarism, SIADH, adrenal gland cortical sclerosis
Various	Intrauterine or postnatal growth failure, short stature, atresia of the choanae, dysmorphic features (e.g., heart/conotruncal defects), cardiomyopathy, various facial anomalies like eyelid changes, broad and depressed nasal tip or bridge, low-set ears, velopharyngeal insufficiency, tracheoesophageal fistulae, asplenia, early-onset arteriosclerotic changes, hepatic veno-occlusive disease, esophageal dysmotility, Hirschprung disease, exocrine pancreatic insufficiency, vascular/ cerebral aneurysms

If sentinel clinical findings are found in a patient suspected to have PID, consulting standard general textbooks on PIDs, pediatric PID specialist, and clinical geneticist are strongly advisable

refers to incomplete mutation(s) in a typical SCID gene leading to small numbers of functional circulating B- and T-cells missing in classical SCIDs. In leaky SCID, the patient may also have a later age of onset of clinical symptoms [31]. Among typical associated autoimmune manifestations, hematologic cytopenias, hepatitis, vitiligo, and villous atrophy have been reported most commonly [32]. Severe early-onset

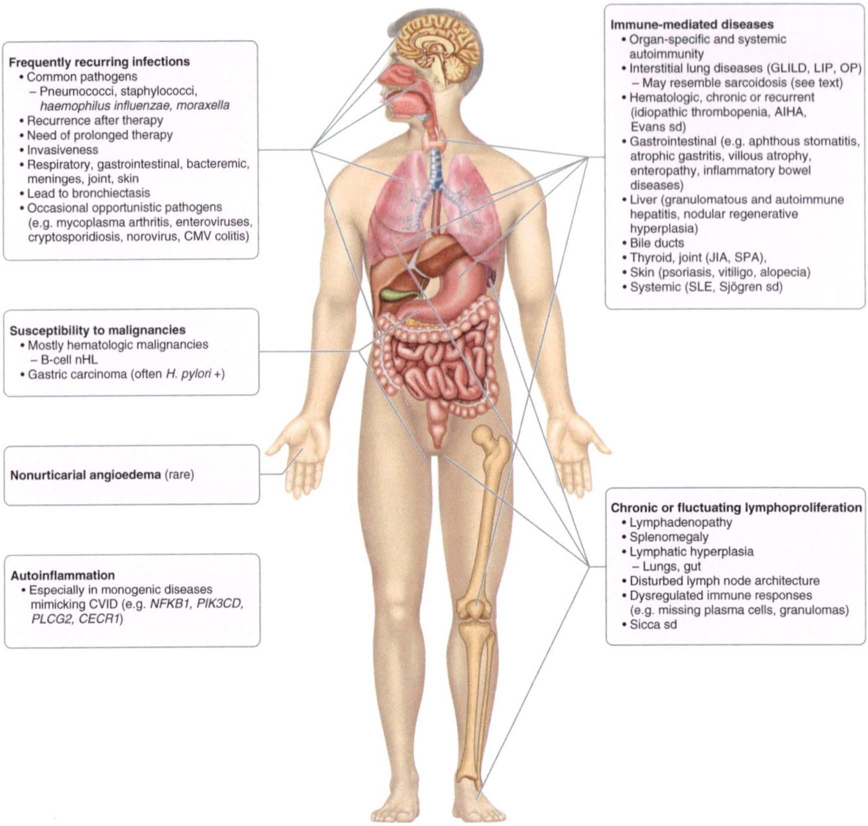

Fig. 1.2 Common features in common variable immunodeficiency (CVID). Usually ≥2 features present. Similar infections seen in other antibody deficiencies. GLILD granulomatous-lymphocytic interstitial lung disease, LIP lymphocytic interstitial pneumonia, OP organizing pneumonia, AIHA autoimmune hemolytic anemia, JIA juvenile idiopathic arthritis, SPA spondylarthropathy, SLE systemic lupus erythrematosus

allergy and atopy (or features resembling these) are among prominent presenting features in a variety of PIDs and are often accompanied by eosinophilia and/or increased concentrations of IgE in blood. These include hyper-IgE syndromes (HIES) like dominant negative (DN) *STAT3* mutations, Comel-Netherton syndrome, and PGM3 deficiency, as well as WAS and DOCK8, RLTPR, ARPC1B, and ERBIN deficiencies [6]. Also, rare monogenic disorders causing severe allergy as well as impaired keratinocyte-specific immunity or barrier function like SAM (severe dermatitis, multiple allergies, and metabolic wasting; *DSP*, *DSG1*) and Loeys-Dietz syndromes (TGFR1/2, SMAD3) may cause differential diagnostic challenges [33]. Each of these diseases has typical associated features and/or predisposes to severe opportunistic infections.

An increasing number of known PIDs display no or negligible infection susceptibility, while various inflammatory, also pulmonary, complications predominate

(Fig. 1.1, Table 1.3). Inflammatory pulmonary complications are reported in most PID categories, bronchiectasis in all of these. However, invasive sampling required for an exact diagnosis and targeted therapy in many of these complications might have been avoided, thus precluding exact diagnosis. Aiding in suspicion, recurrent or chronic infectious and inflammatory complications are frequently found at further sites like the gastrointestinal tract, blood, skin, and various organs but need to be looked for.

Especially in diseases causing immune dysregulation, there is great phenotypic, genotypic, and intrafamilial variability in penetrance, nature, and severity of complications. Also in PIDs with T-cell deficiency, even the observed opportunistic pathogens within a family may differ. Familial polygenic and monogenic traits may thus be difficult to tell apart, unless the index case presents clearly aberrant leukocyte subset counts or function in the used screening tests. Positive family history increases the probability that a patient has PID over tenfolds of a normal person. Family history should be obtained systematically, and any premature deaths in the family should alert the attending physician [34]. Family history may seem negligible due to factors like de novo mutations, incomplete penetrance, or X-linked inheritance, which may not always be apparent if family history has been obtained only for the immediate family. Factors like skewed X inactivation, uniparental disomy, or genetic anticipation may further complicate the assessment of family history [35]. In genetic anticipation, after the appearance of the mutation, each generation displays a more severe phenotype. In PIDs, this is seen in dyskeratosis congenita (DKC).

1.2 Pulmonary and Airway Manifestations in Primary Immunodeficiency Diseases

1.2.1 Upper Airway Infections

Recurrent upper respiratory tract infections (URTIs) like otitis media and rhinosinusitis are common in the general population and in, for example, atopic individuals. It is normal for a small child to have 6–8 episodes, with predisposing factors like atopy and frequent exposure to smokers or to circulating viral pathogens in day care, even 10–15 yearly URTIs [36]. In normal adults, 2–4 and with predisposing factors up to 5–8 yearly URTIs are common. Smoking impairs, for example, airway mucociliary clearance and antigen presentation by MHC molecules. Due to additional commonly seen factors impairing sinus drainage through narrow or closed osteomeatal complexes, even doctor-diagnosed chronic recurrent rhinosinusitis (CRRS) is seen in 1–2.4% of population, in most without any evident PID [37]. Thus, even chronic and recurrent noninvasive URTIs may poorly screen for PIDs. Moreover, the acronym SPUR (severe, persistent, unusual, or recurrent) has been suggested as an indication to check for primary and secondary antibody deficiency [38]. Early-onset nasal polyposis may point to PID; it has been described in cartilage-hair hypoplasia, hypogammaglobulinemia, TAP1/TAP2, and CD3γ deficiency [39]. However, highly recurrent URTIs and CRRS often precede or coincide with invasive lower respiratory tract infections (LRTIs) in PID patients. As a rule, PIDs mostly render patients susceptible to a variety of infections in multiple organs.

Recurrent, early-onset deep tissue upper airway infections like mastoiditis or severe tonsillitis do suggest antibody, MyD88, or IRAK4 deficiency [40]. MyD88-/IRAK4-deficient patients usually also suffer from early-onset episodes of bacterial meningitis, sepsis, arthritis, osteomyelitis caused by *Staphylococcus aureus*, streptococci, gram-negative bacteria, and occasionally septic pneumococcal pneumonias. A significant subset of antibody deficient patients suffers almost exclusively from respiratory infections that untreated may lead to complications like generalized bronchiectasis – they do usually suffer from recurrent pneumonias as well [36].

1.2.2 Recurrent Pneumonias

Infections, only in the respiratory tract or always recurring in the same anatomic regions of the lungs, foremost suggest local impairment of immunity due to, for example, cystic fibrosis, immotile cilia, localized bronchiectasis, middle lobe syndrome, tracheobronchial fistulae, tracheobronchial foreign bodies, or pulmonary sequestration. Also gastroesophageal reflux and tracheobronchomalacia may predispose to recurrent LRTIs, bronchiectasis, and parenchymal changes, especially in children [41]. Finding effective prophylactic treatment to prevent recurring pneumonia in these latter two presents a true challenge.

In the most common PIDs, antibody deficiencies, as well as in rare complement factor C2 and C3 deficiencies, invasive respiratory infections are mostly caused by common virulent encapsulated extracellular bacteria (Table 1.2). Thus, a single episode of pneumonia in the acute phase does not necessarily appear suspicious though may in PIDs recur early and heal slowly. In invasive pneumococcal disease, up to 15% of children have PID. In recurrent such infections, approximately 50% of both children and adults have either primary or secondary immunodeficiency (e.g., chronic lymphocytic leukemia, multiple myeloma), while a few have chronic renal disease or asplenia [42, 43]. Recurrent *Streptococcus pneumoniae*, *haemophilus*, or *Moraxella catarrhalis* pneumonias are also commonly seen in combined immunodeficiencies affecting antibody formation (e.g., *NFKB1*/*NFKB2*, *PIK3CD*/*PIK3R1*, *STAT3* GOF, *LRBA*, *CTLA4*) and in idiopathic or secondary bronchiectasis.

If recurrent pneumonias are caused by *Staphylococcus aureus* leading to pulmonary abscesses, one should check for clinical features of dominant negative (DN) *STAT3* mutations (autosomal dominant (AD) hyper-IgE syndrome, often leading to pneumatocele), *GATA2* mutations, and phagocyte deficiencies. However, pyogenic recurrent pneumonia and bacteremia caused by a wide range of gram-positive and gram-negative bacteria are common in a wide range of combined, severe combined, and T-cell deficiencies. Thus, any signs for a broader susceptibility to opportunistic pathogens should be sought for and lead to appropriate investigations (Tables 1.1

Table 1.5 Tests for immune function of suspected PID patient

Arm of immunity suspected to be deficient	Quantitative tests (cell subsets by flow cytometry)	Qualitative tests	Advanced tests in highly specialized laboratories
Primarily antibody deficiency[a]	*Complete blood count (CBC)* *IgG, IgA, IgM, IgE levels* CD19+ or CD20+ B-cell differential T_{FH} cells If any clinical signs to suggest combined immunodeficiency, T-cell differential (e.g., CD4+/CD8 + RTE, naïve, TEMRA, Tγ/δ, Treg) and qualitative T-cell studies	Specific antibody responses to, e.g., tetanus toxoid, diphtheria toxoid, pneumococcal/salmonella polysaccharide pre- and postvaccination Peripheral blood smear (to exclude asplenia/functional hyposplenism in recurrent bacteremias)	Class switching In vitro antibody production KRECs
T-cell deficiency	*CBC* *Lymphocyte differential (CD19+,CD3 ± CD4+, CD3 ± CD8+, CD16 ± CD56+/NK)* T-cell differential Th17 cells, other Th subsets TRECs	Delayed type hypersensitivity (DTH) skin test (candidin, tetanus toxoid, PPD) Lymphocyte proliferation assays (PHA, ConA, PWM, CD3/CD28, allo-/recall antigens)	CD40L, CD127 (IL-7Rα), CD132 (cγ chain) Treg function Vβ TCR repertoire (immunophenotype/spectratype) In vitro cytokine production ADA/PNP activity Radiosensitivity testing CTL cytolytic activity and degranulation Anticytokine autoantibodies
NK/NKT-cell deficiency	*CBC* *Lymphocyte differential* CD3+, CD16+, CD56+	NK cytolytic activity and degranulation	Expanded NK/NKT phenotyping NK assays on antibody-dependent cellular cytotoxicity and cytokine production

(continued)

Table 1.5 (continued)

Arm of immunity suspected to be deficient	Quantitative tests (cell subsets by flow cytometry)	Qualitative tests	Advanced tests in highly specialized laboratories
Phagocyte deficiency	*CBC*	*Peripheral blood smear* *Dihydrorhodamine test (DHR)* Nitroblue tetrazolium test (NBT)	Phagocyte cell immunophenotyping Adherence Chemotaxis Bactericidal activity
Complement deficiency	C3, C4 C1 inhibitor levels Protein electrophoresis (acquired angioedema)	CH50 AH50 Activity of MBL pathway C1 inhibitor biochemical activity Peripheral blood smear (see above)	Other circulating complement component levels C3 nephritic factor C1q autoantibodies
Signaling defects			Plethora, for example, CD62L shedding/TLR signaling, IL-12 production in response to IFN-γ
Cell death defects[b]	Vitamin B12 + sFasL		Apoptosis assays Autophagy assays

[a]Screening tests underlined. *KRECs* K-deleting recombination excision circles, *RTE* recent thymic emigrants, *TEMRA* "exhausted senescent" terminally differentiated effector memory cells reexpressing CD45RA, *TRECs* T-cell receptor excision circles, *CTL* cytotoxic T lymphocytes

[b]Lead to, for example, autoimmune lymphoproliferative syndromes (ALPS), ALPS-like disorders due to impaired apoptosis, or severe congenital neutropenias (SCN) due to dysregulated autophagy and/or endosomal stress response (ESR)

and 1.5). Early-onset *Pseudomonas aeruginosa* pneumonias in a non-CF patient should make one suspect not only bronchiectasis but also severe congenital neutropenia and other PIDs causing symptomatic neutropenia, specific granule deficiency, and, if other suggestive features are present, *MyD88/IRAK4* deficiencies (Tables 1.1 and 1.2). *TLR5* deficiency is found in up to 10% of Europeans and predisposes to *Legionella* pneumonia, but its phenotype is mild [44].

Lung infections by opportunistic viral and fungal pathogens are mostly seen in PIDs impairing cellular immunity by T-cells or phagocytes (Tables 1.1 and 1.2). An opportunistic lung infection in a child or an adult who is apparently non-immunocompromised or following only mild immunosuppression should always lead to studies to detect PID; one should not wait for a second episode. In an infant, an urgent assessment of potential SCID by a PID physician and appropriate testing are mandatory – without further delay. There are now numerous PIDs, which cause early- or delayed-onset pulmonary *Pneumocystis jirovecii*, other fungi, opportunistic viruses, and nontuberculous systemic and pulmonary mycobacteriosis (Table 1.1). Pneumocystis pneumonia should always alert to the possibility of immunodeficiency. Excluding a *Mycobacterium avium-intracellulare* complex cervical lymph node infection, other nontuberculous mycobacteria (NTM) infections are highly suspicious of PID or secondary immunodeficiency. If pulmonary NTM infection is found in younger individuals, one should thus always exclude a systemic infection (bone marrow, blood, gut). See below for advice on how to differentiate between NTM secondary to bronchiectasis and PIDs in adults. Patients suffering from systemic or clearly opportunistic infections not explained by local factors in the lungs should be remitted to colleagues who are well-versed with PIDs and secondary immunodeficiencies.

1.2.3 Bronchiectasis and Bronchiolitis

Chronic and abnormal dilation or ectasia of the airways and bronchus defines bronchiectasis. It leads to recurrent, chronic, or refractory infections, purulent productive cough especially in the mornings, hemoptysis, chronic airway obstruction, and progressive impairment of breathing. Chronic infection and inflammation in the lungs lead to the influx of neutrophils and ensuing dilatation of the bronchus. Bronchiectasis is exacerbated by locally released neutrophil elastase and other neutrophil proteases, cathepsins, proteinase-3, and matrix metalloproteinases causing epithelial cell damage, mucous hypersecretion, inhibited ciliary function, and impaired phagocytosis of apoptotic neutrophils. Secondarily, both alveolar macrophage function and opsonization by complement, secretory IgA, and intraluminal IgG1 and IgG3 become impaired, creating a vicious cycle. This is potentially further accelerated by increased colonization of the airways by various predominantly gram-negative bacteria and biofilm formation. With the advent of high-resolution computed tomography (HRCT), bronchiectasis is relatively straightforward to diagnose [45]. In PIDs, bronchiectasis is in general bilateral, diffuse, and cylindrical, while localized traction bronchiectasis suggests more local changes. However, widespread fibrotic changes due to advanced granulomatous or interstitial processes and ensuing multifocal traction as well as varicose and cystic bronchiectasis are seen in PIDs [46].

Bronchiectasis is a local complication of acute pneumonia and in, for example, middle lobe syndrome. Bronchiectatic changes are seen in recumbent areas of the lung due to recurrent aspiration. Bronchiectasis is widespread due to inhalation accidents or various rather common genetic traits like cystic fibrosis, primary ciliary dyskinesia, and alpha$_1$-antitrypsin anomalies. Most likely primary weakness of the airways impairing air flow during cough reflexes in pediatric-onset Mounier-Kuhn and Williams-Campbell as well as Marfan syndromes is mechanistically linked to bronchiectasis [45].

Bronchiectasis is seen in all PID categories (Table 1.3). In PIDs, the presence of bronchiectasis at diagnosis predicts poorer prognosis, while early diagnosis and aggressive management predict good outcome [46]. Thus, at PID diagnosis, it is customary to obtain HRCT. As bronchiectasis progresses, airways become colonized by typical bacteria such as *Haemophilus* sp., *S. pneumoniae*, and *Moraxella catarrhalis*, a microbial spectrum also seen with smoking and chronic bronchitis. Consequently, it is imperative to understand that, like seen from chronic bronchitis patients and many examples above, colonization of the airways in itself is not sufficient to cause true bronchiectasis [45]. Also, systemic and local susceptibility conditions should be looked for. After careful systematic assessment, only 10–26% of bronchiectasis cases have remained idiopathic. A large etiologic group is inflammatory and autoimmune diseases including sarcoidosis, rheumatoid arthritis, SLE, Sjögren syndrome, inflammatory bowel disease, and relapsing polychondritis, some of which also may have PID as an underlying cause. In most available studies on etiology of bronchiectasis, screening for PID appears to have been limited and often somewhat random. After cystic fibrosis and idiopathic inflammatory diseases, the most common predisposing factor for bronchiectasis in often potentially selection-biased studies appears to be PIDs, found in up to 7% of adult and up to 10% of pediatric bronchiectasis patients [47]. However, in single-center studies, frequency of antibody deficiencies has been as high as 37.5% of all bronchiectasis patients [48]. Bronchiectasis is also seen in secondary immunodeficiencies like HIV infection, multiple myeloma, chronic lymphocytic leukemia, and lymphoma as well as due to graft-versus-host disease after stem cell transplantation [47, 49].

A subset of asthma and chronic obstructive pulmonary disease (COPD) patients suffer from bronchiectasis; and surprisingly, similar airflow obstruction is seen in PIDs. Even allergic asthma is seen in CVID but requires bronchial allergen provocation tests to diagnose due to the inability to produce IgE displayed by approximately 90% of CVID patients [48, 50].

Considering that aspergilli are ubiquitous saprophytic molds producing airborne spores, which every human inhales by hundreds each day, variability in aspergillus-associated diseases is hardly surprising [51–53]. Recurrent pneumonias in an asthmatic patient with increased IgE and bronchiectasis should alert to the possibility of allergic bronchopulmonary aspergillosis (ABPA). ABPA patients have high titers of IgE and precipitating IgG antibodies against filamentous fungi, most commonly *Aspergillus* [51, 52]. Rarely, ABPA has been reported in *DOCK8* deficiency as well [54]. Multiple fungal balls by aspergillus, bronchiectasis, typical cavitating and necrotizing changes in CT, and aspergillus-specific IgG antibodies are seen in adults with chronic pulmonary aspergillosis (CPA), another seemingly polygenic trait [53]. In the autosomal dominant (AD) hyper-IgE syndrome (HIES) caused by DN *STAT3* mutations, aspergillosis may however start like CPA [55]. AD-HIES patients display early-onset severe eczema and, with advancing age, also typical structural features (Chap. 2).

The prevalence of NTM and bronchiectasis is 0.1–0.4: 10,000, which is highest among persons over 50 years old. In middle-aged and older individuals, idiopathic NTM together with bronchiectasis may be seen together with structural features of Lady Windermere syndrome [45]. Besides, this also appears to be a polygenic trait [56]. Overall, prevalence of NTM in non-cystic fibrosis bronchiectasis is around 2–10% [45]. Especially in early-onset cases, one should look for systemic mycobacteriosis and an underlying PID [57]. Other infrequent idiopathic causes for bronchiectasis include Swyer-James-MacLeod, yellow nail, and Young's syndromes [49].

Most often, bronchiectasis is found in patients with antibody deficiencies, who usually do not display severe opportunistic infections by pathogens with low virulence in normal population (fungi, viruses) [58]. Since screening for antibody deficiency is economical and early diagnosis radically alters patient's treatment and prognosis, in the authors' opinion, it is highly recommendable to screen for these by measuring serum IgG, IgA, IgM, and IgE levels in every bronchiectasis patient. If two of these isotypes are at below reference, remittal to a PID physician is highly recommendable.

Commonly in reviews, only antibody deficiencies and chronic granulomatous disease are listed as PIDs causing bronchiectasis. Prevalence of bronchiectasis in AD hyper-IgE syndrome seems rare (<2.5% in children, very rare in adults), while it is very common in phenotypically somewhat similar *DOCK8* and *PGM3* mutations [59]. While bronchiectasis is a common complication in antibody deficiencies, seen in 17–76% in published series and in over 20% in most, excluding antibody deficiency is too insensitive if there are features that suggest other PIDs [48, 60]. In fact, bronchiectasis is seen in most other PID categories, with the exception of most (but not all) monogenic autoinflammatory diseases (AID) and severe congenital neutropenias (SCN). In AID, bronchiectasis is mainly seen in patients who also display hypogammaglobulinemia as one of the manifestations. In SCN, bronchiectasis has been reported in *G6PC3* deficiency (Table 1.3). Thus, if a bronchiectasis patient displays systemic features that suggest PIDs other than antibody deficiencies, a more thorough clinical assessment and laboratory workup seems warranted.

There are no high-quality trials on supportive treatment of bronchiectasis in PID patients; thus therapy is mainly based on current general guidelines [61]. In antibody deficiencies, long-term use of inhaled corticosteroid +/− long-acting muscarinic antagonist and macrolide together with increased IgG replacement dosage and pulmonary rehabilitation has been suggested [62]. Vitamin D deficiency, common in CVID, may aggravate the risk and length of respiratory infections and bronchiectasis and is often substituted [46]. Vaccination strategies follow those recommended to PID patients [63–65]. In antibody-deficient bronchiectasis patients, airway clearance techniques and exercise seem very helpful, if IgG substitution therapy alone does not keep symptoms at bay. Importantly, smoking is not recommended.

While bronchiolitis obliterans is rarely seen in confirmed PIDs, respiratory and follicular bronchiolitis-like changes in HRCT and pulmonary nodular lymphoid hyperplasia are commonly seen in a wide range of PIDs associated with persistent lymphadenopathy, chronic lymphoproliferation, and interstitial lung diseases (e.g., CVID, *PIK3CD*, autoinflammatory and autoimmune PIDs) [58]. Often, interstitial manifestations predominate in these patients and are thus discussed in more detail below.

1.3 Interstitial Lung Diseases

If interstitial lung diseases (ILDs) are suspected in PID patients, HRCT often gives limited information on the specific nature of such changes, and one should strive to obtain both bronchoalveolar lavage (BAL) and lung biopsies. Since PID patients often have highly aberrant blood counts and systemically highly Th1/Th2/Th17-skewed immune responses, the interpretation of BAL findings may be challenging. Bronchoscopy and BAL are of course required if opportunistic pulmonary infections are suspected. Often, ILDs in PID patients are complex. Patchy granulomatous, fibrotic, lymphocytic, and nonspecific interstitial foci findings may be seen at the same time, if multiple biopsies by video-assisted thoracoscopy (VATS) or open biopsies are obtained [66, 67]. Such procedures may not always be safe in PID patients. As a result, despite the fact that interstitial lung changes are commonly seen in PIDs, few reports either describe the exact form of ILD or the biopsy findings may sometimes also seem somewhat atypical compared to commonly defined ILDs (Table 1.3).

Interstitial lung changes are common in SCID patients and in a wide range of combined immunodeficiencies. In these patients, such changes may also be caused by opportunistic pathogens like adenovirus, respiratory syncytial virus, cytomegalovirus, or *Pneumocystis jirovecii*. However, idiopathic interstitial pneumonitis is also seen (Table 1.3). Early-onset interstitial pneumonias are seen in surfactant protein (SP) deficiencies [68]. Interestingly, ILDs have not been reported in CD40, CD40L, AID, or UNG deficiencies ("hyper-IgM syndromes") and appear to be rare in genetic agammaglobulinemias [62]. Pulmonary nodules have however been reported in AID deficiency [54].

1.3.1 Granulomatous Lung Inflammation

ILDs including granulomatous lung disease, lymphocytic interstitial pneumonia (LIP), idiopathic pulmonary fibrosis (IPF), follicular bronchiolitis, and organizing pneumonia (OP) are seen in at least 10–25% of patients suffering from CVID [62, 69]. These superimposed features have been coined as granulomatous and lymphocytic interstitial lung disease (GLILD) [66, 67]. Sarcoidosis-like features in CVID patients include the systemic nature of the disease, frequent mediastinal and hilar adenopathy, and noncaseating granulomas in various organs. Unlike in sarcoidosis where hypergammaglobulinemia is a rule, CVID patients display hypogammaglobulinemia, and frequently also concomitant autoimmune cytopenias, splenomegaly, nodular regenerative hyperplasia of the liver, LIP, follicular bronchiolitis, recurrent infections, low percentages of memory B-cells, and CD4/CD8 ratio are rarely high in BAL [27, 62]. Antibody-deficient patients with LIP/GLILD seem to tolerate long-term high-dose glucocorticoid treatment poorly and may succumb to fatal opportunistic infections. Thus, measurement of antibody levels in a suspected sarcoidosis patient with recurrent infections or other inflammatory diseases seems prudent before such therapy is started. Frequency of GLILD in CVID varies between 5% and 20% in various cohorts and associates with various autoimmune manifestations [48, 62, 69]. Management of GLILD is rapidly evolving. It includes the use of systemic corticosteroids as the first-line and azathioprine, rituximab, and/or mycophenolate as the second-line therapies. If second-line therapy is contemplated, obtaining representative lung biopsies – if not previously available – by VATS is recommendable, since differential diagnosis of GLILD is demanding [70]. GLILD has also been reported in monogenic diseases somewhat resembling CVID like CTLA4, LRBA, XIAP, and GATA2 deficiencies and Kabuki syndrome. Similar changes may be seen in a small subset of IgA deficiency patients, usually with IgG2 deficiency. Therefore, the diagnosis of each disease will change the treatment strategy to more targeted [62]. Early-onset lung granulomas are typical in, for example, Rhoh deficiency and Blau syndrome (*CARD15*); patients suffering from the latter may even develop interstitial pneumonitis [71]. Granulomas are a frequent feature in many phagocyte, combined, and T-cell deficiencies; in the latter two, lymphopenia usually predates the onset of granulomas, and granulomas sometimes appear to be associated with chronic rubella virus infections by vaccine strain rubella [72, 73]. Granulomatous lesions mimicking granulomatous polyangiitis have been reported in TAP1/TAP2 deficiency [74].

1.3.2 Lymphocytic and Nonspecific Interstitial Pneumonias

In common variable immunodeficiency, the biopsy findings of LIP and NSIP usually seem to represent GLILD in follow-up and in VATS-obtained multiple biopsies [75]. LIP has been reported in monogenic autoimmune diseases (e.g., APECED,

STAT3 GOF, STAT5b deficiency) and ataxia-telangiectasia [48, 54, 58]. Pulmonary lymphoid hyperplasia, follicular and respiratory bronchiolitis, as well as nodular changes in CT may be seen in a wide range of PIDs associated with lymphoproliferation, autoimmunity, or chronic EBV viremia [76]. Many of the reported interstitial radiologic changes probably represent nonspecific interstitial pneumonia (NSIP) or usual interstitial pneumonia (UIP), seen also in autoinflammatory diseases like AD STING (*TMEM173*) deficiency, deficiency of IL-1 receptor antagonist (DIRA, *IL1RN*), autoinflammation, PLCγ2-associated antibody deficiency, and immune dysregulation (APLAID, *PLCG2*) [58, 76, 77]. Since LIP, NSIP, and UIP are treated differently, lung biopsies should be obtained to confirm the underlying lung pathology [75].

1.3.3 Organizing Pneumonia

Organizing pneumonia (OP) may frequently be seen both in primary or secondary antibody deficiencies and occasionally in *CATCH22*, severe combined immunodeficiencies, idiopathic CD4 lymphopenia, and *GATA-2*, *LRBA*, and *UNC119* deficiencies [48, 75, 78–81]. Transbronchial biopsy is usually sufficient to show OP.

1.3.4 Early-Onset Desquamative Pneumonia

Early-onset desquamative interstitial pneumonia without apparent exposure to smoke may be caused by surfactant protein SP-A2, SP-B, SP-C, and ABCA3 deficiencies and *STAT3* gain-of-function (GOF) mutations [82, 83]. In PID patients, smoking seems to further expedite the progression of ILDs.

1.3.5 Pulmonary Fibrosis

In late stages of GLILD, UIP, and other ILDs, fibrotic changes may predominate also in PID patients. Familial pulmonary fibrosis is seen in dyskeratosis congenita [84, 85]. DKC is clinically diagnosed when the mucocutaneous triad of nail dysplasia, skin pigmentation changes, and oral leukoplakia are present. Also, the presence of one feature of the triad in combination with bone marrow failure and two other DKC-associated findings suffices for diagnosis [86]. In most DKC patients, skin hypo- and hyperpigmentation are superimposed with atrophic and telangiectatic changes as so-called poikiloderma and are most pronounced around the neck and head. Since DKC displays genetic anticipation, exact genetic diagnosis and genetic counseling seem mandatory. DKC can be caused by more than ten different genes with autosomal dominant (AD), autosomal recessive (AR), and X-linked modes of inheritance; however not all DKC-associated genes are known yet. Patients with DKC are at very high risk of bone marrow failure, immunodeficiency, pulmonary and liver fibrosis, premature hair graying, leukemia, and squamous cell cancer of the head, neck, or anogenital regions [86]. However, DKC may be tricky to diagnose without high index of suspicion [87]. Rare variants of DKC genes and/or shortened telomere length seem to be associated with sporadic idiopathic pulmonary fibrosis, risk of UIP/NSIP, and lung adenocarcinoma [88–90]. Pulmonary fibrosis is also associated with ataxia-telangiectasia, *STAT3* GOF, Hermansky-Pudlak syndrome type 2, and Somech syndrome or may develop due to prolonged pulmonary alveolar proteinosis (PAP), for example, in GATA2 deficiency [58, 91–94].

1.3.6 Mulch Pneumonitis

Chronic granulomatous disease (CGD) patients may develop a fulminant hypersensitivity pneumonitis-like "mulch pneumonitis" after inhalation of aerosolized decaying organic matter like hay, mulch, or dead leaves and require emergency care, corticosteroids, and antimicrobial treatment [95].

1.3.7 Pulmonary Alveolar Proteinosis

Pulmonary alveolar proteinosis (PAP) is a rare syndrome characterized by abnormal alveolar surfactant accumulation and hypoxemic respiratory insufficiency, caused by impaired surfactant production or clearance. Early-onset pulmonary alveolar proteinosis is most commonly caused by colony-stimulating factor (CSF) receptor deficiencies (*CSF2RA*, *CSFR2B*) but also seen in SCID caused by adenosine deaminase (*ADA*) deficiency and seems likely in *IRF8* deficiency (Table 1.3) [6]. While PAP has only been described in *ITCH*-deficient mice, humans deficient in ITCH seem to develop NSIP [96]. Later-onset PAP is most commonly caused by cytokine autoantibodies against GM-CSF, most often in smoking males. Acquired PAP is also seen as the result of somatic mutations in common beta chain of GM-CSF, IL-3, and IL-5 receptors in AML. Furthermore, it has been reported in a number of other myeloid and B-cell malignancies, often leading to secondary immunodeficiency, as well as in secondary immune dysregulatory states caused by organ transplantation, HIV, amyloidosis, juvenile dermatomyositis, and renal tubular acidosis [97]. However, later-onset PAP is also frequently seen in the surprisingly common GATA-2 deficiency, which causes the absence of pulmonary macrophages, and occasionally reported in *CD40L*, AR agammaglobulinemia, Fanconi anemia, lysinuric protein intolerance, and *CSF2RA* deficiencies [97, 98]. Correction of PAP in GATA-2 deficiency by stem cell transplant together with a high risk of severe pneumonias suggests proceeding to it without further delay [99]. PAP may also manifest acutely by prolonged inhalation of fumes, inorganic or organic dusts, and infections by cytomegalovirus, *Proteus*, *Nocardia*, *Aspergillus*, *Histoplasma*, and *Cryptococcus*; all these infections may be seen in PIDs. PAP patients also have increased susceptibility to opportunistic pathogens and increased mortality [97].

1.3.8 Malignancies in the Lungs

Germ line *SFTPA2* mutations predispose to familial lung cancer; also somatic indels are common in lung adenocarcinoma [100]. Despite the occasional lung adenocarcinoma and leiomyoma reports from PID patients, these appear to be rare [46, 101, 102]. Malignancies associated with systemic PIDs include B- and T-cell lymphoma, Hodgkin lymphoma (myelodysplastic syndrome-related), leukemia, various often skin carcinomas, and, rarely, melanoma, medulloblastoma, neuroblastoma, or other tumors [46, 101, 102]. PIDs thus primarily predispose to malignancies of the hematopoietic tissue [101]. The etiopathogenetic mechanisms leading to malignancies in PIDs and an extensive list of PIDs associated with malignancy are outside the scope of this chapter. These have however been recently extensively reviewed [103]. Various PIDs exhibit radiosensitivity [6]. In radiosensitive PIDs, radiologic follow-up is thus problematic unless lung MRI is used; secondary carcinomas in these frequently metastasize the lungs [48, 104, 105]. In CVID, there is an increased risk of gastric carcinoma, which frequently metastasizes into lungs [46]. Thymoma may cause secondary hypogammaglobulinemia (see below).

B-cell lymphomas associated with susceptibility to EBV-associated lymphoproliferation and non-Hodgkin lymphomas (NHL) commonly affect the lungs and may lead to superior vena cava syndrome [48]. PIDs associated with a clearly increased risk of NHL include CVID, ataxia-telangiectasia, Nijmegen breakage syndrome, constitutive mismatch repair deficiencies, *SH2D1A* deficiency, Wiskott-Aldrich syndrome, autoimmune lymphoproliferative syndrome, cartilage-hair hypoplasia, *STK4* deficiency, *CD40L* deficiency, and AD hyper-IgE syndrome [102, 106]. In some of these diseases, fever, fatigue weight loss, and adenopathy may occur due to other causes as well. Lymph node biopsies in PIDs may suggest lymphoma without clinical progression. Consequently, treatment and follow-up of such patients should be planned together with clinical immunologists and hematologists familiar with PIDs [58, 103].

1.3.9 Other Airway and Pulmonary Manifestations

Angioedema without urticaria, often affecting the respiratory tract, is seen in hereditary angioedema types I–III. Acquired urticaria has been reported in CVID and IgA deficiency [48]. Patients with a recently discovered autoinflammatory disease with autoimmunity, Copa defect, predominantly present with extensive neutrophilic capillaritis in the alveolar septa, pulmonary hemorrhage, and ILD, together with arthritis and renal disease [107]. Pulmonary vasculitis may also be seen in, for example, WAS, TAP1/2, and STING deficiencies. Alveolar hemorrhage and pulmonary graft-versus-host disease may also occur after stem cell transplant in PID [54]. Pulmonary arterial hypertension (PAH) without end-stage ILD may be seen in CVID, GATA-2, and ADA2 deficiencies together with chronic CD3+CD8+ large granular lymphocyte (LGL) lymphoproliferation or leukemia [108, 109]. CD8+ T-LGL cells are known to be able to attack against pulmonary epithelial cells [110, 111]. In GATA-2 deficiency, PAH may also be the result of pulmonary fibrosis due to long-standing PAP [112, 113]. PAH has also been reported in Caspase-8 deficiency [114]. GATA-2 deficiency is also associated with cholesterol pneumonia [115]. Pulmonary dysgenesis and structural airway anomalies like laryngeal web and subglottic stenosis are occasionally seen in 22q11 deletion (velocardiofacial/DiGeorge syndrome) [46, 54]. Pulmonary embolism may be seen in antiphospholipid syndrome (often together with SLE) associated with phagocyte, complement, IgA, and DOCK8 deficiencies [48, 116].

1.4 Diagnostic Immunology Workup

A well-grounded clinical suspicion of primary immunodeficiency based on thoroughly taken lifelong patient and family history focused on common PID manifestations (Figs. 1.1 and 1.2, Tables 1.1, 1.2, 1.3, and 1.4) should always lead to either proper screening for PIDs and HIV or to the consultation of a clinical immunologist. If the patient has previously received prolonged immunomodulatory and immunosuppressive medication, it is often wise to leave the final assessment to a specialist in PIDs. Typical screening tests are listed in Table 1.5. Especially in PIDs that present mostly with autoimmune or autoinflammatory manifestations, common screening tests are insensitive [6, 8]. Also, many signaling defects require a highly specialized immunology laboratory from the start. Often, highly specialized flow cytometry and functional and genetic studies will be required and give cause for early consultation. Since PIDs without stem cell or gene therapy are lifelong, invasive testing to accurately assess associated organ-specific complications is often advisable. Some monogenic hematologic diseases causing bone marrow failure (e.g., DKC, Fanconi anemia, Blackfan-Diamond anemia) may be classified as PIDs or hematologic disorders and should also be remembered when testing PID patients with compatible findings.

Since many of the required tests need freshly isolated cells, also controlled environment during shipping and reliability and availability of fast transport often prevent problems. Elaborate flow and functional studies may also be cost prohibitive (Table 1.5). With the advent of relatively low-cost next-generation sequencing (NGS, including large targeted panels, whole exome and whole genome sequencing), choosing NGS at an early stage in pursuit of diagnosis may be well cost-effective (Table 1.6). In all tests, interpretation however requires expertise, reasonable control populations, and experience as well as thorough knowledge

Table 1.6 Examples of genetic testing of suspected PID patient

Genetic tests	Scenario	Further genetic testing	Note
Cytogenetic analysis (karyotyping)	Structural features suggesting abnormality of chromosome number, ring chromosome or very large deletions, insertions or inversions associated with PID	In Bloom sd, cytogenetic test of dermal fibroblasts may be necessary In Nijmegen breakage sd, testing of PHA-stimulated lymphocytes	Typically includes, for example, trisomy 21 (Down) and Turner (XO, iso X, ring X) syndromes, ring chromosome 21
Array-based comparative genomic hybridization (CGH, molecular karyotyping) or fluorescence in situ hybridization (FISH)	Structural abnormalities suggesting copy number variation (CNV) including deletions	For example, whole genome sequencing to detect small microdeletions or complex rearrangements	Typical examples include 22q11.2 del and other DiGeorge sd-associated deletions like 10p13-p14 del, 11qter del/Jacobsen sd, *DOCK8* del, 4p16 del/Wolf-Hirschhorn sd, 18p- and 22q13 del, 2q37 del
Southern blot analysis of satellite DNA methylation	Features suggest immunodeficiency, centromeric instability, and facial dysmorphism sd	DNTM3B and ZBTB24 capillary or panel sequencing	Chromosomal aberrations often easier to detect with increasing culture time
Telomere length, for example, by flow-FISH	Suspicion of dyskeratosis congenita	NGS to detect responsible pathogenic mutation	Short telomeres reported in myelodysplasias (e.g., *CTC1, STN1, SAMD9, SAMD9L*), radiosensitive PIDs (e.g., *NBN, ATM*), and other PIDs (e.g., CHH, CORO1A def)
Targeted capillary sequencing	Typical features and a single candidate gene	If negative and thus novel disease suspected, WES/WGS	Labor intensive and easily costly
Next-generation sequencing panel	Typical features and multiple candidate genes	If negative and thus novel disease suspected, WES/WGS	Great depth of sequencing, detects introns and smaller CNVs. Great clinical and immunophenotypic as well as genotypic heterogeneity causes problems, potential somewhat overlapping genes may be missed; novel genes will be missed

(continued)

Table 1.6 (continued)

Genetic tests	Scenario	Further genetic testing	Note
Whole exome sequencing[a]	Atypical features, novel genes, or multiple genes suspected with no suitable panel available. Regionally, well-covered in-house controls needed. Panels and targeted approaches frequently do not find causative genes in the region	WES needs to cover the suspected genes. Suspected genes are not highly homologous. Thus, gaps in the coverage of the used WES platform need to be known. (NGS panels/ WGS?)	Requires relatively large population-based in-house and international control cohorts to assess frequent polymorphisms and VUSs. Detection of, for example, deep intronic, regulatory region, noncoding exon mutation, small CNVs, or complex rearrangements impaired. Mutations in highly homologous genes often not detected reliably (e.g., CGD). Depth may be suboptimal. Prediction algorithms lack power and data analysis demanding
Whole genome sequencing[a]	Much like WES, also if complex rearrangements or small microdeletions in multiple genes suspected	Data analysis is the bottleneck, thus interpretation often difficult; too many potential candidates	Relatively large population-based in-house and international control cohorts to assess frequent polymorphisms and VUSs still largely missing. Depth may be suboptimal. Prediction algorithms lack power and data analysis very demanding

NGS next-generation sequencing, *WES* whole exome sequencing, *WGS* whole genome sequencing, *VUS* variant of unknown significance

[a]For a more in-depth discussion on caveats and reliability of WES/WGS, see, for example, *J Allergy Clin Immunol*. 2016;138:957–69

about the pitfalls of all approaches [117]. Often, remit of the patient for diagnostic evaluation and centralization of such evaluation to large PID services seems reasonable, especially in those patients who display signs other than predominantly antibody deficiency (Tables 1.5 and 1.6).

1.4.1 *Differential Diagnosis*

If a patient presents with recurrent infections suggesting immunodeficiency, one should also test for HIV and obtain a careful medication history. In addition to chemotherapeutic, immunosuppressive, and biologic drugs, also certain anti-convulsants, anti-psychotic medications, antimicrobial and antimalarial drugs, and NSAIDs may occasionally induce clinically relevant T- or B-cell immunodeficiency [47]. Long-term proton pump inhibitor use may also predispose to recurrent pneumonias [118].

Various primary pulmonary diseases that mimic PIDs have been discussed above. Particularly challenging is the differential diagnosis between adult idiopathic or atopic severe asthma and COPD patients suffering from bronchiectasis, recurrent pneumonias, long-term high-dose systemic and inhaled glucocorticoid treatment-induced secondary hypogammaglobulinemia, and primary forms of late-onset antibody deficiency, where patients may also suffer from asthma and bronchiectasis [119]. Asthmatic patients without true PIDs do not benefit from immunoglobulin therapy [120]. And, there are yet no large controlled studies to guide us when to expect glucocorticoid-induced changes. As a rule of thumb, the equivalent of more than 1 g daily inhaled fluticasone seems in its metabolic effects equal to approximately 5 mg of daily oral prednisone. In practice, if the total cumulative glucocorticoid use in previous 18 months in an adult exceeds a dose equivalent to or larger than 7.5 mg of prednisone/prednisolone daily, one may expect to see some extent of both hypogammaglobulinemia and sluggish antipneumococcal responses [121–123]. Aiding in assessment, glucocorticoid use also induces changes into B- and T-cell subsets that would be unexpected in PIDs [124]. One should also use well-studied cutoff points to define impaired anti-polysaccharide responses [125, 126]. Both vitamin A and vitamin B12 deficiencies have been associated with secondarily impaired anti-polysaccharide responses in sporadic case reports.

In its report on PIDs, IUIS concisely lists also secondary immunodeficiencies caused by autoantibodies or somatic mutations or clones that greatly mimic PIDs [6]. Of these, GM-CSF autoantibodies in PAP and LGL leukemia in PAH have been mentioned above. Autoantibodies against interferon-γ are seen in late-onset generalized NTM infections. In upper airway angioedema, besides hereditary forms, also a form induced by anti-C1 inhibitor autoantibodies is known. In thymoma with hypogammaglobulinemia (Good syndrome), a patient may develop cytokine autoantibodies and variable hypo-/agammaglobulinemia and completely lack circulating antibodies and B-cells as well as develop opportunistic infections [6].

1.5 Assessment and Follow-Up

When autoimmune manifestations or invasive infections like pneumonias are suspected in PID patients, one should avoid serologic testing at least in antibody, combined, and severe combined immunodeficiencies. Serologic tests in these patient groups are frequently falsely negative or may just reflect the antibodies from immunoglobulin substitution therapy. Direct staining, cultures, antigen, or polymerase chain reaction tests should be performed whenever possible. This usually requires invasive testing.

Since many rare combined immunodeficiencies display defective chromosome stability, telomere maintenance, and DNA repair, they also render patients radiosensitive [6]. A degree of radiosensitivity has been noted even in CVID [105]. The combined use of lung ultrasound and chest X-ray has been suggested as a potential approach in reducing the need of HRCT in ILD. Frequent monitoring of ILD in PID is safest by using diffusion capacity studies [48]. One should avoid injudicious use of radiologic studies especially in PIDs and often consider invasive testing instead [69].

Respiratory insufficiency is still one of the leading causes of death in PIDs. Progressive lung disease is due to underlying subclinical infection and inflammation, best documented in antibody deficiencies. Viral and bacterial pathogens have been detected in secretions from the airways of patients with various PIDs with persistent and/or recurrent infections and from PID patients with no apparent infections at the time of testing. Currently, screening and follow-up measures used in PID centers include frequent monitoring of respiratory infection and antibiotic use; lung function tests such as forced expiratory volume at 1 s (FEV1), forced vital capacity (FVC), and transfer factor for carbon monoxide (TLCO); imaging with HRCT and MRI; cultures from induced sputum; blood gas analysis; and exercise testing [127]. Prophylactic systemic or inhaled antibiotics are given to selected patient groups. To detect impeding decline in lung function, exercise tests like 6-minute walking test and reduced gas transfer capacity seem the most sensitive but appear to be used too infrequently [69, 127].

Regular lung function testing, which may be demanding in the youngest age groups, requires close collaboration between PID doctors, specialists supervising as well as nurses, and technicians running the testing facilities. Impulse oscillometry, which is effort-independent unlike spirometry and conventional diffusion studies, has shown promise in the follow-up of young children with PIDs [128].

Some endemic and emerging infections pose a threat to PID patient's health during travel [129]. Oral polio, smallpox, live attenuated influenza, yellow fever, and live bacterial vaccines should be avoided in severe humoral immunodeficiencies, while all live vaccines should be avoided in combined immunodeficiencies. Also live bacterial vaccines should not be used in phagocyte deficiencies or BCG in interferon-γ/IL-12 pathway defects. In partial T-cell deficiencies, like partial DiGeorge syndrome and CVID, patients however often seem to tolerate at least some live vaccines [63–65, 130]. Therapy of respiratory manifestations in PIDs, including immunoglobulin replacement, transplantation, and gene and adjunct therapies, is covered in Chap. 10.

1.6 Pulmonologist and Care of PID Patients

PIDs are mostly systemic diseases that greatly benefit from multidisciplinary approach. Since many pulmonary complications have special features and therapeutic approaches in PIDs, a joint team effort by pulmonologists and PID doctors benefits both. Frequently, the help of chest physicians and pulmonary radiologists is needed during the evaluation of an acutely ill PID patient. Such help includes the often unavoidable invasive microbial and biopsy sampling as well as the interpretation of radiologic studies. In rehabilitation and evaluation of long-term respiratory impairment and disability, respiratory medicine specialist, clinical physiology specialist, and respiratory physiotherapist's help is indispensable [46, 60].

There is scarce data on the long-term natural history and evolution of respiratory impairment and disability in most PIDs; therefore, this will require much collaborative systematic study and follow-up [20, 130].

References

1. Armstrong J, Gluck EH, Crapo RO, Jones HA, Hughes JM. Lung tissue volume estimated by simultaneous radiographic and helium dilution methods. Thorax. 1982;37(9):676–9.
2. Borges I, Sena I, Azevedo P, Andreotti J, Almeida V, Paiva A, et al. Lung as a niche for hematopoietic progenitors. Stem Cell Rev. 2017;13(5):567–74.
3. Mercer RR, Russell ML, Roggli VL, Crapo JD. Cell number and distribution in human and rat airways. Am J Respir Cell Mol Biol. 1994;10(6):613–24.
4. Mason RJ, Dobbs LG. Alveolar epithelium and pulmonary surfactant. Murray and Nadel's textbook of respiratory medicine. 6th ed. Philadelphia: Elsevier; 2016. p. 134–49. e5.
5. Netea MG, Balkwill F, Chonchol M, Cominelli F, Donath MY, Giamarellos-Bourboulis EJA-O, et al. A guiding map for inflammation. Nat Immunol. 2017;18(8):826.
6. Picard C, Gaspar HB, Al-Herz W, Bousfiha A, Casanova J-L, Chatila T, et al. International union of immunological societies: 2017 primary immunodeficiency diseases committee report on inborn errors of immunity. J Clin Immunol. 2018;38(1):96–128.
7. Kaustio M, Haapaniemi E, Goos H, Hautala T, Park G, Syrjanen J, et al. Damaging heterozygous mutations in NFKB1 lead to diverse immunologic phenotypes. J Allergy Clin Immunol. 2017;140(3):782–96.
8. Bousfiha A, Jeddane L, Picard C, Ailal F, Gaspar HB, Al-Herz W, et al. The 2017 IUIS phenotypic classification for primary immunodeficiencies. J Clin Immunol. 2018;38(1):129–43.
9. Pai SY, Logan BR, Griffith LM, Buckley RH, Parrott RE, Dvorak CC, Kapoor N, et al. Transplantation outcomes for severe combined immunodeficiency, 2000–2009. N Engl J Med. 2014;271(5):434–46.
10. Joshi AY, Iyer VN, Hagan JB, St Sauver JL, Boyce TG. Incidence and temporal trends of primary immunodeficiency: a population-based cohort study. Mayo Clin Proc. 2009;84(1):16–22.
11. Ludviksson BR, Sigurdardottir ST, Johannsson JH, Haraldsson A, Hardarson TO. Epidemiology of Primary Immunodeficiency in Iceland. J Clin Immunol. 2015;35(1):75–9.
12. The U.S. Immunodeficiency Network (USIDNET), a program of the Immune Deficiency Foundation (IDF), is supported by a cooperative agreement, U24AI86837, from the National Institute of Allergy and Infectious Diseases (NIAID). https://usidnet.org/registry-data/.
13. Al-Mousa H, Al-Saud B. Primary immunodeficiency diseases in highly consanguineous populations from Middle East and North Africa: epidemiology, diagnosis, and care. Front Immunol. 2017;8:678.
14. Immunodeficiencies ESf. Registry Working Party ESID Database Statistics; Update June 19, 2018. 2018. https://esid.org/Working-Parties/Registry-Working-Party/ESID-Database-Statistics.
15. Leiva LE, Zelazco M, Oleastro M, Carneiro-Sampaio M, Condino-Neto A, Costa-Carvalho BT, Grumach AS, et al. Primary immunodeficiency diseases in Latin America: the second report of the LAGID registry. J Clin Immunol. 2007;27(1):101–8.

16. Modell V, Quinn J, Orange J, Notarangelo LD, Modell F. Primary immunodeficiencies worldwide: an updated overview from the Jeffrey Modell Centers Global Network. Immunol Res. 2016;64(3):736–53.
17. Trotta L, Hautala T, Hamalainen S, Syrjanen J, Viskari H, Almusa H, et al. Enrichment of rare variants in population isolates: single AICDA mutation responsible for hyper-IgM syndrome type 2 in Finland. Eur J Hum Genet. 2016;24(10):1473.
18. Selenius JS, Martelius T, Pikkarainen S, Siitonen S, Mattila E, Pietikäinen R, et al. Unexpectedly high prevalence of common variable immunodeficiency in Finland. Front Immunol. 2017;8:1190.
19. Griffith LM, Cowan MJ, Notarangelo LD, Puck JM, Buckley RH, Candotti F, Conley ME, et al. Improving cellular therapy for primary immune deficiency diseases: recognition, diagnosis, and management. J Allergy Clin Immunol. 2009;124(6):1152–60.
20. Gennery AR, Holland SM. Primary immunodeficiencies: not just paediatric diseases. Eur Respir J. 2015;45:1521–3.
21. Gathmann B, Mahlaoui N, Gerard L, Oksenhendler E, Warnatz K, Schulze I, et al. Clinical picture and treatment of 2212 patients with common variable immunodeficiency. J Allergy Clin Immunol. 2014;134(1):116–26.
22. Lucas M, Lee M, Lortan J, Lopez-Granados E, Misbah S, Chapel H. Infection outcomes in patients with common variable immunodeficiency disorders: relationship to immunoglobulin therapy over 22 years. J Allergy Clin Immunol. 2010;125(6):1354–60.
23. Netea MG, van der Meer JW. Trained immunity: an ancient way of remembering. Cell Host Microbe. 2017;21(3):297–300.
24. Arkwright PD, Gennery AR. Ten warning signs of primary immunodeficiency: a new paradigm is needed for the twenty-first century. Ann N Y Acad Sci. 2011;1238(1):7–14.
25. Al-Herz W, Aldhekri H, Barbouche MR, Rezaei N. Consanguinity and primary immunodeficiencies. Hum Hered. 2014;77(1–4):138–43.
26. Wood P, Network UPI. Primary antibody deficiencies: recognition, clinical diagnosis and referral of patients. Clin Med (Lond). 2009;9(6):595–9.
27. Arnold DF, Wiggins J, Cunningham-Rundles C, Misbah SA, Chapel HM. Granulomatous disease: distinguishing primary antibody disease from sarcoidosis. Clin Immunol. 2008;128(1):18.
28. Verbsky JW, Routes JM, editors. Sarcoidosis and common variable immunodeficiency: similarities and differences. Seminars in respiratory and critical care medicine. Stuttgart: Thieme Medical Publishers; 2014.
29. Juhn YJ. Risks for infection in patients with asthma (or other atopic conditions): is asthma more than a chronic airway disease? J Allergy Clin Immunol. 2014;134(2):247–57.
30. Jung JA, Kita H, Yawn BP, Boyce TG, Yoo KH, McGree ME, Weaver AL, et al. Increased risk of serious pneumococcal disease in patients with atopic conditions other than asthma. J Allergy Clin Immunol. 2010;125(1):217–21.
31. Shearer WT, Dunn E, Notarangelo LD, Dvorak CC, Puck JM, Logan BR, et al. Establishing diagnostic criteria for severe combined immunodeficiency disease (SCID), leaky SCID, and Omenn syndrome: the Primary Immune Deficiency Treatment Consortium experience. J Allergy Clin Immunol. 2014;133(4):1092–8.
32. Griffith LM, Cowan MJ, Notarangelo LD, Kohn DB, Puck JM, Pai S-Y, et al. Primary immune deficiency treatment consortium (PIDTC) report. J Allergy Clin Immunol. 2014;133(2):335–47. e11.
33. McAleer MA, Pohler E, Smith FJ, Wilson NJ, Cole C, MacGowan S, et al. Severe dermatitis, multiple allergies, and metabolic wasting syndrome caused by a novel mutation in the N-terminal plakin domain of desmoplakin. J Allergy Clin Immunol. 2015;136(5):1268–76.
34. Luk ADW, Lee PP, Mao H, Chan K-W, Chen XY, Chen T-X, et al. Family history of early infant Death correlates with earlier age at Diagnosis But not shorter Time to Diagnosis for severe combined immunodeficiency. Front Immunol. 2017;8:808.
35. Nelson KS, Lewis DB. Adult-onset presentations of genetic immunodeficiencies: genes can throw slow curves. Curr Opin Infect Dis. 2010;23(4):359.

36. Woroniecka M, Ballow M. Office evaluation of children with recurrent infection. Pediatr Clin N Am. 2000;47(6):1211–24.
37. Immunology EAoAaC. European position paper on rhinosinusitis and nasal polyps. Rhinol Suppl. 2005;18:1–87.
38. Wood P, Peckham D. Investigating recurrent respiratory infections in primary care. BMJ (CR)-print. 2009;339(2):b4118.
39. Gokturk B, Keles S, Kirac M, Artac H, Tokgoz H, Guner S, et al. CD3G gene defects in familial autoimmune thyroiditis. Scand J Immunol. 2014;80(5):354–61.
40. von Bernuth H, Picard C, Puel A, Casanova JL. Experimental and natural infections in M y D 88-and IRAK-4-deficient mice and humans. Eur J Immunol. 2012;42(12):3126–35.
41. Yalçın E, Doğru D, Özçelik U, Kiper N, Aslan AT, Gözaçan A. Tracheomalacia and bronchomalacia in 34 children: clinical and radiologic profiles and associations with other diseases. Clin Pediatr. 2005;44(9):777–81.
42. Einarsdottir H, Erlendsdottir H, Kristinsson K, Gottfredsson M. Nationwide study of recurrent invasive pneumococcal infections in a population with a low prevalence of human immunodeficiency virus infection. Clin Microbiol Infect. 2005;11(9):744–9.
43. Gaschignard J, Levy C, Chrabieh M, Boisson B, Bost-Bru C, Dauger S, et al. Invasive pneumococcal disease in children can reveal a primary immunodeficiency. Clin Infect Dis. 2014;59(2):244–51.
44. Netea MG, van der Meer JW. Immunodeficiency and genetic defects of pattern-recognition receptors. N Engl J Med. 2011;364(1):60–70.
45. Chan ED, Iseman MD. Bronchiectasis. In: Broaddus VC, Ernst JD, Gotway MB, King TE, Lazarus SC, Mason RJ, et al., editors. Murray and Nadel's textbook of respiratory medicine. 6th ed. Philadelphia: Elsevier - Health Sciences Division; 2016. p. 853–76.
46. Jesenak M, Banovcin P, Jesenakova B, Babusikova E. Pulmonary manifestations of primary immunodeficiency disorders in children. Front Pediatr. 2014;2:77.
47. Truong T. The overlap of bronchiectasis and immunodeficiency with asthma. Immunol Allergy Clin North Am. 2013;33(1):61–78.
48. Yazdani R, Abolhassani H, Asgardoon M, Shaghaghi M, Modaresi M, Azizi G, et al. Infectious and noninfectious pulmonary complications in patients with primary immunodeficiency disorders. J Investig Allergol Clin Immunol. 2017;27(4):213–24.
49. McShane PJ, Naureckas ET, Tino G, Strek ME. Non–cystic fibrosis bronchiectasis. Am J Respir Crit Care Med. 2013;188(6):647–56.
50. Agondi R, Barros M, Rizzo L, Kalil J, Giavina-Bianchi P. Allergic asthma in patients with common variable immunodeficiency. Allergy. 2010;65(4):510–5.
51. Knutsen AP, Bush RK, Demain JG, Denning DW, Dixit A, Fairs A, et al. Fungi and allergic lower respiratory tract diseases. J Allergy Clin Immunol. 2012;129(2):280–91.
52. Muldoon EG, Strek ME, Patterson KC. Allergic and noninvasive infectious pulmonary aspergillosis syndromes. Clin Chest Med. 2017;38(3):521–34.
53. Denning DW, Chakrabarti A. Pulmonary and sinus fungal diseases in non-immunocompromised patients. Lancet Infect Dis. 2017;17(11):e357–66.
54. Owayed A, Al-Herz W. Sinopulmonary complications in subjects with primary immunodeficiency. Respir Care. 2016. https://doi.org/10.4187/respcare.04479.
55. Rezaei N, de Vrie E, Gambineri E, Haddad E. Common presentations and diagnostic approaches. In: Sullivan K, Stiehm ER, editors. Stiehm's immune deficiencies. 1st ed. Amsterdam: Academic Press; 2014. p. 3–59.
56. Szymanski EP, Leung JM, Fowler CJ, Haney C, Hsu AP, Chen F, et al. Pulmonary nontuberculous mycobacterial infection. A multisystem, multigenic disease. Am J Respir Crit Care Med. 2015;192(5):618–28.
57. Aksamit TR, O'donnell AE, Barker A, Olivier KN, Winthrop KL, Daniels MLA, et al. Adult patients with bronchiectasis: a first look at the US bronchiectasis research registry. Chest. 2017;151(5):982–92.

58. Nonas S. Pulmonary manifestations of primary immunodeficiency disorders. Immunol Allergy Clin North Am. 2015;35(4):753–66.
59. Freeman AF, Olivier KN. Hyper-IgE syndromes and the lung. Clin Chest Med. 2016;37(3):557–67.
60. Wood P, Stanworth S, Burton J, Jones A, Peckham D, Green T, et al. Recognition, clinical diagnosis and management of patients with primary antibody deficiencies: a systematic review. Clin Exp Immunol. 2007;149(3):410–23.
61. Pasteur MC, Bilton D, Hill AT. British Thoracic Society guideline for non-CF bronchiectasis. Thorax. 2010;65(Suppl 1):i1–i58.
62. Schussler E, Beasley MB, Maglione PJ. Lung disease in primary antibody deficiencies. J Allergy Clin Immunol Pract. 2016;4(6):1039–52.
63. Sobh A, Bonilla FA. Vaccination in primary immunodeficiency disorders. J Allergy Clin Immunol Pract. 2016;4(6):1066–75.
64. Shearer WT, Fleisher TA, Buckley RH, Ballas Z, Ballow M, Blaese RM, et al. Recommendations for live viral and bacterial vaccines in immunodeficient patients and their close contacts. J Allergy Clin Immunol. 2014;133(4):961–6.
65. Kroger A, Duchin J, Vázquez M. Best practices guidance of the Advisory Committee on Immunization Practices (ACIP). Atlanta, GA: US Department of Health and Human Services, CDC; 2017.
66. Bates CA, Ellison MC, Lynch DA, Cool CD, Brown KK, Routes JM. Granulomatous-lymphocytic lung disease shortens survival in common variable immunodeficiency. J Allergy Clin Immunol. 2004;114(2):415–21.
67. Wheat WH, Cool CD, Morimoto Y, Rai PR, Kirkpatrick CH, Lindenbaum BA, et al. Possible role of human herpesvirus 8 in the lymphoproliferative disorders in common variable immunodeficiency. J Exp Med. 2005;202(4):479–84.
68. van Moorsel CH, ten Klooster L, van Oosterhout MF, de Jong PA, Adams H, Wouter van Es H, et al. SFTPA2 mutations in familial and sporadic idiopathic interstitial pneumonia. Am J Respir Crit Care Med. 2015;192(10):1249–52.
69. Verma N, Grimbacher B, Hurst JR. Lung disease in primary antibody deficiency. Lancet Respir Med. 2015;3(8):651–60.
70. Hurst JR, Verma N, Lowe D, Baxendale HE, Jolles S, Kelleher P, et al. British Lung Foundation/United Kingdom primary immunodeficiency network consensus statement on the definition, diagnosis, and management of granulomatous-lymphocytic interstitial lung disease in common variable immunodeficiency disorders. J Allergy Clin Immunol Pract. 2017;5(4):938–45.
71. Becker ML, Martin TM, Doyle TM, Rosé CD. Interstitial pneumonitis in Blau syndrome with documented mutation in CARD15. Arthritis Rheum. 2007;56(4):1292–4.
72. Bodemer C, Sauvage V, Mahlaoui N, Cheval J, Couderc T, Leclerc-Mercier S, et al. Live rubella virus vaccine long-term persistence as an antigenic trigger of cutaneous granulomas in patients with primary immunodeficiency. Clin Microbiol Infect. 2014;20(10):O656–O63.
73. Perelygina L, Plotkin S, Russo P, Hautala T, Bonilla F, Ochs HD, et al. Rubella persistence in epidermal keratinocytes and granuloma M2 macrophages in patients with primary immunodeficiencies. J Allergy Clin Immunol. 2016;138(5):1436–9. e11.
74. Gadola S, Moins-Teisserenc H, Trowsdale J, Gross W, Cerundolo V. TAP deficiency syndrome: IMMUNODEFICIENCY REVIEW. Clin Exp Immunol. 2000;121(2):173–8.
75. Rao N, Mackinnon AC, Routes JM. Granulomatous and lymphocytic interstitial lung disease: a spectrum of pulmonary histopathologic lesions in common variable immunodeficiency—histologic and immunohistochemical analyses of 16 cases. Hum Pathol. 2015;46(9):1306–14.
76. Allenspach E, Torgerson TR. Autoimmunity and primary immunodeficiency disorders. J Clin Immunol. 2016;36(1):57–67.
77. Aksentijevich I, Nowak M, Mallah M, Chae JJ, Watford WT, Hofmann SR, et al. De novo CIAS1 mutations, cytokine activation, and evidence for genetic heterogeneity in patients with

neonatal-onset multisystem inflammatory disease (NOMID): a new member of the expanding family of pyrin-associated autoinflammatory diseases. Arthritis Rheum. 2002;46(12):3340–8.
78. Kaufman J, Komorowski R. Bronchiolitis obliterans organizing pneumonia in common variable immunodeficiency syndrome. Chest. 1991;100(2):552–3.
79. Shokri S, Nabavi M, Hirschmugl T, Aghamohammadi A, Arshi S, Bemanian MH, et al. LPS-responsive beige-like anchor gene mutation associated with possible Bronchiolitis Obliterans organizing pneumonia associated with Hypogammaglobulinemia and normal IgM phenotype and low number of B cells. Acta Med Iran. 2016;54(10):620–3.
80. Tamada T, Nara M, Tomaki M, Ashino Y, Hattori T. Secondary bronchiolitis obliterans organising pneumonia in a patient with carbamazepine-induced hypogammaglobulinemia. Thorax. 2007;62(1):100.
81. Pohl W, Armbruster C, Bernhardt K, Drlicek M, Vetter N. Idiopathic CD4+ T-lymphocytopenia in 2 patients without indications for HIV infection. Wien Klin Wochenschr. 1995;107(3):95–100.
82. Mason RJ, Dobbs LG. Alveolar epithelium and pulmonary surfactant. In: Broaddus VC, Ernst JD, Gotway MB, King TE, Lazarus SC, Mason RJ, et al., editors. Murray and Nadel's textbook of respiratory medicine. 6th ed; 2016. p. 134–49.
83. Haapaniemi EM, Kaustio M, Rajala HL, van Adrichem AJ, Kainulainen L, Glumoff V, et al. Autoimmunity, hypogammaglobulinemia, lymphoproliferation and mycobacterial disease in patients with dominant activating mutations in STAT3. Blood. 2014. https://doi.org/10.1182/blood-2014-04-570101.
84. Snetselaar R, Van Moorsel CH, Kazemier KM, Van Der Vis JJ, Zanen P, Van Oosterhout MF, et al. Telomere length in interstitial lung diseases. Chest. 2015;148(4):1011–8.
85. Newton CA, Batra K, Torrealba J, Kozlitina J, Glazer CS, Aravena C, et al. Telomere-related lung fibrosis is diagnostically heterogeneous but uniformly progressive. Eur Respir J. 2016;48(6):1710–20.
86. Ballew BJ, Savage SA. Updates on the biology and management of dyskeratosis congenita and related telomere biology disorders. Expert Rev Hematol. 2013;6(3):327–37.
87. Speckmann C, Sahoo SS, Rizzi M, Hirabayashi S, Karow A, Serwas NK, et al. Clinical and molecular heterogeneity of RTEL1 deficiency. Front Immunol. 2017;8:449.
88. Petrovski S, Todd JL, Durheim MT, Wang Q, Chien JW, Kelly FL, et al. An exome sequencing study to assess the role of rare genetic variation in pulmonary fibrosis. Am J Respir Crit Care Med. 2017;196(1):82–93.
89. Stella GM, Balestro E, Lacedonia D, Baraldo S. Telomeropathies: an emerging spectrum of disorders with important implications for patients with interstitial lung disease. Minerva Med. 2016;107(1 Suppl 1):9–14.
90. Haycock PC, Burgess S, Nounu A, Zheng J, Okoli GN, Bowden J, et al. Association between telomere length and risk of cancer and non-neoplastic diseases: a Mendelian randomization study. JAMA Oncol. 2017;3(5):636–51.
91. Bhatt JM, Bush A, van Gerven M, Nissenkorn A, Renke M, Yarlett L, et al. Ataxia telangiectasia: why should the ERS care? Eur Respir J. 2015;46(6):1557–60.
92. Vicary GW, Vergne Y, Santiago-Cornier A, Young LR, Roman J. Pulmonary fibrosis in Hermansky–Pudlak syndrome. Ann Am Thorac Soc. 2016;13(10):1839–46.
93. Somech R, Somers GR, Chitayat D, Grunebaum E, Atkinson A, Kolomietz E, et al. Fatal lung fibrosis associated with immunodeficiency and gonadal dysgenesis in 46XX sisters—a new syndrome. Am J Med Genet A. 2008;146(1):8–14.
94. Ballerie A, Nimubona S, Meunier C, Gutierrez FL, Desrues B, Delaval P, et al. Association of pulmonary alveolar proteinosis and fibrosis: patient with GATA2 deficiency. Eur Respir J. 2016. https://doi.org/10.1183/13993003.00252-2016.
95. Siddiqui S, Anderson VL, Hilligoss DM, Abinun M, Kuijpers TW, Masur H, et al. Fulminant mulch pneumonitis: an emergency presentation of chronic granulomatous disease. Clin Infect Dis. 2007;45(6):673–81.

96. Lohr NJ, Molleston JP, Strauss KA, Torres-Martinez W, Sherman EA, Squires RH, et al. Human ITCH E3 ubiquitin ligase deficiency causes syndromic multisystem autoimmune disease. Am J Hum Genet. 2010;86(3):447–53.
97. Trapnell BC, Luisetti M. Pulmonary alveolar proteinosis syndrome. In: Broaddus VC, Ernst JD, Gotway MB, King TE, Lazarus SC, Mason RJ, et al., editors. Nadel's textbook of respiratory medicine. 6th ed; 2015. p. 1260–74.
98. Ito M, Nakagome K, Ohta H, Akasaka K, Uchida Y, Hashimoto A, et al. Elderly-onset hereditary pulmonary alveolar proteinosis and its cytokine profile. BMC pulmonary medicine. 2017;17(1):40.
99. Hsu AP, McReynolds LJ, Holland SM. GATA2 deficiency. Curr Opin Allergy Clin Immunol. 2015;15(1):104.
100. Imielinski M, Guo G, Meyerson M. Insertions and deletions target lineage-defining genes in human cancers. Cell. 2017;168(3):460–72. e14.
101. Mayor PC, Eng KH, Singel KL, Abrams SI, Odunsi K, Moysich KB, et al. Cancer in primary immunodeficiency diseases: cancer incidence in the United States immune deficiency network registry. J Allergy Clin Immunol. 2018;141(3):1028–35.
102. Mortaz E, Tabarsi P, Mansouri D, Khosravi A, Garssen J, Velayati A, et al. Cancers related to immunodeficiencies: update and perspectives. Front Immunol. 2016;7:365.
103. Hauck F, Voss R, Urban C, Seidel MG. Intrinsic and extrinsic causes of malignancies in patients with primary immunodeficiency disorders. J Allergy Clin Immunol. 2018;141(1):59–68. e4.
104. Milito C, Pulvirenti F, Serra G, Valente M, Pesce AM, Granata G, et al. Lung magnetic resonance imaging with diffusion weighted imaging provides regional structural as well as functional information without radiation exposure in primary antibody deficiencies. J Clin Immunol. 2015;35(5):491–500.
105. Serra G, Milito C, Mitrevski M, Granata G, Martini H, Pesce AM, et al. Lung MRI as a possible alternative to CT scan for patients with primary immune deficiencies and increased radiosensitivity. Chest. 2011;140(6):1581–9.
106. Attarbaschi A, Carraro E, Abla O, Barzilai-Birenboim S, Bomken S, Brugieres L, et al. Non-Hodgkin's lymphoma and pre-existing conditions: spectrum, clinical characteristics and outcome in 213 children and adolescents. Haematologica. 2016. https://doi.org/10.3324/haematol.2016.147116.
107. Vece TJ, Watkin LB, Nicholas SK, Canter D, Braun MC, Guillerman RP, et al. Copa syndrome: a novel autosomal dominant immune dysregulatory disease. J Clin Immunol. 2016;36(4):377–87.
108. Johnston S, Hill S, Lock R, Dwight J, Unsworth D, Gompels M. Echocardiographic abnormalities in primary antibody deficiency. Postgrad Med J. 2004;80(942):214–8.
109. Spinner MA, Sanchez LA, Hsu AP, Shaw PA, Zerbe CS, Calvo KR, et al. GATA2 deficiency: a protean disorder of hematopoiesis, lymphatics, and immunity. Blood. 2013. https://doi.org/10.1182/blood-2013-07-515528.
110. Rossoff LJ, Genovese J, Coleman M, Dantzker DR. Primary pulmonary hypertension in a patient with CD8/T-cell large granulocyte leukemia: amelioration by cladribine therapy. Chest. 1997;112(2):551–3.
111. Grossi O, Horeau-Langlard D, Agard C, Haloun A, Lefebvre M, Neel A, et al. Low-dose methotrexate in PAH related to T-cell large granular lymphocyte leukaemia. Eur Respir J. 2012;39(2):493–4.
112. Jouneau S, Ballerie A. Haemodynamically proven pulmonary hypertension in a patient with GATA2 deficiency-associated pulmonary alveolar proteinosis and fibrosis. Eur Respir J. 2017;49(5).
113. Sanges S, Prévotat A, Fertin M, Terriou L, Lefèvre G, Quesnel B, et al. Haemodynamically proven pulmonary hypertension in a patient with GATA2 deficiency-associated pulmonary alveolar proteinosis and fibrosis. Eur Respir J. 2017;49(5):1700178.

114. Niemela J, Kuehn HS, Kelly C, Zhang M, Davies J, Melendez J, et al. Caspase-8 deficiency presenting as late-onset multi-organ lymphocytic infiltration with granulomas in two adult siblings. J Clin Immunol. 2015;35(4):348–55.
115. Griese M, Zarbock R, Costabel U, Hildebrandt J, Theegarten D, Albert M, et al. GATA2 deficiency in children and adults with severe pulmonary alveolar proteinosis and hematologic disorders. BMC Pulm Med. 2015;15(1):87.
116. Jouhadi Z, Khadir K, Ailal F, Bouayad K, Nadifi S, Engelhardt KR, et al. Ten-year follow-up of a DOCK8-deficient child with features of systemic lupus erythematosus. Pediatrics. 2014. https://doi.org/10.1542/peds.2013-1383.
117. Meyts I, Bosch B, Bolze A, Boisson B, Itan Y, Belkadi A, et al. Exome and genome sequencing for inborn errors of immunity. J Allergy Clin Immunol. 2016;138(4):957–69.
118. Ho SW, Teng YH, Yang SF, Yeh HW, Wang YH, Chou MC, et al. Association of proton pump inhibitors usage with risk of pneumonia in dementia patients. J Am Geriatr Soc. 2017;65(7):1441–7.
119. Gelfand EW, Ochs HD, Shearer WT. Controversies in IgG replacement therapy in patients with antibody deficiency diseases. J Allergy Clin Immunol. 2013;131(4):1001–5.
120. Kishiyama J, Valacer D, Cunningham-Rundles C, Sperber K, Richmond G, Abramson S, et al. A multicenter, randomized, double-blind, placebo-controlled trial of high-dose intravenous immunoglobulin for oral corticosteroid-dependent asthma. Clin Immunol. 1999;91(2):126–33.
121. Borgers H, Jeurissen A, Flamaing J, Peetermans W, Moens L, Verhaegen J, et al. Elderly subjects do not show impaired pneumococcal capsular polysaccharide serotype-specific antibody responses as assessed by a multiplexed bead assay. Clin Immunol. 2010;135(3):501–2.
122. Borgers H, Moens L, Picard C, Jeurissen A, Raes M, Sauer K, et al. Laboratory diagnosis of specific antibody deficiency to pneumococcal capsular polysaccharide antigens by multiplexed bead assay. Clin Immunol. 2010;134(2):198–205.
123. Cunningham-Rundles C. Key aspects for successful immunoglobulin therapy of primary immunodeficiencies. Clin Exp Immunol. 2011;164:16–9.
124. Wirsum C, Glaser C, Gutenberger S, Keller B, Unger S, Voll RE, et al. Secondary antibody deficiency in glucocorticoid therapy clearly differs from primary antibody deficiency. J Clin Immunol. 2016;36(4):406–12.
125. Beck SC. Making sense of serotype-specific pneumococcal antibody measurements. London, England: SAGE Publications Sage UK; 2013.
126. Schaballie H, Bosch B, Schrijvers R, Proesmans M, De Boeck K, Boon MN, et al. Fifth percentile cutoff values for antipneumococcal polysaccharide and anti-Salmonella typhi Vi IgG describe a normal polysaccharide response. Front Immunol. 2017;8:546.
127. Jolles S, Sánchez-Ramón S, Quinti I, Soler-Palacín P, Agostini C, Florkin B, et al. Screening protocols to monitor respiratory status in primary immunodeficiency disease: findings from a European survey and subclinical infection working group. Clin Exp Immunol. 2017;190(2):226–34.
128. Komarow HD, Sokolic R, Hershfield MS, Kohn DB, Young M, Metcalfe DD, et al. Impulse oscillometry identifies peripheral airway dysfunction in children with adenosine deaminase deficiency. Orphanet J Rare Dis. 2015;10(1):159.
129. Sullivan KE, Bassiri H, Bousfiha AA, Costa-Carvalho BT, Freeman AF, Hagin D, et al. Erratum to: emerging infections and pertinent infections related to travel for patients with primary immunodeficiencies. J Clin Immunol. 2017;37(7):693.
130. Heimall J, Buckley RH, Puck J, Fleisher TA, Gennery AR, Haddad E, et al. Recommendations for screening and management of late effects in patients with severe combined immunodeficiency after allogenic hematopoietic cell transplantation: a consensus statement from the second Pediatric Blood and Marrow Transplant Consortium international conference on late effects after pediatric HCT. Biol Blood Marrow Transplant. 2017;23(8):1229–40.

Chapter 2
Pulmonary Manifestations of Combined T- and B-Cell Immunodeficiencies

Andrew R. Gennery

2.1 Introduction

The immune system has evolved in coexistence with microbes over billions of years with the purpose of providing efficient but self-limited host defense against the biotic and abiotic environment, during which self-tolerance is maintained. Therefore, while infectious agents initiate many presentations, the presentation may be of an infectious nature, but symptoms of inflammation or autoimmunity may be present or predominate. The immune system is composed of three elements: effective physical and mechanical barriers, nonspecific innate immunity, and specific, personalized adaptive immunity. The system is a complex interconnected network of proteins and cells, functional throughout the body. Throughout evolutionary history, different elements have been developed as microbes have evolved, so that there is some overlap and redundancy. The three key components of human immune defense are (i) barriers, (ii) innate immune response, and (iii) adaptive immune response.

The key elements of the adaptive response are T-lymphocytes and B-lymphocytes, and defects in T-lymphocytes alone or both T- and B-lymphocytes give rise to combined immunodeficiency. Because the lung is a major interface between the internal and external environment, so pulmonary infection is a frequent consequence of combined immunodeficiency, but other pulmonary manifestations are also recognized. This chapter will concentrate on clinical patterns of presentation, as well as describe specific diseases in detail, as the clinical presentation of respiratory infection due to *Pneumocystis jirovecii*, for instance, is similar for all genetic defects.

A. R. Gennery (✉)
Institute of Cellular Medicine, Newcastle University, Newcastle upon Tyne, UK

Paediatric Immunology and Haematopoietic Stem Cell Transplantation Unit, Great North Childrens' Hospital, Newcastle upon Tyne, UK
e-mail: a.r.gennery@ncl.ac.uk; andrew.gennery@newcastle.ac.uk

S. A. Mahdaviani, N. Rezaei (eds.), *Pulmonary Manifestations of Primary Immunodeficiency Diseases*, https://doi.org/10.1007/978-3-030-00880-2_2

Specific respiratory syndromes associated with specific diseases will be highlighted.

(For further information you may see: Deist FL, Moshous D, Villa A, Al-Herz W, Roifman CM, Fischer A, and Notarangelo LD. Combined T- and B-Cell Immunodeficiencies. In: Rezaei N, Aghamohammadi A, Notarangelo LD. editors. *Primary immunodeficiency diseases: definition, diagnosis, and management.* 2nd ed. p. 83–182.)

2.2 Severe Combined Immunodeficiencies

2.2.1 Background

Severe combined immunodeficiencies (SCID) are the most acute combined immunodeficiencies. First presentation is within the first few months of life, and they are generally fatal within the first 18–24 months of life without curative treatment. They comprise a group of inherited disorders that are characterized by deficient T-lymphocyte differentiation due to genetic defects causing interruption in lymphocyte development [1, 2]. Depending on the genetic defect, B-lymphocytes may be affected: they may be absent or intrinsically nonfunctioning, but even in those that are present and intrinsically functional, the absence of CD4+ T-lymphocytes in SCID prevents generation of normal antibody responses (Table 2.1). This leads to a coexistent or combined deficit of cellular and humoral immunity. Natural killer (NK) cells may be present or absent.

Infection is a common manifestation of SCID – persistent respiratory tract infection is frequently encountered – with a failure to clear viruses accompanied by persistent bronchiolitis-like signs. Often patients are considered to have recurrent infection, when in reality they have never cleared the infection. Respiratory signs may include tachypnea, nasal flaring, subcostal and intercostal recession with widespread crepitation and rales, and cyanosis. Insidiously progressive respiratory symptoms with a creeping oxygen requirement and with radiological evidence of interstitial pneumonitis and hyperinflation suggest *Pneumocystis jirovecii* infection. In these patients, coexistent respiratory viral infection is common (Fig. 2.1) [3]. Other frequent coexisting features include persistent viral diarrhea with failure to thrive. Although patients with SCID are often initially well and growing normally, they fall away from the growth centile after a few months, when infection occurs, because intestinal villous atrophy leads to malabsorption, which in severe cases results in malnutrition [4]. There may be evidence of oral or perineal candidiasis and other superficial infections. There is no clinically detectable lymphoid tissue, although detecting this in young infants is not easy because lymph nodes and tonsils in normal infants are often very small.

Immunization with the live attenuated Bacillus Calmette-Guérin (BCG) vaccine can lead to disseminated BCG infection. In countries where BCG is routinely offered, the vaccine is normally administered within the first few days of birth,

Table 2.1 Types of severe combined immunodeficiency

Disorder	Disease	Phenotype	Inheritance
Cytokine signaling	CγC	T^-B^+	XL
	JAK3	T^-B^+	AR
	IL7Rα	T^-B^+	AR
Nucleotide biosynthesis salvage pathway defects	ADA deficiency	T^-B^-	AR
Defects affecting signaling through the T-lymphocyte antigen receptor	CD45	$T^{-/low}B^+$	AR
	CD3δ	$T^{-/low}B^+$	AR
	CD3ε	$T^{-/low}B^+$	AR
	CD3ζ	$T^{-/low}B^+$ $T^{-/low}B^{low}$	AR AR
VDJ recombination defects	RAG1/RAG2	T^-B^-	AR
	DCLRE1C (artemis)	T^-B^-	AR
	DNA-PKcs	T^-B^-	AR
	DNA ligase 4	$T^{low}B^{low}$	AR
	NHEJ1 (Cernunnos-XLF)	$T^{low}B^{low}$	AR
Mitochondrial defect	*AK2* deficiency (Reticular dysgenesis)	$T^-B^{+/-}$	AR
	RMRP (Cartilage haïr hypoplasia)	T^-B^+	AR
Other	Coronin-1A deficiency	T^-B^+	AR
Thymic defects	DiGeorge syndrome	T^-B^+	AD
	CHARGE syndrome	T^-B^+	AD
	FOXN1 (winged helix)	T^-B^+	AR

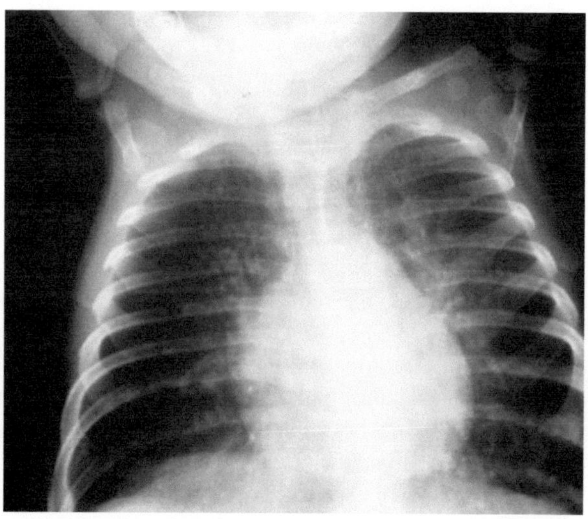

Fig. 2.1 Chest radiograph from an infant with severe combined immunodeficiency showing hyperinflated lungs with midline pleural borders of the upper lobes visible in the absence of a thymic shadow and interstitial pneumonitis secondary to *Pneumocystis jirovecii* pneumonia and parainfluenzae type 3 infection

before a diagnosis of SCID is apparent – vaccinated infants can present with widespread BCG infection – affecting the bones, marrow, liver, and brain as well as the respiratory tract, which is the third most commonly affected site after the lymph nodes and skin [5]. Treatment with appropriate anti-mycobacterial antibiotics reduces the risk of mortality, even in asymptomatic infants.

Bacterial infections of the respiratory tract are less common in patients with SCID partly because of the presence of maternal IgG in early infancy. Prolonged otitis media and invasive bacterial infections, such as staphylococcal or pseudomonas septicemia and pneumonia, may rarely occur, which may respond poorly to appropriate treatment.

2.2.1.1 Adenosine Deaminase Deficiency

This form of SCID is due to a systemic metabolic defect. Adenosine deaminase (ADA) is an essential enzyme of the purine salvage pathways: deficiency caused by loss-of-function mutations in the ADA gene results in one of the most common causes of autosomal recessive SCID, accounting for approximately 10–15% of cases in outbred populations [6]. Adenosine deaminase is required for the irreversible deamination of adenosine and 2'deoxyadenosine to inosine and 2'deoxyinosine, respectively. Absent or impaired ADA function consequently results in both intracellular and extracellular accumulation of these substrates.

Absent or deficient ADA function causes accumulation of the toxic metabolites adenosine, 2'deoxyadenosine and deoxyadenosine triphosphate (dATP). ADA-deficient SCID is characterized by severe lymphocytopenia affecting T- and B-lymphocytes and NK cells. The infectious complications seen in these patients are the same as other forms of SCID. However, because of the ubiquitous nature of the enzyme, non-immunological manifestations are also observed, including neurodevelopmental deficits [7], sensorineural deafness [8], and skeletal abnormalities, particularly of the scapulae and ribs (Fig. 2.2) [9, 10].

Additionally, these patients may experience severe respiratory problems due to direct toxicity of adenosine metabolites on the lung. The role of ADA and the sequelae due to accumulation of toxic substrate in the lungs has been shown in experimental models: ADA$^{(-/-)}$ mice display severe pulmonary inflammation, with associated accumulation of activated macrophages and eosinophils leading to airway remodeling, which can be reversed with polyethylene-glycosylated ADA enzyme replacement therapy [11]. Murine models have demonstrated that prolonged exposure of lung tissue to high concentrations of adenosine due to treatment with low dose enzyme replacement therapy leads to pulmonary fibrosis, changes which were reversed upon reducing pulmonary adenosine levels [12]. Similar pulmonary manifestations are seen in ADA-deficient patients: noninfectious pulmonary disease, including pneumonitis and pulmonary alveolar proteinosis, is found more frequently in ADA-deficient patients than in other genetic forms of SCID [13]. Almost half of patients with ADA-deficient SCID had pulmonary alveolar proteinosis in one study, which rapidly resolved upon initiating treatment with polyethylene-

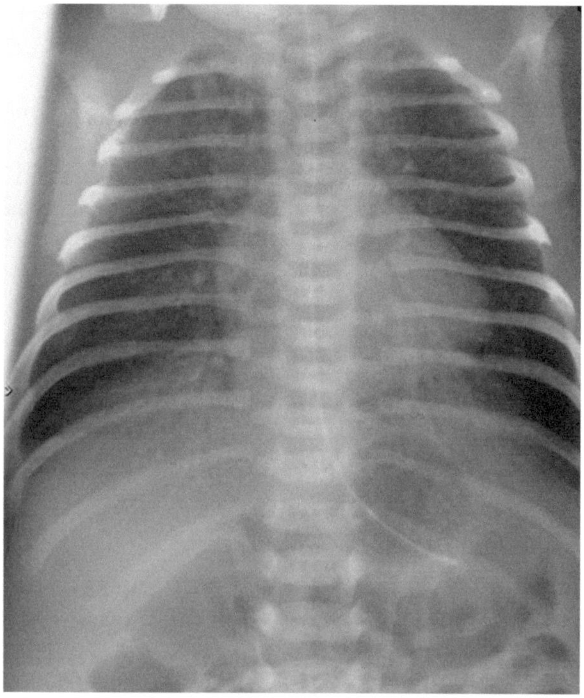

Fig. 2.2 Chest radiograph from an infant with adenosine deaminase-deficient severe combined immunodeficiency showing abnormal scapulae and cupping deformities at the ends of the ribs

glycosylated ADA [14]. Coexistence of adenosine-induced pulmonary toxicity with infection is likely, and chest radiographs do not distinguish the pathology – accordingly patients with ADA-deficient SCID presenting with pulmonary symptoms should receive appropriate antimicrobial treatment and polyethylene-glycosylated ADA enzyme replacement therapy.

2.2.1.2 Reticular Dysgenesis

Patients with loss-of-function mutations in *AK2* encoding adenylate kinase 2 have a particular form of SCID characterized by agranulocytosis as well as absence of T- and B-lymphocytes and NK cells. Patients are usually born before term or are small for gestational age and have associated sensorineural deafness. While most infants with SCID present in the first few months of life, the associated agranulocytosis in *AK2* deficiency confers an unusually severe phenotype, and patients present in the first few days or weeks of life. Aside from lymphocytes and granulocytes, other hematological indices may be low, including hemoglobin or thrombocytes, and a bone marrow examination may show evidence of hypoplasia or hyperplasia. Invasive bacterial infection is the most common presentation, usually bacterial sepsis, often with respiratory features – omphalitis is frequently coexistent. Implicated bacteria include *S. aureus*, streptococcal commensal species, *K. pneumonia*, and *E. coli*. Candida sepsis is also described [15].

2.2.1.3 Omenn Syndrome and Atypical SCID

Omenn syndrome is a form of SCID with a characteristic clinical and immunological phenotype, due to the presence of a few autologous clonally expanded autoreactive T-lymphocytes. Patients present with a widespread, thickened rash, often with scaling and with erythematous exfoliation, and a protein-losing erythroderma, which develops a "leathery" consistency. Hair, often including eyebrows and eyelashes, is lost as the rash evolves. The rash can be present at birth or shortly afterward or evolve over the first few weeks of life. Associated with this is lymphadenopathy, particularly of the axillary and inguinal nodes. Hepatosplenomegaly is a frequent finding [16]. The immunophenotype is also characteristic and quite different to classic SCID (Table 2.2). A high T-lymphocytosis with a highly activated phenotype is apparent, dominated by a restricted oligoclonal expansion of a few TCRVβ families with absence of other families [17– 19]. Markers of thymopoiesis, such as CD4 + CD45RA + CD31+ T-lymphocytes, or T-lymphocytes bearing T-lymphocyte receptor excision circles (episomal DNA formed during T-lymphocyte receptor rearrangement, indicative of a recent thymic emigrant and absent in SCID, also known as TREC), are absent. B-lymphocytes are absent, and NK cells are generally present in normal numbers. T-lymphocytes fail to proliferate in response to stimulation with phytohemagglutinin. Although serum immunoglobulins IgM, IgA, and IgG are absent, with the absence of vaccine

Table 2.2 Clinical and immunological features of Omenn syndrome and maternofetal engraftment

Omenn syndrome	Maternofetal GVHD
Diagnostic clinical features	
Thickened, scaly, exfoliating erythroderma	Similar tp Omenn syndrome but generally less severe
Partial or total alopecia	Partial or total alopecia
Widespread generalized lymphadenopathy	Lymphadenopathy, usually not so marked as Omenn syndrome
Hepatosplenomegaly	Hepatosplenomegaly
Inflammatory features	
Hepatitis	Hepatitis
Pneumonitis	Pneumonitis
Enteritis	Enteritis
Cerebritis	Cerebritis
Immunophenotype	
Autologous T-lymphocytosis, absent B-lymphocytes, normal NK cell numbers	Maternal T-lymphocytosis, B-lymphocyte variable, NK cell numbers variable
Extreme T-lymphocyte oligoclonality, abnormal spectrotype, and Vβ repertoire	Extreme T-lymphocyte oligoclonality, abnormal spectrotype, and Vβ repertoire
Highly activated T-lymphocytes, absent naïve cells	Highly activated T-lymphocytes, absent naïve cells
Agammaglobulinaemia with raised IgE	Agammaglobulinaemia with raised IgE
Eosinophilia	Eosinophilia

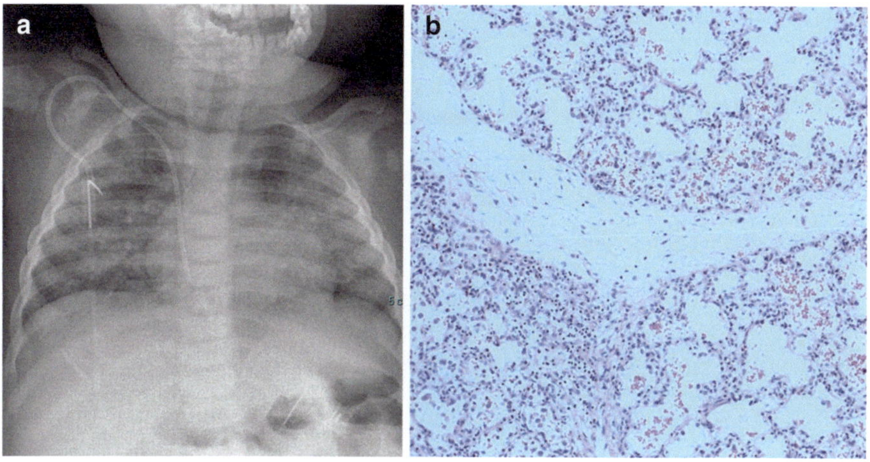

Fig. 2.3 Chest radiograph (**a**) and lung biopsy (**b**) from an infant with Omenn syndrome showing interstitial pneumonitis due to autologous T-lymphocyte infiltration – no microorganisms were detected

antigen responses, the serum IgE is usually very high, with an associated eosinophilia.

An important difference between Omenn syndrome and classical SCID is the presence of intense autoinflammation. An inflammatory enteritis, hepatitis, or pneumonitis (Fig. 2.3) may be present [20], and there may also be coexisting infection with conventional or opportunistic pathogens. The clinico-immunophenotype is similar to that found in patients with classical SCID and maternofetal engraftment with graft-versus-host disease (GVHD) (Table 2.2) [21] or classical SCID and blood transfusion-associated GVHD [22].

While most patients with a clinical diagnosis of SCID and mutations in the genes listed in Table 2.1 demonstrate absent circulating T-lymphocytes, SCID patients may rarely present with normal or elevated T-lymphocyte numbers, particularly those patients that harbor hypomorphic mutations in SCID-causing genes, which permit residual T-lymphocyte development. These patients are said to have "atypical SCID." The most common presentation of these patients is severe recurrent pneumonia, often not due to opportunistic microorganisms such as *Pneumocystis jirovecii* [23].

2.2.1.4 Other Presentations

Although infection is the most common respiratory presentation in patients with SCID, other rare presentations have been described (Table 2.3). Hemophagocytic lymphohistiocytosis, a life-threatening hyperinflammatory syndrome, is more usually associated with defects in genes of the cytotoxic granule-mediated cell death pathway but has been described in patients with SCID, sometimes in association

Table 2.3 Clinical features of classic severe combined immunodeficiency

Common presentations	Common pathogens	Rare presentations
Persistent viral enteritis	Rotavirus	Bacterial septicemia
	Norovirus	Disseminated BCG infection
	Astrovirus	Autoimmune cytopenias
	Adenovirus	Maternofetal engraftment
Persistent viral upper respiratory tract infection	Respiratory syncytial virus	Lymphoid malignancy
	Parainfluenza viruses	Hemophagocytosis
	Cytomegalovirus	
Pneumocystis jirovecii pneumonitis	*Pneumocystis jirovecii*	
Recurrent or recalcitrant candidiasis		
Failure to thrive		

with engraftment of maternal T-lymphocytes [24]. Nonspecific respiratory features, particularly associated with uncontrolled fever in the young infant, may include tachypnea, nasal flaring, and costal recession.

Very rarely, polymorphous lymphoproliferative lesions, resembling B-lymphocyte lymphoma, have been described, which may be associated with Epstein-Barr viral infection – described lesions may involve the thoracic cage as well as soft tissue (Fig. 2.4) [25].

2.2.2 *Management*

The specific management will depend on the cause of respiratory disease. Humidified oxygen may be required if the infant is hypoxic, and if severe respiratory compromise is present, mechanical ventilation may be required. Appropriate investigations include chest radiography, or more detailed imaging with computerized tomography or magnetic resonance imaging may be required.

Accurate identification of microbial organisms is critical for appropriate antimicrobial management. Microbial testing of nasopharyngeal secretions may be helpful in identifying viruses causing infection of the lower respiratory tract, such as respiratory syncytial virus, but isolates from these samples may indicate upper respiratory tract colonization or infection only (e.g., rhinovirus, although in the severely immunocompromised this may rarely cause lower respiratory tract infection), and so bronchoalveolar lavage is recommended in these patients – non-bronchoscopic examination is adequate for most patients – but directed fiber-optic bronchoscopy may be indicated in patients with isolated lesions identified on chest imaging [26]. An open lung biopsy should be seriously considered in the presence of respiratory symptoms if no pathogen is identified by the above procedures [27]. The isolation of one pathogen from the respiratory tract should not deter investigation for a co-pathogen, which may be coexistent in these patients [3].

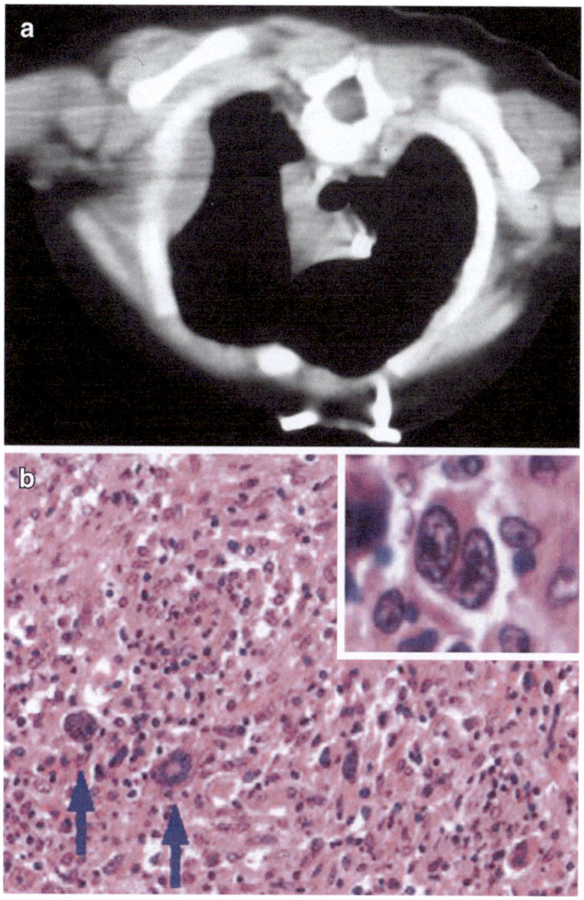

Fig. 2.4 Thoracic computerized tomography (**a**) of an infant with IL2Rγ-deficient severe combined immunodeficiency, showing a mass causing boney erosion of the 3rd rib. (**b**) Morphologic and phenotypic characteristics from a biopsy of the lymphoproliferative lesion showing large cells with large hyperchromatic nuclei, set in a background of reactive cells including histiocytes, fibroblasts, and lymphocytes. Multinucleate forms are seen (arrowed), and some cells of more typical Hodgkin Reed-Sternberg cell morphology were also present (inset)

Careful liaison with the microbiology specialist is key in extracting maximum information from the obtained specimens – including seeking pathogens generally considered not to cause severe lower respiratory infection in healthy individuals – such as parainfluenza type 4 or enterovirus [28, 29].

Appropriate microbial therapy should be directed at the specific pathogen – an appropriate antibacterial for bacterial infection or in the case of *Pneumocystis jirovecii*, at least 3 weeks of high-dose co-trimoxazole, 5 mg/kg body weight/dose of the trimethoprim component, and 19–25 mg/kg body weight/dose of the sulfamethoxazole component administered intravenously every 6 h if the infant is sick or orally if this route is tolerated [30], often combined with methylprednisolone at a dose of 2 mg/kg during the initial treatment phase to counter inflammatory symptoms – the methylprednisolone can be weaned as there is symptomatic improvement. Intravenous pentamidine isethionate (4 mg/kg body weight) once daily is recommended for patients who cannot tolerate co-trimoxazole or who demonstrate clinical treatment failure after 5–7 days of treatment with co-trimoxazole [31]. Viral infection is more problematic to treat, and without restoration of T-lymphocyte function, viral clearance will not be achieved [29]. Some control of infection may be gained with antiviral agents – cidofovir (or brincidofovir) can control the viral load in cases with adenovirus infection – although there may be significant renal side effects. Cytomegalovirus may be controlled with ganciclovir or foscarnet – generally it is advisable to switch ganciclovir for foscarnet at time of transplant – as ganciclovir has significant myelosuppressive properties. However, foscarnet is nephrotoxic, and there may be significant interactions with other nephrotoxic agents used through the transplant process – particularly calcineurin inhibitors used to prevent GVHD. In severe cases, donor or third-party adenovirus- or cytomegalovirus-specific cytotoxic T-lymphocytes may be administered [32], but an intense inflammatory pneumonitis may result, and so administration of concomitant corticosteroids is prudent. Treatment of other respiratory viruses is more difficult – aerosolized ribavirin may be used to treat respiratory syncytial virus – but it is not particularly effective in the absence of functioning T-lymphocytes. Palivizumab, an anti-respiratory syncytial virus monoclonal antibody, is effective at preventing respiratory syncytial virus infection in high-risk infants and should be given to infants with SCID who present during the winter months. The role of palivizumab in treating infants with established lower respiratory tract respiratory syncytial virus infection is less clear – it appears safe to give [33] – but efficacy has yet to be demonstrated, either alone or in combination with ribavirin [34]. All infants with SCID should receive immunoglobulin replacement therapy until B-lymphocyte function is restored – the value of nebulized immunoglobulin to treat viral respiratory infection has yet to be demonstrated.

Respiratory impairment results a significant adverse outcome following hematopoietic stem cell transplantation (HSCT) [35], particularly in infants with active infection at time of transplantation [36]. Every effort should be made to optimize the physical condition of infant prior to the transplant procedure – early diagnosis before infection has occurred gives the best outcomes [37], which is why newborn screening for SCID is being introduced in increasing numbers of countries [38].

2.3 Combined Immunodeficiencies

2.3.1 Background

Patients with combined immunodeficiency (CID) usually present with recurrent respiratory and gastrointestinal tract infections, caused by a wide range of pathogens. Although the clinical presentation shares feature with those of patients with SCID, particularly atypical SCID presentations, typically because of residual T-lymphocyte function, patients with CID have a less severe presentation with later onset (>1 year of age). Because of impaired T-lymphocyte function, viral infections can be particularly severe, but depending on the specific immunodeficiency, many different infectious agents are described. The latest International Union of Immunology Societies classification lists 30 different genes associated with non-syndromic CID [39].

2.3.2 *Immunoglobulin Class Switch Recombination Deficiencies Affecting CD40-CD40L (CD40LG Deficiency, CD40 Deficiency)*

Defects in a number of different genes are described that disrupt the ability of B-lymphocytes to switch from making IgM immunoglobulin to isotypes with different constant regions (IgA, IgE, IgG) (Table 2.4). These defects may be extrinsic to the B-lymphocyte signaling pathway or affect the intrinsic B-lymphocyte switch pathway. Accurate identification of the defect is important, as the management approach will be targeted, according to the specific gene involved [40]. CD40 ligand (CD40L) deficiency [X-linked hyper-IgM syndrome type 1], the most common isotype class switch defect, is a rare X-linked primary immunodeficiency caused by mutations in CD40LG, on chromosome Xq26.3-Xq27.1, encoding the transmembrane CD40L glycoprotein (CD154) found on the surface of activated CD4 T-lymphocytes. Mutations in CD40LG result in altered co-stimulatory T-lymphocyte function, which impairs B-lymphocyte isotype switching and dendritic cell signaling, leading to increased susceptibility to intracellular and bacterial pathogens. Patients commonly present in infancy or early childhood with recurrent upper and

Table 2.4 Immunodeficiencies associated with raised IgM

Disease	Genetic defect	Affected cell type	Inheritance
CD40 ligand deficiency	*CD40LG*	CD4+ T-lymphocytes	X-linked
CD40 deficiency	*CD40*	B-lymphocytes, monocytes, dendritic cells	Autosomal recessive
Ataxia telangiectasia	*ATM*	B-lymphocytes	Autosomal recessive
DNA ligase IV deficiency	*LIG4*	B-lymphocytes	Autosomal recessive
Cernunnos-XLF deficiency	*NHEJ1*	B-lymphocytes	Autosomal recessive
Nijmegen breakage syndrome	*NBN*	B-lymphocytes	Autosomal recessive
NF-KAPPA-B essential modulator (NEMO) deficiency	*IKBKG*	Polymorphonuclear cells, monocytes, dendritic cells, lymphocytes	X-linked
Activation-induced cytidine deaminase deficiency	*AICDA*	B-lymphocytes	Autosomal recessive
Activation-induced cytidine deaminase deficiency, C-terminus variant	*AICDA*	B-lymphocytes	Autosomal dominant
uracil-DNA glycosylase deficiency	*UNG*	B-lymphocytes	Autosomal recessive
IL21R deficiency	*IL21R*	T-lymphocytes, B-lymphocytes, NK cells	Autosomal recessive

lower respiratory tract infections, including *Pneumocystis jirovecii* interstitial pneumonia [41]. Cryptosporidium infection is a common cause of acute or chronic diarrhea and may lead to severe biliary tract disease, including sclerosing cholangitis and cirrhosis and rarely cholangiocarcinoma, hepatocellular carcinoma, and adenocarcinoma [42]. Less commonly, central nervous system infections, particularly enteroviral meningoencephalitis, or JC virus progressive multifocal leukoencephalopathy, causing progressive neurodegeneration, has been reported [43, 44].

Although long-term survival with conservative therapy of immunoglobulin replacement and cryptosporidial prophylaxis has been historically poor, with only 20–50% of patients surviving to the third decade [41, 45], recent data show an improved median survival time from diagnosis of 25 years in 109 patients with XHIM [46]. HSCT is curative: a European retrospective analysis of 38 patients undergoing HSCT demonstrated a survival of 68%, curative in 58% of patients. Infection-related complications, particularly severe cryptosporidiosis were the predominant cause of death [47]. Pre-existing lung disease was the most important adverse risk factor. A more recent multicenter study of 130 patients revealed an overall survival after transplantation of 80%, with improved outcome especially in those transplanted before 10 years of age or transplanted early after diagnosis. The use of myeloablative conditioning regimens was associated with higher overall and disease-free survival, while the use of reduced-intensity and non-myeloablative conditioning associated with poor donor cell engraftment [48]. Transplant survivors experienced significantly better well-being, as measured by using Karnofsky/Lansky scales, than those not transplanted [46]. For those with severe liver disease, liver transplant may be performed prior to HSCT [49].

Mutations in the gene encoding CD40, the receptor for CD40L, give rise to similar phenotype as patients with CD40L deficiency. The disease is inherited in an autosomal recessive fashion and is much less frequently encountered – females may be affected. Monocytes and B-lymphocytes demonstrate absent or faulty CD40, whereas CD40L expression is normal. The clinical features overlap with those of CD40L deficiency and include bacterial sinopulmonary infection due to antibody deficiency, as well as infection with opportunistic microorganisms such as *Pneumocystis jirovecii*. Severe lung damage due to bronchiectasis can develop [50, 51]. Liver disease due to cryptosporidium is also reported [52]. Similar to CD40L deficiency, severe neutropenia may occur. The treatment approach is the same as for patients with CD40L deficiency – immunoglobulin replacement and antibiotic prophylaxis to prevent *Pneumocystis jirovecii* and *Cryptosporidium* infection. HSCT has been successfully performed [53].

2.3.3 IKAROS Deficiency

Ikaros family zinc finger 1 (*IKZF1*) encodes a transcription factor, which by recruiting target DNA to proteins that modify chromatin regulates gene transcription during hematopoietic cell development in the bone marrow [54].

Heterozygous mutations in *IKZF1* have been associated with numerous immune defects including pancytopenia with anemia, thrombocytopenia, and neutropenia presaging B-lymphocytopenia and diminished NK cells [55]. Progressive B-lymphocytopenia with associated hypogammaglobulinemia, inherited in an autosomal dominant fashion with incomplete penetrance and giving rise to a common variable immunodeficient-type clinical picture, is also described [56, 57]. Variable abnormalities in T-lymphocyte subsets are described including increased $CD8^+$ T-lymphocyte counts reduced regulatory T-lymphocyte numbers, a skewed T-lymphocyte receptor repertoire, and increased T-lymphocyte receptor $\alpha\beta^+CD4^-CD8^-$ double-negative T-lymphocyte counts, as well as impaired proliferation to mitogens [58]. Abnormalities in dendritic cell subsets leading to decreases in plasmacytoid dendritic cell numbers and expansion in conventional dendritic cells 1 are described in these patients [59].

Clinical features are variable but include severe bacterial infection, with recurrent sinopulmonary infection described, and infection with *Pneumocystis jirovecii*. Autoimmunity is described with hematological cytopenias, vasculitis, and systemic lupus erythematosus. B-cell leukemia is also an associated feature [56]. Treatment is replacement immunoglobulin and appropriate management of autoimmune features. The place of HSCT in selected patients is yet to be determined [58].

2.3.4 DOCK8 Deficiency

Previously classified as autosomal recessive Hyper IgE syndrome [60, 61], patients with bi-allelic mutations in dedicator of cytokinesis 8 (*DOCK8*) are better considered to have a combined immunodeficiency [62, 63]. DOCK8 is highly expressed in immune cells, activates CDC42 and RAC. Failure of DOCK8 function impairs T-lymphocyte proliferation and production of antiviral T_H1 cytokines, decreased production of T_H17 cytokines, and increased production of T_H2 cytokines, associated with allergic responses [64]. Immune synapse formation is also impaired with loss of DOCK8 expression interfering with antiviral NK cell cytotoxicity.

Patients can present from infancy with severe bacterial, viral, and fungal infections. Herpes simplex, severe molluscum contagiosum, and severe human papilloma virus infections are common. Common bacterial pathogens include *Staphylococcus aureus* and *Streptococcus pneumonia*. *Pneumocystis jirovecii* can cause interstitial pneumonitis and *Cryptosporidium* is associated with severe liver disease and sclerosing cholangitis. Mucocutaneous candidiasis is frequently reported. Severe food allergies are common and may be associated with anaphylaxis. Vasculitis is well described, including cerebral vasculitis. Malignancies are common and include lymphoma and squamous cell carcinoma. Severe eczema is one of the most common complications, with recurrent respiratory infection, which may lead to bronchiectasis. Asthma is also common.

Immunological features include a highly elevated IgE and eosinophilia. IgG and IgA levels can be normal or high; IgM levels are often progressively reduced.

Vaccine antibody responses may be subnormal and isohemagglutinins diminished or absent. T-lymphocyte subsets are diminished, and B-lymphocyte counts reduced with low or absent class-switched memory B-lymphocytes. NK cell counts can be reduced [62, 63]. Some patients with DOCK8 deficiency may be detected at birth by newborn screening for SCID, due to a low number or absent TRECs [65].

Aggressive treatment of infection is important, and antimicrobial prophylaxis is required. Immunoglobulin replacement is recommended. However, even with these conservative measures, survival is less than 40% by 30 years of age and event-free survival (life-threatening infection, cerebral stroke, vasculitis or encephalitis, malignancy, or death) only 4% by 30 years of age [63]. For these reasons, HSCT should be considered the treatment of choice for these patients. A recent report demonstrated 84% survival in a large multicenter cohort [66]. However, although infection susceptibility and skin manifestations responded well to transplantation, resolution of food allergy was variable [66, 67].

2.3.5 MHC II Deficiency

MHC class II molecules are transmembrane glycoprotein heterodimers constructed from α and β chains, the genes for which are encoded on the short arm of chromosome 6. MHC class II molecules present exogenous peptides to CD4 T-lymphocyte receptors to initiate the normal adaptive response. The expression of MHC II molecules on thymic epithelial cells leads to the positive selection of CD4+ T-lymphocytes during thymic development. MHC II deficiency is caused by mutations in one of four regulatory genes (*CIITA*, *RFX5*, *RFXANK*, *RFXAP*) that encode transacting regulatory factors that are critical for the expression of MHC II molecules on the cell surface. Mutations in any of these genes lead to a similar clinical picture.

Patients classically present later than patients with SCID. However, severe, persistent gastrointestinal or respiratory infections are the hallmark of the disease, with infections caused by bacterial, viral, fungal, or protozoal pathogens including *Pneumocystis jirovecii*. Severe sinopulmonary infections are common, as is growth failure secondary to viral gastrointestinal infection. Cryptosporidial liver disease is well described. Enteroviral infections are frequent and may cause meningoencephalitis. Autoimmunity is a distinct feature in some patients, particularly autoimmune cytopenias [68–70].

Immunological findings include a CD4+ lymphocytopenia, with diminished immunoglobulin levels and impaired vaccine antibody responses. T-lymphocyte proliferative responses to phytohemagglutinin may be normal. Most patients will not be detected by newborn screening for SCID as some TRECs are present.

Treatment of choice is HSCT. Historically, results have been less good for this disease compared with other immunodeficiencies [35], in part because of increased mortality from viral infection or GVHD [71]. Recent results are more encouraging [72].

2.3.6 MHCI Deficiency

MHC class I molecules are also transmembrane glycoprotein heterodimers constructed from α chains, the genes for which are encoded on the short arm of chromosome 6 and a β2-microglobulin protein. MHC class I molecules present peptides derived from protein synthesized within the cell to CD8 T-lymphocyte receptors to initiate the cytotoxic T-lymphocyte response and are thus important in countering intracellular pathogens. The expression of MHC I molecules on thymic epithelial cells leads to the positive selection of CD8+ T-lymphocytes during thymic development. MHC I deficiency is caused by defects in the genes encoding one of the proteins essential for transporting the peptide to the endoplasmic reticulum and loading it onto the MHC I molecule, namely, transporter associated with antigen processing (TAP) 1 and TAP2 and tapasin proteins. Without antigen loading, the MHC I molecule is not presented at the cell surface [73].

The clinical presentation is usually during childhood with recurrent upper respiratory tract disease causing sinusitis, otitis media, nasal disease, and pharyngitis. Lower respiratory tract bacterial infections lead to chronic inflammatory lung disease and bronchiectasis. Additionally, sterile necrotizing granulomatous skin lesions resembling Wegener's granulomatosis are described in some patients and may cause midface deformities. Immunological findings include diminished CD8+ TCRαβ lymphocyte numbers. MHC I expression is severely diminished or absent. Natural killer cell numbers may be increased. Treatment is supportive with aggressive use of prophylactic antibiotics – immunoglobulin replacement may be necessary. Treatment of the granulomata can be extremely challenging and include immunosuppression with local topical steroid [74].

2.3.7 Combined Immunodeficiency with Alopecia Totalis (FOXN1 Deficiency)

Defects in *FOXN1* cause a phenotype similar to that in the nude mouse, the so-called winged-helix-nude deficiency. It is a rare immunodeficiency characterized by athymia with congenital alopecia and nail dystrophy. *FOXN1* is a critical transcription factor for the development of thymic epithelial cells, the skin, hair, and nails [75] and is important for thymic epithelial cell differentiation, maintenance, and function [76]. T-lymphocyte development is arrested during the intra-thymic positive and negative selection of thymocytes. Patients present with features of SCID, including viral infection of the respiratory and intestinal tract and *Pneumocystis jirovecii* interstitial pneumonia, as well as the characteristic phenotypic features of skin, hair, and nail dystrophy [77]. Immunological investigations show failure of efficient thymopoiesis with an increase in circulating double-negative (CD4-CD8-) T-lymphocytes in the peripheral blood [78] and a low number or absent TRECs or CD31+ recent thymic emigrants. There is an oligoclonal TCR repertoire with reduced in vitro proliferation [79, 80]. Patients may present with an Omenn syndrome phenotype with associated eosinophilia, elevated serum IgE, and activated oligoclonal T-lymphocytes [81]. HSCT may be attempted [80], but as the genetic defect resides in thymic epithelial cells rather than hematopoietic stem cells, thymic transplantation is the treatment of choice [79].

2.3.8 Combined Immunodeficiency with Immuno-Osseous Dysplasias

Immuno-osseous dysplasias encompass a number of disorders, some of which remain undefined. Six disorders are well characterized, with identified gene defects.

2.3.8.1 Schimke Syndrome

Schimke immune-osseous dysplasia is inherited in an autosomal recessive fashion and is due to bi-allelic pathogenic variants in *SMARCAL1*. It is a multisystem disorder characterized by spondyloepiphyseal dysplasia leading to short stature, nephropathy, and T-lymphocyte immunodeficiency. The gene encodes an ATP-dependent annealing helicase, SWI/SNF-related, matrix-associated, actin-dependent regulator of chromatin, subfamily a-like 1 (SMARCAL1), which has roles in DNA repair, telomere maintenance, and DNA replication fork stability during DNA replication stress [82]. Clinical features include prenatal and postnatal disproportionate growth failure due to spondyloepiphyseal dysplasia with a reduction in trunk length significantly more than that for leg length. Characteristic radiographic manifestations of Schimke immune-osseous dysplasia include ovoid and mildly flattened vertebral bodies, with small deformed capital femoral epiphyses, and shallow dysplastic acetabular fossa. Most patients develop steroid-resistant nephrotic syndrome and renal failure due to focal glomerulosclerosis, which progresses to end-stage renal disease. Opportunistic infection due to a T-lymphocyte deficiency occurs in some individuals. There is an increased risk of frequent and severe bacterial infection, including pneumonia. Fulminant EBV infection has been reported. Autoimmune enteropathy with vomiting, diarrhea, and malabsorption has been reported [83]. Hyperpigmented macules, commonly on the trunk and less frequently on the limbs, head, and neck, occur. The hair is fine or thin, and teeth small or missing. Dysmorphic features include a broad, low nasal bridge, bulbous nasal tip, lumbar lordosis, and protuberant abdomen. Other less common features include bone marrow failure in about 10% of patients [84].

Schimke immune-osseous dysplasia represents a spectrum of disease that ranges from an infantile or severe early-onset form with death early in life to a juvenile or milder later-onset form with survival into adulthood. Severe disease phenotypes are associated with nonsense, frameshift, or splicing mutations, whereas affected individuals with milder disease have missense mutations [85].

Management of the immunodeficiency consists of antibiotic and antiviral prophylaxis. Immunosuppression should be given to those with autoimmune manifestations. Granulocyte colony-stimulating factor may be required to treat neutropenia. Other measures include consideration of renal transplantation for end-stage renal disease and hip replacement for femoral dysplasia.

2.3.8.2 Cartilage Hair Hypoplasia

Cartilage hair hypoplasia is a rare autosomal recessive metaphyseal chondrodysplasia, (short-limbed dwarfism), associated with T-lymphocyte deficiency. It is relatively more common in the Old Order Amish and the Finnish populations. Bi-allelic pathogenic changes in the ribonuclease mitochondrial RNA-processing (*RMRP*) gene, encoding for the 267 nucleotide-long RNA component of the mitochondrial RNA-processing endonuclease, cause the disease through disruption of ribosomal processing and disruption of cell cycle progression in rapidly dividing cells such as lymphocytes and chondrocytes [86]. There is a spectrum of clinical phenotypes. The classical presentation is of short stature with radiographic findings of variable metaphyseal dysplasia, epiphyseal and vertebral dysplasia, and short tubular bones with widened, scalloped, and sclerotic metaphyses most notable in knees and ankles [87].

Other features include T-lymphocyte-mediated immunodeficiency, bone marrow dysplasia and particularly erythrocyte aplasia, and Hirschsprung's disease. Sparse and fine scalp, eyebrow, and eyelash hair, with a reduction of the diameter of the hair shaft, which lacks a central pigmented core of the hair shaft cause the distinctive appearance of the hair [88, 89]. The features are variable, depending on the mutations present, but within families, clinical variability is observed [89, 90]. Sterile cutaneous granulomata are described in this condition [91].

Up to half of patients have increased susceptibility to infection, with exquisite risk of severe varicella infection [92]. Humoral immunodeficiency can lead to a high frequency of bronchiectasis [93]. However, the immune defect is variable, ranging from a SCID immunophenotype [94, 95] through to normal immunity. Autoimmune disease is described, including enteropathy, hypothyroidism, hemolytic anemia, and inflammatory skin disease, and patients have an increased risk of developing malignancy [96]. Not all patients with an immunophenotype have the skeletal features [95]. Immunological investigations reveal T-lymphocytopenia, including CD4+ and CD8+ subsets. Proliferative responses to concanavalin A, phytohemagglutinin, and pokeweed mitogen are often reduced. B-lymphocytes are usually normal. While immunoglobulin levels are usually normal, IgG and IgA levels may be low. Antibody responses to vaccine protein antigens are usually normal but may be impaired to polysaccharide vaccine antigens [88].

Management is dependent on the degree of immunodeficiency. Immunoglobulin therapy should be instituted if significant humoral deficiency is present. Varicella vaccine should be considered if T-lymphocyte function is normal. Varicella infection should be treated with antiviral drugs. Profound T-lymphocyte defects are correctable by HSCT, although non-immunological features will not be cured [95, 97].

2.3.8.3 Roifman Syndrome

Bi-allelic changes in *RNU4ATAC* cause the rare immuno-spondyloepiphyseal dysplasia known as Roifman syndrome [98, 99]. *RNU4ATAC* is a small nuclear RNA gene, which is an essential component of the minor spliceosome, critical for the correct splicing of about 800 genes carrying minor introns. Roifman syndrome is characterized by spondyloepiphyseal dysplasia with platyspondyly and flattened proximal femoral epiphyses, growth retardation, facial dysmorphism, retinal dystrophy, mental retardation, and immunodeficiency [100]. Patients have had recurrent bacterial ear and pulmonary infections including pneumonia, lymphadenopathy, and hepatosplenomegaly. Patients have an isolated B-lymphocytopenia, with developmental interruption at the transitional B-lymphocyte stage [101]. Immunoglobulin levels are variably low, normal, or increased, but there are impaired antibody responses to vaccination. Treatment is with antibiotic prophylaxis and immunoglobulin replacement as indicated.

2.3.8.4 Spondyloenchondrodysplasia with Immune Dysregulation

Spondyloenchondrodysplasia associated with combined immunodeficiency and autoimmunity has been described in patients with bi-allelic mutations and deletions of the *ACP5* gene [102]. Other non-immunological features described include spasticity, mental retardation, and cerebral calcifications.

Immunological manifestations most commonly include autoimmunity, particularly immune-mediated thrombocytopenia, hemolytic anemia, thyroiditis, and lupus erythematosus. Inflammatory bowel disease is described. Other immune features include recurrent upper and lower respiratory infection. The immunophenotype demonstrates CD4+ lymphocytopenia, reduced T-lymphocyte mitogenic response, and reduced specific antibody titers. Treatment is directed at the specific immune manifestation including immunosuppression and chemoprophylaxis [103, 104].

2.3.8.5 MYSM1 Deficiency

The histone H2A deubiquitinase, MYSM1, is essential for maintaining hematopoietic and mesenchymal stem cell quiescence and survival. Few patients are described with mutations in *MYSM1*. Clinical features include short stature with microcephaly and developmental delay, recurrent infections, congenital bone marrow failure, and myelodysplasia. The immunophenotype includes B-alymphocytosis and T-lymphocytopenia with agammaglobulinemia. Treatment is supportive with antibiotic prophylaxis and immunoglobulin replacement – one patient had resolution of immunological features following a spontaneous in vivo genetic reversion in a hematopoietic stem cell [105, 106].

2.3.8.6 EXTL3 Deficiency

Exostosin-like glycosyltransferase 3, encoded by *EXTL3*, is an *N*-acetylglucosaminyltransferase, important in heparan sulfate (HS) and heparan sulfate proteoglycan (HSPG) biosynthesis. Heparan sulfate proteoglycans modulate the activity of numerous developmental proteins that are critical in skeletal and hematopoietic development. A few patients have been reported with autosomal recessive EXTL3 deficiency. Predominant non-immunological manifestations comprise platyspondyly, brachydactyly, kyphosis, variable skeletal dysplasias, and developmental delay. The immunophenotype is variable, ranging from T-alymphocytosis with normal B-lymphocytes and hypogammaglobulinemia, an Omenn syndrome-like picture, to apparent normal immunity. Early mortality in infancy is documented, but other patients have survived to adulthood, with seeming recovery of lymphocyte numbers [107–109].

2.3.9 Combined Immunodeficiency with Intestinal Atresias (TTC7A Deficiency)

The tetratricopeptide repeat domain-containing protein 7A (TTC7A) encoded by *TTC7A* consists of nine tetratricopeptide repeat domains that mediate protein-protein interactions and assemble multi-protein complexes to regulate cell cycle, transcription, and protein transport. Bi-allelic mutations in *TTC7A* lead to dysregulation of the distribution of α6-integrin and actin in the epithelial surface [110]. To establish and maintain multicellular epithelial tissues, each cell requires apicobasal polarization to establish the correct orientation. The protein TTC7A is critical in this signaling pathway to coordinate epithelial cell polarity, growth, and differentiation. An inverted bipolarity displaces intestinal epithelia and thymocytes resulting in constant apoptotic enteropathy and lymphocyte depletion [111].

The clinical phenotype is variable. Null mutations result in intestinal atresia, while hypomorphic variants give rise to early-onset inflammatory bowel disease, which may be associated with alopecia and may resolve with increasing age [112, 113]. Patients may present with a severe infectious phenotype equivalent to that of patients with SCID. Furthermore, as many require intestinal surgery, infection with enteric organisms is common. Autoimmunity is described in older patients with hypomorphic mutations [113].

The immunodeficiency may be profound, with T-alymphocytosis, absent thymic emigrants, and absent lymphocyte proliferations to mitogens. Panhypogammaglobulinemia may be present. In less severe patients, lymphocyte numbers may be normal.

Nutritional support is a significant element of management. For patients with a severe immunophenotype, HSCT may reverse the T-lymphocyte immunodeficiency, although not the intestinal atresia [114]. For less severely affected patients, prophylactic antibiotics and immunoglobulin should be administered.

2.3.10 ZAP-70 Deficiency

The zeta-chain associated protein kinase 70 kDa (ZAP-70) is important for effective T- and B-lymphocyte receptor signaling and critical for T-lymphocyte differentiation and function [115]. Mutations in *ZAP70* cause an autosomal recessive combined immunodeficiency characterized by CD8+ T-lymphocytopenia. The majority of patients present in the first year of life with severe infections including *Pneumocystis jirovecii* infection and failure to thrive [116, 117]. However, patients with hypomorphic mutations may present later [118], when autoimmunity may be predominant [119].

Classically, patients present with normal or elevated peripheral lymphocyte numbers, associated with normal or increased CD4+ T-lymphocytes but low or absent CD8+ T-lymphocytes, which may increase over time suggesting development of limited thymic output, although TREC levels are very low [120]. CD4+ T-lymphocyte numbers are normal, but cells do not proliferate in response to T-lymphocyte mitogens, although by-passing stimulation of the T-lymphocyte receptor with PMA and ionomycin does induce a proliferative response [116]. Although B-lymphocyte numbers are normal, most patients have hypogammaglobulinemia.

Management of patients with ZAP-70 kinase deficiency is as for other patients with a SCID – antimicrobial prophylaxis and immunoglobulin replacement. HSCT is curative [121].

2.3.11 CD8α Chain Deficiency

The CD8 T-lymphocyte co-receptor is expressed on the cell surface as αα homodimers or αβ heterodimers. The expression of CD8β on the cell surface is dependent on expression of CD8α, without which CD8β remains in the endoplasmic reticulum and is degraded. CD8 expression is required for positive thymocyte selection in the thymus, without which CD8+ T-lymphocytes are not released into the periphery. Few cases of CD8α chain deficiency have been described to date [122–124]. Pulmonary complications are a particular feature in some of the cases described, although younger family members sharing the same genetic defect and immunotype were reported as asymptomatic. Affected patients had a history of recurrent viral and bacterial sinopulmonary infections from early childhood, progressing to severe bronchiectasis. Immunological evaluation demonstrated a normal number of lymphocytes, with normal CD4+ and CD19+ values and normal numbers of NK cells but completely absent CD8+ T-lymphocytes. A high percentage of CD4-CD8-TCRαβ+ T-lymphocytes has been demonstrated. Proliferation to mitogens was normal, and there were normal levels of immunoglobulin, with positive antibody responses to vaccine antigen. There was in one patient, incomplete seroconversion to EBV. Optimal treatment has yet to be determined, but benefit from antibiotics and immunoglobulin replacement has been reported.

2.3.12 CD4+ Deficiency

The syndrome of idiopathic CD4 lymphopenia was initially described by the Centers for Disease Control and Prevention in the United States and defined as a syndrome of persistent absolute CD4+ T-lymphocytes less than 300 cells/μL or 20% of total T-lymphocytes in the absence of HIV infection or other recognized immunosuppressing infections or medication [125]. The first described patients experienced opportunistic infections reminiscent of HIV infection that prompted lymphocyte phenotyping, which demonstrated CD4+ lymphocytopenia, consistent with HIV infection despite negative HIV testing [126]. Subsequently, asymptomatic individuals with abnormalities noted on routine full blood counts have been described [127].

For many patients, a genetic cause of the immunotype has yet to be determined, although a few genetic causes have been identified. Some are variants of previously identified genes involved in immune function. One patient presenting with hemorrhagic varicella zoster associated with pneumonitis and subsequent recurrent fever and pneumonia was found to have CD4+ lymphocytopenia, with normal humoral immunity, caused by bi-allelic heterozygous missense mutations in *RAG1* [128]. In other patients, new genetic etiologies have been revealed (Table 2.5) (vide infra).

While most of the patients described to date have presented with severe or opportunistic infection, an emerging cohort is being identified through newborn screening for SCID [129]. Less than 3% of infants identified as having low TRECs will have idiopathic CD4+ lymphopenia, but these infants will be asymptomatic [130] – careful evaluation of their immune system with appropriate safeguards regarding live vaccines and antibiotic prophylaxis is required, until a decision can be made about the requirement for definitive treatment or the lymphocyte count normalizes [131].

Table 2.5 Genetic immune deficiencies associated with CD4+ T-lymphocytopenia

Disease	Gene
MHC II deficiency	*CIITA, RFX5, RFXANK, RFXAP*
Hypomorphic mutation in recombinase activating gene 1	*RAG1*
Lck deficiency	*LCK*
RASGRP1 deficiency	*RASGRP1*
ITK deficiency	*ITK*
MAGT1 deficiency	*MAGT1*
MST1 deficiency	*STK4*

2.3.12.1 UNC119 Deficiency

There is a single report of a 32-year-old female with a history of recurrent sinusitis, otitis media, and zoster. The patient experienced persistent severe fungal nail infections, fungal dermatitis, and oral herpetic lesions. Two episodes of bacterial pneumonia were reported followed by bronchiolitis obliterans organizing pneumonia and oral herpetic lesions [132, 133]. The patient had persistent CD4+ lymphocytopenia of less than 300 cells/μL with associated CD3+ lymphocytopenia. Serum levels of IgM, IgA, and IgG were normal with normal vaccine antigen responses. The patient had a heterozygous mutation in *UNC119*, which interfered with the normal subcellular localization of Lck, leading to reduced T-lymphocyte proliferation following T-lymphocyte receptor stimulation. Management was not indicated, but early use of prophylactic antibiotics and antivirals is likely to be useful.

2.3.12.2 Lck Deficiency

The lymphocyte-specific protein-tyrosine kinase, Lck, encoded by *LCK*, is a protein-tyrosine kinase of the SRC oncogene family, important in signal transduction through the T-lymphocyte receptor. The p56 (LCK) protein is bound to the plasma membrane and interacts with intracellular domains of CD4+ and CD8+ co-receptors. There are few reports of mutations in *LCK* in patients. A young female with homozygous changes in *LCK* is reported who, from age 15 months, had protracted diarrhea, resulting in failure to thrive. She presented with recurrent upper and lower respiratory tract infections, including a pneumonia complicated by a pneumatocele. By the age of 22 months, she had daily fevers associated with multiple nodular skin lesions identified as neutrophilic panniculitis and interphalangeal joint inflammation [134]. The immunophenotype demonstrated a profound CD4+ T-lymphocytopenia with a reduction in proportion of TCRαβ+ T-lymphocytes and rise in TCRγδ+ T-lymphocytes. B-lymphocytes and NK cell counts were normal or slightly low. Optimal management is not clear – the patient underwent HSCT – but succumbed to complications [135]. A further patient with common variable immunodeficiency and CD4+ lymphocytopenia has been described with CD4+ T-lymphocytopenia and an aberrantly spliced lck transcript lacking the entire exon 7 of *LCK* [136]. The same defect was found in an infant with SCID, presenting with oral candidiasis and rotavirus-associated loose stools and poor weight gain [137]. *Enterobacter cloacae* was isolated from the blood and cytomegalovirus from the urine and intestinal biopsies. HSCT was successful.

2.3.12.3 RASGRP1 Deficiency

Ras proteins actively switch between inactive GDP-bound and active GTP-bound conformation and are critical to coordinate the cellular response to growth factors or extracellular stimuli. RASGRP1 is a guanine-nucleotide exchange factor that converts Ras-GDP to Ras-GTP permitting activation of the RAS-REF-MAPK-ERK pathway, which is involved in lymphocyte development and function.

Several patients have now been described with bi-allelic loss-of-function mutations in *RASGRP1* who presented with pleiotropic manifestations, associated with a CD4+ T-lymphocytopenia [138–142]. Symptoms encompass infection, including opportunistic infection from *Pneumocystis jirovecii*, as well as recurrent pneumonias from infancy with development of bronchiectasis, and enteral infection causing growth failure. Severe recurrent EBV infection is a characteristic feature, which predisposes to lymphoma – other malignancies including smooth muscle tumors are described. Human papilloma virus can cause epidermodysplasia verruciformis. Autoimmunity is an important associated feature – autoimmune hemolytic anemia and immune-mediated thrombocytopenia are described in several patients – as well as autoimmune hepatitis.

The immunophenotype characteristically demonstrates normal numbers of CD3+ T-lymphocytes associated with CD4+ T-lymphocytopenia. CD8+ T-lymphocyte numbers are normal, as are B-lymphocyte and NK cells. Mucosal-associated invariant T-lymphocytes and invariant NKT lymphocytes are also reported as very low or absent. Immunoglobulin levels and vaccine response are variably low to normal.

Treatment is supportive including antibiotic and antiviral chemoprophylaxis. Specific treatment should be directed at treating autoimmune or malignant complications. HSCT is reported as successful and recommended.

2.3.12.4 Interleukin-2- Inducible T-lymphocyte Kinase Deficiency

Interleukin-2-inducible T-lymphocyte kinase (ITK), encoded by *ITK*, is involved in lymphocyte signaling and development. When the T lymphocyte receptor is activated, ITK is recruited to the cell membrane and activates PLCγ1, which causes intracellular calcium release and activation of the NFκB, mTOR, and MAPK/ERK intracellular pathways.

Patients with mutations in *ITK* characteristically present with EBV-associated lymphoproliferation and are highly susceptible to developing EBV-related lymphoma – 9 of 16 developed lymphomas in a recent review of ITK-deficient patients [143]. Other features included CMV or varicella infection and EBV-driven hemophagocytic lymphohistiocytosis in two. Autoimmune features were documented in three patients. Specific pulmonary manifestations included pulmonary lymphoproliferation or lymphoma (Fig. 2.5), and pulmonary interstitial nodules were present in most patients. Pulmonary infection was documented in some patients including *Pneumocystis jirovecii*. One patient experienced progressive pulmonary infections and bronchiectasis [144–153]. A CD4+ T-lymphocytopenia was present in most patients, although CD3+ and CD8+ lymphocyte values were normal. Natural killer T-lymphocytes, when measured, were reduced. Progressive hypogammaglobulinemia was documented in some patients. Of the 16 patients reported, 6 had died without definitive therapy. HSCT seems curative and should be offered to these patients once any malignancy has been controlled [143].

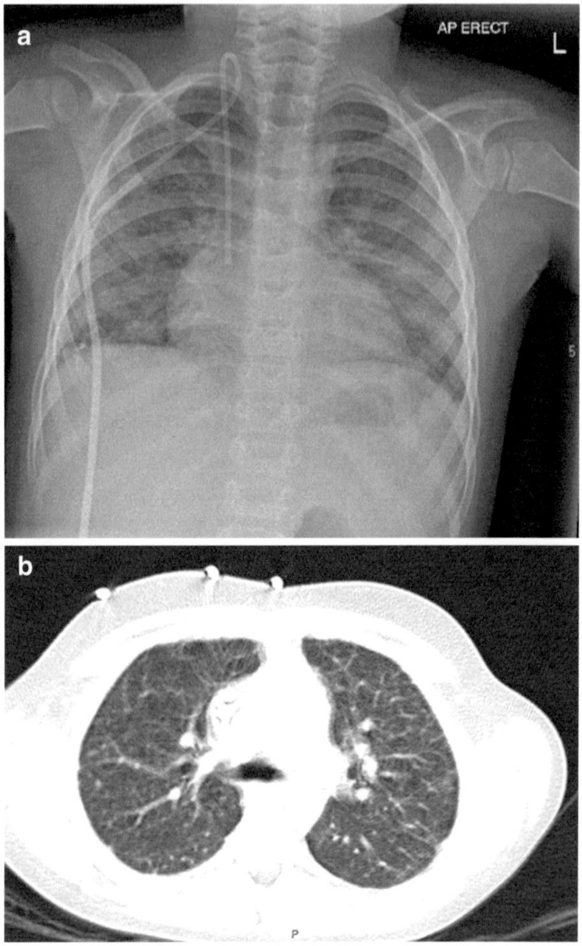

Fig. 2.5 Chest radiograph (**a**) of a 4-year-old child with ITK deficiency demonstrating extensive bilateral pulmonary nodules of variable sizes, confirmed on thoracic computerized tomography with contrast (**b**). Biopsy of the nodules demonstrated an EBV-driven lymphoproliferative disorder

2.3.12.5 Magnesium Transporter 1 Deficiency

Magnesium is an essential cofactor for ATP, nucleic acids, and many enzymes. Magnesium also acts as a second messenger following T-lymphocyte activation through the T-lymphocyte receptor. Magnesium transporter 1 (MAGT1) mediates a transient, magnesium influx immediately after T-lymphocyte receptor stimulation to facilitate downstream signaling and intracellular calcium release. Few patients with mutations in *MAGT1*, located on the X-chromosome, have been described to date [154, 155]. Characteristic clinical features are an X-linked inheritance associated with chronic infection with EBV and B-lymphocyte lymphoma in some. Other viral infections are described, including molluscum contagiosum and recurrent varicella zoster. Viral pneumonia has been documented. A few patients have experienced autoimmune cytopenias. The immunophenotype includes CD4+

T-lymphocytopenia with normal CD3+, CD8+ and CD19+ counts, but with evidence of diminished thymic output evidenced by low CD4 + CD27+ or CD31+ T-lymphocytes. A variable dysgammaglobulinemia is described with intermittent impairment of vaccine antibody responses. Lymphocyte proliferations are diminished when mitogens that act through the T-lymphocyte receptor are employed, but normal after stimulation with PMA and ionophore. Optimum treatment has yet to be demonstrated, but it is likely that HSCT will be curative and should be recommended.

2.3.13 TCRα Subunit Constant Chain Deficiency

The majority of T-lymphocytes express an extracellular and transmembrane T-lymphocyte receptor heterodimer consisting of α and β peptides in association with transmembrane and intracellular subunits of the CD3 complex. During T-lymphocyte development in the thymus, the antigen-capture (variable) region of the T-lymphocyte receptor is constructed following stochastic recombination events of specific coding segments in the V (variable), D (diversity), and J (joining) regions of the T-lymphocyte receptor loci and this joins with the constant subunit of the T-lymphocyte receptor α and β chains. Two patients from the unrelated families have been described who harbored a mutation at the last base of exon 3 following the translational termination codon, causing abnormal splicing and a leaky termination signal. Clinical features comprised recurrent upper and lower sinopulmonary infection leading to chronic lung damage, candidiasis, diarrhea, and growth failure. One child exhibited chronic varicella, EBV and human herpesvirus 6 infection. Hepatosplenomegaly and lymphadenopathy were evident. There was evidence of autoimmunity with vitiligo, alopecia and hemolytic anemia [156].

The immunotype was similar between patients and showed normal CD3+ T-lymphocytes, which expressed the γδ T-lymphocyte receptor. An abnormal population of $CD3^{lo}$ cells was present, which expressed the αβ T-lymphocyte receptor at extremely low levels. Proliferation of lymphocytes in response to phytohemagglutinin was variably impaired. Class-switched memory B-lymphocytes were present, immunoglobulin levels were normal (although IgE was elevated), and vaccine responses were present. Autoantibodies were also documented.

The infections responded to conventional antimicrobial treatment and did not recur upon institution of antibacterial and antifungal prophylaxis. Both patients responded favorably to HSCT.

2.3.14 Ca^{2+} Selective Release-Activated Ca^{2+} Channelopathies

Channelopathies are a diverse group of diseases caused by dysfunctional ion channels and transporters due to mutations in the pore-forming alpha subunits or in accessory proteins that regulate function. Store-operated Ca^{2+} entry is the major method of restoration of intracellular Ca^{2+} in cells in reaction to the depletion of Ca^{2+} stores in the endoplasmic reticulum, primarily facilitated by the Ca^{2+}-selective release-activated Ca^{2+} (CRAC) channel The CRAC channel is constructed from the pore-forming subunits ORAI1,2,3 and the Ca^{2+} sensors, STIM1 and STIM2. Recessive loss-of-function mutations in STIM1 or ORAI1 result in immune deficiency.

2.3.14.1 ORAI1 Deficiency

Few patients are described with ORAI1 deficiency [157–160]. Classical features include growth failure, severe infections including BCGitis, interstitial pneumonia, sepsis, chronic diarrhea, chronic candidiasis, pneumonia, pyelonephritis, otitis and toxoplasma encephalitis. One patient developed autoimmune cytopenia. Non-immune manifestations include myotonia, anhidrotic ectodermal dysplasia and amelogenesis imperfecta. Immunological findings are characterized by normal lymphocyte numbers of all subsets. T-lymphocyte activation is severely diminished. HSCT has been successfully performed.

2.3.14.2 STIM-1 Deficiency

Like ORAI1 deficiency, immunodeficiency due to defects in STIM-1 is rare, with few patients described [161–164]. Patients present during infancy, with infection and autoimmunity. Infectious presentations may be recurrent and involve upper and lower respiratory tract, and sepsis. Bacterial and viral infections are described, including chronic EBV infection with lymphomatoid granulomatosis in the lungs and enteroviral encephalitis. Colitis is reported in two patients and autoimmunity is a common feature. One patient is described with Kaposi sarcoma. Non-immunological features include partial iris hypoplasia, myopathy or hypotonia and defective enamel dentition. Immunological findings include normal lymphocyte numbers but low or absent invariant natural killer T-lymphocytes and decreased number of mucosal-associated invariant T-lymphocytes. Immunoglobulins are variably low, normal or raised. Lymphocyte proliferations are diminished. HSCT has been successfully performed in a few patients.

2.3.15 Serine-Threonine Protein Kinase 4 Deficiency (Mammalian Sterile 20-like Protein Deficiency)

The serine/threonine kinase 4 gene (*STK4*) encodes Mammalian sterile 20-like protein (MST1), which is important in regulating lymphocyte homing and cell survival and proliferation. Bi-allelic loss-of-function mutations have been described in a few individuals [165–169]. Clinical features are varied, but severe lower respiratory infection with bacterial agents, including extensive molluscum contagiosum, eczema, recurrent skin abscesses, and significant human papillomavirus infection is described. In some patients, mucocutaneous candida infection was a feature. Autoimmune cytopenias were documented in a few patients.

The immune phenotype consistently showed lymphocytopenia, which was variable, but in some patients, CD4+ lymphocytopenia was remarkable. Low numbers of naïve T-lymphocytes were present. B-lymphocyte numbers were generally normal, and immunoglobulin levels were normal or high. Autoantibodies were present in some patients. Intermittent neutropenia was a significant feature in several patients.

Treatment with antimicrobial prophylaxis and immunoglobulin replacement was effective for some patients, but given the severity of the combined immunodeficiency, HSCT seems a reasonable approach and was successful for some patients.

2.3.16 CARD11/BCL10/MALT1 (CBM) Complex Deficiencies

Nuclear factor kB (NF-kB) is a key component of lymphocyte activation, survival, proliferation, and production of inflammatory cytokines. Physiological regulation of NF-kB activation is performed by a protein complex constituted from caspase activation and recruitment domain 11 (CARD11), B-cell CLL/lymphoma 10 (BCL10), and mucosa-associated lymphoid tissue lymphoma translocation protein 1 (MALT1), the CBM complex. Loss-of-function and gain-of-function mutations in the *CARD11*, *BCL10*, and *MALT1* genes encoding these protein constituents have been described in a few patients [170–180].

Autoimmune features are prominent in these diseases, particularly severe inflammatory bowel disease in *MALT1* and *BCL10* deficiency, but severe eczematous disease is also reported. Infection is also a prominent feature – particularly sinopulmonary infections due to bacterial, viral, and fungal pathogens – infection with *Pneumocystis jirovecii* is reported in one patient with *CARD11* mutations. EBV infection has not been significant, and lymphoproliferative disease has not been reported in this group of disorders.

The immunotype shows wide variation. The lymphocyte numbers are generally normal, although B-lymphocytopenia has been described in a patient with MALT1 deficiency. Regulatory T-lymphocytes and T_H17 lymphocytes are generally reduced in CARD11-deficient patients but normal in MALT1-deficient patients. The patient with BCL10 deficiency showed a profound hypogammaglobulinemia, and progressive hypogammaglobulinemia is found in CARD11 deficiency, with absent antibody responses to vaccine antigens. In MALT1-deficient patients, immunoglobulin levels are normal, and antibody response to vaccine antigen is variable.

Optimum treatment is yet to be determined – antimicrobial prophylaxis and immunoglobulin replacement may be of some value – but there are a few reports of successful HSCT.

2.3.17 RHOH Deficiency

The Ras homolog family member H is an important negative regulator of hematopoietic cell growth and survival. Two adult patients have been described with biallelic loss-of-function mutations in *RHOH*, whose main clinical phenotype was severe persistent epidermodysplasia verruciformis from early childhood, with less severe molluscum in one patient [181]. One patient developed a Burkitt lymphoma. Significant pulmonary complications included development of a lobar granulomatous lesion and emphysema. The immunological investigations revealed normal T-lymphocyte counts but with slightly low CD4+ T-lymphocytes and high CD8+ T-lymphocytes. However, recent thymic emigrants were very low, and there was restricted TCR usage with clonal expansion of certain Vβ families. There was impaired lymphocyte proliferation after stimulation through the T-lymphocyte receptor. There were no major abnormalities in the immunoglobulin levels or vaccine antibody responses. Treatment was symptomatic; however, the T-lymphocytopenia was corrected in mice after HSCT, suggesting that this treatment modality may have utility in human patients.

2.3.18 IL21R Deficiency

The interleukin-21 receptor (IL21R) binds to the common γ chain to transmit signals through the JAK-signal transducer and activator of transcription (STAT) pathways. IL-21 also regulates lymphocyte proliferation, B-lymphocyte cell differentiation, NK cell cytotoxicity, and T_H17 lymphocyte differentiation. Loss-of-function mutations in *IL21R* have recently been identified in a few patients [182–184]. The clinical presentation often begins in childhood – respiratory infection and gastrointestinal disease predominate. Chronic upper and lower respiratory infection is frequently described, leading in some cases to bronchiectasis, and *Pneumocystis jirovecii* infection appears to occur frequently. Atypical mycobacterial lung infection is described. Progressive cholangitis secondary to cryptosporidial infection also occurs frequently, leading to cirrhosis and end-stage liver disease. Candidial infection was documented in several patients.

Immunological findings were variable. T-lymphocyte numbers were in the normal range. Some patients demonstrated raised B-lymphocytes, but class-switched memory B-lymphocyte numbers were reduced. Immunoglobulin levels were variably low or normal, except IgM and IgE which were often raised.

Immunoglobulin replacement was offered as treatment, but the severity of the immune defect and risk of serious lung and liver disease suggest that HSCT should be offered early in the course of disease.

2.3.19 *MTHFD1 Deficiency*

Methylenetetrahydrofolate dehydrogenase 1, encoded by *MTHFD1*, is a protein that catalyzes three reactions involved in cellular folate metabolism and is essential for the generation of formyltetrahydrofolate and methylenetetrahydrofolate and important for nucleotide and homocysteine metabolism. To date, only one patient has been described with bi-allelic loss-of-function mutations in *MTHFD1* [185, 186]. The infant presented as a patient with SCID, with poor feeding within a few weeks of birth, associated with pallor. By 8 weeks of age she required an erythrocyte transfusion and had *Pneumocystis jirovecii* pneumonitis associated with pancytopenia and elevated lactate dehydrogenase. She was profoundly pan-lymphocytopenic with absent lymphocyte proliferations and reduced IgG but normal IgM and IgA. A bone marrow examination showed giant bands and nuclear-cytoplasmic dyssynchrony with hypersegmented neutrophils and on a peripheral blood smear showed hypersegmented neutrophils. She had elevated serum homocysteine and slightly low serum methionine. She exhibited mild bilateral sensorineural hearing loss and epilepsy.

Treatment of the *Pneumocystis jirovecii*, commencement of immunoglobulin, and addition of hydroxocobalamin, oral folate, and betaine resulted in improved hematopoiesis and partial immune reconstitution with rising lymphocyte counts and improved proliferations. The patient remained on methylfolate, methylcobalamin, and immunoglobulin replacement and at 6 years of age had experienced no further serious or opportunistic infection but has a refractory seizure disorder and mild to moderate intellectual disability.

2.3.20 *CARMIL2/RLTPR Deficiency*

RGD-, leucine-rich repeat-, tropomodulin domain-, and proline-rich domain-containing (RLTPR) protein, encoded by *CARMIL2*, is important for T-lymphocyte co-stimulation mediated through CD28. A few patients have been described with bi-allelic loss-of-function mutations [187–190]. Typical clinical features described affect the skin, gastrointestinal tract, and sinopulmonary system. Additionally, for some patients, EBV is persistent, and a number have developed smooth muscle tumors. Skin involvement was common and affected most patients – dermatitis, warts, and molluscum were most frequent manifestations, but varicella infection was well described. Less common were psoriatic lesions and hyperkeratotic lesions. Upper airway infections were common, as well as pneumonias, and several patients developed bronchiectasis. Growth failure associated with diarrhea was common, and few patients developed inflammatory bowel disease. One patient developed hemophagocytic lymphohistiocytosis.

The immunotype demonstrated normal CD3+, CD4+, and CD8+ T-lymphocyte counts with normal B-lymphocyte and NK cell counts. However, there was an increase in the CD4+ naïve T-lymphocyte pool and decrease in the memory pool. There was a reduction in FOXP3+ regulatory T-lymphocytes. Proliferative responses were generally impaired but not absent, particularly of naïve CD4+ T-lymphocytes. Immunoglobulins and antigen-specific antibody levels were variably normal or reduced.

A number of the described patients have reached adulthood. Appropriate treatment of infection, possibly with antimicrobial prophylaxis, appears to be adequate. Patients with hypogammaglobulinemia may benefit from immunoglobulin replacement. The role of hematopoietic stem cell treatment has not been explored for this disease.

2.4 Conclusion

Much has been learnt over the last 50 years about the clinical manifestations of many combined immunodeficiencies. The elucidation of immune function pathways from the discovery of new genetic defects causing disease enables prediction of other uncharacterized diseases as our understanding of the immune connectome broadens. For those diseases that have been recognized and identified for the longest periods of time or for which there are larger patient cohorts, the functional defect, natural history, and current optimal treatment are well established. However, as new information becomes available, we may need to modify our management approach. For the more newly described diseases, much more information is required before we can confidently recommend the best investigative and treatment approach – when only a few patients are described, it is not clear if these represent the dominant clinical and immunological phenotype or rather are extremely severe or mild examples of disease manifestation. Additionally, we should be mindful of the impact that environment plays on disease manifestation – for the newly described diseases, a number of patients come from specific ethnic and geographical backgrounds, and so the disease manifestation may not represent that of patients with the same disease in other parts of the world.

References

1. Fischer A, Notarangelo LD, Neven B, Cavazzana M, Puck JM. Severe combined immunodeficiencies and related disorders. Nat Rev Dis Primers. 2015;1:15061.
2. Picard C, Bobby Gaspar H, Al-Herz W, et al. International Union of Immunological Societies: 2017 primary immunodeficiency diseases committee report on inborn errors of immunity. J Clin Immunol. 2018;38:96–128.
3. Berrington JE, Flood TJ, Abinun M, Galloway A, Cant AJ. Unsuspected Pneumocystis carinii pneumonia at presentation of severe primary immunodeficiency. Arch Dis Child. 2000;82:144–7.
4. van der Burg M, Gennery AR. The expanding clinical and immunological spectrum of SCID. Eur J Pediatr. 2011;170:561–71.
5. Marciano BE, Huang CY, Joshi G, et al. BCG vaccination in patients with severe combined immunodeficiency: complications, risks, and vaccination policies. J Allergy Clin Immunol. 2014;133:1134–41.
6. Gaspar HB. Bone marrow transplantation and alternatives for adenosine deaminase deficiency. Immunol Allergy Clin N Am. 2010;30:221–36.
7. Rogers MH, Lwin R, Fairbanks L, Gerritsen B, Gaspar HB. Cognitive and behavioral abnormalities in adenosine deaminase deficient severe combined immunodeficiency. J Pediatr. 2001;139:44–50.
8. Albuquerque W, Gaspar HB. Bilateral sensorineural deafness in adenosine deaminase-deficient severe combined immunodeficiency. J Pediatr. 2004;144:278–80.
9. Manson D, Diamond L, Oudjhane K, Hussain FB, Roifman C, Grunebaum E. Characteristic scapular and rib changes on chest radiographs of children with ADA-deficiency SCIDS in the first year of life. Pediatr Radiol. 2013;43(5):589–92.
10. Sauer AV, Mrak E, Hernandez RJ, et al. ADA-deficient SCID is associated with a specific microenvironment and bone phenotype characterized by RANKL/OPG imbalance and osteoblast insufficiency. Blood. 2009;114(15):3216–26.
11. Blackburn MR, Kellems RE. Adenosine deaminase deficiency: metabolic basis of immune deficiency and pulmonary inflammation. Adv Immunol. 2005;86:1–41.
12. Chunn JL, Molina JG, Mi T, et al. Adenosine- dependent pulmonary fibrosis in adenosine deaminase-deficient mice. J Immunol. 2005;175:1937–46.
13. Booth C, Algar VE, Xu-Bayford J, et al. Non- infectious lung disease in patients with adenosine deaminase deficient severe combined immunodeficiency. J Clin Immunol. 2012;32:449–53.
14. Grunebaum E, Cutz E, Roifman CM. Pulmonary alveolar proteinosis in patients with adenosine deaminase deficiency. J Allergy Clin Immunol. 2012;129:1588–93.
15. Hoenig M, Lagresle-Peyrou C, Pannicke U, EBMT Inborn Errors Working Party, et al. Reticular dysgenesis: international survey on clinical presentation, transplantation and outcome. Blood. 2017;129:2928–38.
16. Omenn GS. Familial reticuloendotheliosis with eosinophilia. N Engl J Med. 1965;273:427–32.
17. Rieux-Laucat F, Bahadoran P, Brousse N, et al. Highly restricted human T cell repertoire in peripheral blood and tissue-infiltrating lymphocytes in Omenn's syndrome. J Clin Invest. 1998;102:312–21.
18. Harville TO, Adams DM, Howard TA, et al. Oligoclonal expansion of CD45RO+ T lymphocytes in Omenn syndrome. J Clin Immunol. 1997;17:322–32.
19. de Saint-Basile G, Le Deist F, de Villartay JP, et al. Restricted heterogeneity of T lymphocytes in combined immunodeficiency with hyper- eosinophilia (Omenn's syndrome). J Clin Invest. 1991;87:1352–9.
20. Altmann T, Slack J, Slatter MA, et al. Endothelial cell damage in idiopathic pneumonia syndrome following hematopoietic stem cell transplantation. Bone Marrow Transplant. 2018;53:515–8.

21. Wahn V, Yokota S, Meyer KL, et al. Expansion of a maternally derived monoclonal T cell population with CD3+/CD8+/T cell receptor-gamma/delta+ phenotype in a child with severe combined immunodeficiency. J Immunol. 1991;147:2934–41.
22. Sebnem Kilic S, Kavurt S, Balaban AS. Transfusion-associated graft-versus-host disease in severe combined immunodeficiency. J Investig Allergol Clin Immunol. 2010;20:153–6.
23. Felgentreff K, Perez-Becker R, Speckmann C, et al. Clinical and immunological manifestations of patients with atypical severe combined immunodeficiency. Clin Immunol. 2011;141:73–82.
24. Bode SFN, Ammann S, Al-Herz W, Inborn Errors Working Party of the EBMT, et al. The syndrome of hemophagocytic lymphohistiocytosis in primary immunodeficiencies: implications for differential diagnosis and pathogenesis. Haematologica. 2015;100:978–88.
25. Slatter MA, Angus B, Windebank K, et al. Polymorphous lymphoproliferative disorder with Hodgkin like features in common gamma chain deficient severe combined immunodeficiency. J Allergy Clin Immunol. 2011;127:533–5.
26. Slatter MA, Rogerson EJ, Taylor CE, et al. Value of Bronchoalveolar lavage prior to Haematopoietic stem cell transplantation for primary immunodeficiency. Bone Marrow Transplant. 2007;40:529–33.
27. Hughes WT. Pneumocystis carinii pneumonia: new approaches to diagnosis, treatment and prevention. Pediatr Infect Dis J. 1991;10:391–9.
28. Vachon ML, Dionne N, Leblanc E, et al. Human parainfluenza type 4 infections, Canada. Emerg Infect Dis. 2006;12:1755–8.
29. Crooks BN, Taylor CE, Turner AJ, et al. Respiratory viral infections in primary immune deficiencies: significance and relevance to clinical outcome in a single BMT unit. Bone Marrow Transplant. 2000;26:1097–102.
30. Thea DM, Lambert G, Weedon J, et al. Benefit of primary prophylaxis before 18 months of age in reducing the incidence of Pneumocystis carinii pneumonia and early death in a cohort of 112 human immunodeficiency virus-infected infants. New York City Perinatal HIV Transmission Collaborative Study Group. Pediatrics. 1996;97:59–64.
31. Panel on Opportunistic Infections in HIV-Infected Adults and Adolescents. Guidelines for the prevention and treatment of opportunistic infections in HIV-infected adults and adolescents: Recommendations from the Centers for Disease Control and Prevention, the National Institutes of Health, and the HIV Medicine Association of the Infectious Diseases Society of America. Available at https://aidsinfo.nih.gov/contentfiles/lvguidelines/adult_oi.pdf.
32. Keller MD, Nicholas S, Leen A, et al. Adoptive Immunotherapy for Primary Immunodeficiency Disorders with Virus-Specific Cytotoxic T-lymphocytes. J Allergy Clin Immunol. 2016;137:1498–1505.e1.
33. Boeckh M, Berrey MM, Bowden RA, et al. Phase 1 evaluation of the respiratory syncytial virus-specific monoclonal antibody palivizumab in recipients of hematopoietic stem cell transplants. J Infect Dis. 2001;184:350–4.
34. Chávez-Bueno S, Mejías A, Merryman RA, et al. Intravenous palivizumab and ribavirin combination for respiratory syncytial virus disease in high-risk pediatric patients. Pediatr Infect Dis J. 2007;26:1089–93.
35. Gennery AR, Slatter MA, Grandin L, et al. Transplantation of Haematopoietic Stem Cells and Long Term Survival for Primary Immunodeficiencies in Europe: entering a new century, do we do better? J Allergy Clin Immunol. 2010;126:602–10. e1–11
36. Pai S-Y, Logan BR, Griffith LM, et al. Transplantation outcomes for severe combined immunodeficiency, 2000–2009. N Engl J Med. 2014;371:434–46.
37. Brown L, Xu-Bayford J, Allwood Z, et al. Neonatal diagnosis of severe combined immunodeficiency leads to significantly improved survival outcome: the case for newborn screening. Blood. 2011;117:3243–6.
38. Kwan A, Abraham RS, Currier R, et al. Newborn screening for severe combined immunodeficiency in 11 screening programs in the United States. JAMA. 2014;312:729–38.

39. Picard C, Bobby Gaspar H, Al-Herz W, et al. International Union of Immunological Societies: 2017 primary immunodeficiency diseases committee report on inborn errors of immunity. J Clin Immunol. 2018;38:96–128.
40. Durandy A, Kracker S, Fischer A. Primary antibody deficiencies. Nat Rev Immunol. 2013;13:519–33.
41. Levy J, Espanol-Boren T, Thomas C, et al. Clinical spectrum of X-linked hyper-IgM syndrome. J Pediatr. 1997;131:47–54.
42. Hayward AR, Levy J, Facchetti F, Notarangelo L, et al. Cholangiopathy and tumors of the pancreas, liver, and biliary tree in boys with X-linked immunodeficiency with hyper-IgM. J Immunol. 1997;158:977–83.
43. Cunningham CK, Bonville CA, Ochs HD, et al. Enteroviral meningoencephalitis as a complication of X-linked hyper IgM syndrome. J Pediatr. 1999;3:584–8.
44. Aschermann Z, Gomori E, Kovacs GG, et al. X-linked hyper-IgM syndrome associated with a rapid course of multifocal leukoencephalopathy. Arch Neurol. 2007;64:273–6.
45. Toniati P, Savoldi G, Davies G, et al. Report of the ESID collaborative study on clinical features and molecular analysis in X-LINKED HYPER-IgM syndrome. Clin Exp Immunol. 2008;154(S1):121.
46. de la Morena MT, Leonard D, Torgerson T, et al. Long term outcomes of 176 patients with X-linked hyper IgM syndrome. J Allergy Clin Immunol. 2016;139:1282–92.
47. Gennery AR, Khawaja K, Veys P, et al. Treatment of CD40 ligand deficiency by hematopoietic stem cell transplantation: a survey of the European experience, 1993-2002. Blood. 2004;103:1152–7.
48. Ferrua F, Galimberti S, Courteille V, et al. Hematopoietic stem cell transplantation for CD40 ligand deficiency: results from an EBMT/ESID-IEWP-SCETIDE-PIDTC Study. J Allergy Clin Immunol. 2018.; (in press).
49. Quarello P, Tandoi F, Carraro F, et al. Successful sequential liver and hematopoietic stem cell transplantation in a child with CD40 ligand deficiency and Cryptosporidium-induced liver cirrhosis. Transplantation. 2018;102:823–8.
50. Ferrari S, Giliani S, Insalaco A, et al. Mutations of CD40 gene cause an autosomal recessive form of immunodeficiency with hyper IgM. Proc Natl Acad Sci U S A. 2001;98:12614–9.
51. Lougaris V, Badolato R, Ferrari S, Plebani A. Hyper immunoglobulin M syndrome due to CD40 deficiency: clinical, molecular, and immunological features. Immunol Rev. 2005;203:48–66.
52. Kutukculer N, Moratto D, Aydinok Y, et al. Disseminated cryptosporidium infection in an infant with hyper-IgM syndrome caused by CD40 deficiency. J Pediatr. 2003;142:194–6.
53. Al-Saud B, Al-Jomaie M, Al-Ghonaium A, et al. Haematopoietic stem cell transplant for hyper-IgM syndrome due to CD40 defects: a single-centre experience. Bone Marrow Transplant. 2018.; (in press).
54. John LB, Ward AC. The Ikaros gene family: transcriptional regulators of hematopoiesis and immunity. Mol Immunol. 2011;48:1272–8.
55. Goldman FD, Gurel Z, Al-Zubeidi D, et al. Congenital pancytopenia and absence of B lymphocytes in a neonate with a mutation in the Ikaros gene. Pediatr Blood Cancer. 2012;58:591–7.
56. Kuehn HS, Boisson B, Cunningham-Rundles C, et al. Loss of B cells in patients with heterozygous mutations in IKAROS. N Engl J Med. 2016;374:1032–43.
57. Bogaert DJ, et al. A novel IKAROS haploinsufficiency kindred with unexpectedly late and variable B-cell maturation defects. J. Allergy Clin Immunol. 2017;141:432–435.e7.
58. Hoshino A, Okada S, Yoshida K, et al. Abnormal hematopoiesis and autoimmunity in human subjects with germline IKZF1 mutations. J Allergy Clin Immunol. 2016;140:223–31.
59. Cytlak U, Resteu A, Altmann T, et al. Dendritic cell and monocyte anomalies in human IKZF1 haploinsufficiency. Nat Commun. 2018;9:1239.
60. Zhang Q, Davis JC, Lamborn IT, et al. Combined immunodeficiency associated with DOCK8 mutations. N Engl J Med. 2009;361:2046–55.

61. Engelhardt KR, McGhee S, Winkler S, et al. Large deletions and point mutations involving *DOCK8* in the autosomal recessive form of the hyper-IgE syndrome. J Allergy Clin Immunol. 2009;124:1289–130.
62. Engelhardt KR, Gertz EM, Keles S, et al. The extended clinical phenotype of 58 patients with DOCK8 deficiency. J Allergy Clin Immunol. 2015;136:402–12.
63. Aydin SE, Kilic SS, Aytekin C, inborn errors working party of EBMT, et al. DOCK8 deficiency: clinical and immunological phenotype and treatment options. J Clin Immunol. 2015;35:189–98.
64. Su HC, Jing H, Zhang Q. DOCK8 deficiency. Ann N Y Acad Sci. 2011;1246:26–33.
65. Dasouki M, Okonkwo KC, Ray A, et al. Deficient T cell receptor excision circles (TRECs) in autosomal recessive hyper IgE syndrome caused by DOCK8 mutation: implications for pathogenesis and potential detection by newborn screening. Clin Immunol. 2011;141:128–32.
66. Aydin SE, Freeman AF, Al-Herz W, inborn errors working party of the European Group for Blood and Marrow Transplantation (EBMT) and the European Society for Primary Immunodeficiencies (ESID), et al. Hematopoietic stem cell transplantation as treatment for patients with DOCK8 deficiency. Blood Adv. 2018. (in press).
67. Happel CS, Stone KD, Freeman AF, et al. Food allergies can persist after myeloablative hematopoietic stem cell transplantation in dedicator of cytokinesis 8-deficient patients. J Allergy Clin Immunol. 2016;137:1895–1898.e5.
68. Al-Herz W, Alsmadi O, Melhem M, et al. Major histocompatibility complex class II deficiency in Kuwait: clinical manifestations, immunological findings and molecular profile. J Clin Immunol. 2013;33:513–9.
69. Ben-Mustapha I, Ben-Farhat K, Guirat-Dhouib N, et al. Clinical, immunological and genetic findings of a large tunisian series of major histocompatibility complex class II deficiency patients. J Clin Immunol. 2013;33:865–70.
70. Ouederni M, Vincent QB, Frange P, et al. Major histocompatibility complex class II expression deficiency caused by a RFXANK founder mutation: a survey of 35 patients. Blood. 2011;118:5108–18.
71. Renella R, Picard C, Neven B, et al. Human leukocyte antigen identical hematopoietic stem cell transplantation in major histocompatibility complex class II immunodeficiency: reduce survival correlated with an increase incidence of acute graft versus host disease and pre-existing viral infections. Br J Hematol. 2006;134:510–6.
72. Elfeky R, Furtado-Silva JM, Chiesa R, et al. Umbilical cord blood transplantation without *in vivo* T-cell depletion for children with MHC class II deficiency. J Allergy Clin Immunol. 2018;141:2279–2282.e2.
73. de la Salle H, Donato L, Hanau D. Peptide transporter defects in human leukocyte antigen class I deficiency. In: Ochs H, Smith E, Puck J, editors. Primary immunodeficiency diseases. A molecular and genetic approach. New York: Oxford University Press; 2014. p. 258–68.
74. Gadola SD, Moins-Teisserenc HT, Trowsdale J, et al. TAP deficiency syndrome. Clin Exp Immunol. 2000;121:173–8.
75. Palamaro L, Romano R, Fusco A, et al. FOXN1 in organ development and human diseases. Int Rev Immunol. 2014;33:83–93.
76. Nowell CS, Bredenkamp N, Tetélin S, et al. Foxn1 regulates lineage progression in cortical and medullary Thymic epithelial cells but is dispensable for medullary sublineage divergence. PLoS Genet. 2011;7:e1002348.
77. Pignata C, Fusco A, Amorosi S. Human clinical phenotype associated with FOXN1 mutations. Adv Exp Med Biol. 2009;665:195–206.
78. Albuquerque AS, Marques JG, Silva SL, et al. Human FOXN1-deficiency is associated with alphabeta double-negative and FoxP3+ T-cell expansions that are distinctly modulated upon thymic transplantation. PLoS One. 2012;7:e37042.
79. Markert ML, Marques JG, Neven B, Devlin BH, McCarthy EA, Chinn IK, et al. First use of thymus transplantation therapy for FOXN1 deficiency (nude/SCID): a report of 2 cases. Blood. 2011;117:688–96.

80. Chou J, Massaad MJ, Wakim RH, et al. A novel mutation in FOXN1 resulting in SCID: a case report and literature review. Clin Immunol. 2014;155:30–2.
81. Pignata C, Fiore M, Guzzetta V, et al. Congenital alopecia and nail dystrophy associated with severe functional T-cell immunodeficiency in two sibs. Am J Med Genet. 1996;65:167–70.
82. Lugli N, Sotiriou SK, Halazonetis TD. The role of SMARCAL1 in replication fork stability and telomere maintenance. DNA Repair (Amst). 2017;56:129–34.
83. Kaitila I, Savilahti E, Ormälä T. Autoimmune enteropathy in Schimke immunoosseous dysplasia. Am J Med Genet. 1998;77:427–30.
84. Morimoto M, Lewis DB, Lücke T, et al. Schimke Immunoosseous Dysplasia. In: Adam MP, Ardinger HH, Pagon RA, Wallace SE, LJH B, Stephens K, Amemiya A, editors. GeneReviews®. Seattle (WA): University of Washington, Seattle; 1993-2018.
85. Boerkoel CF, Takashima H, John J, et al. Mutant chromatin remodeling protein SMARCAL1 causes Schimke immuno-osseous dysplasia. Nat Genet. 2002;30:215–20.
86. Ridanpää M, van Eenennaam H, Pelin K, et al. Mutations in the RNA component of RNase MRP cause a pleiotropic human disease, cartilage-hair hypoplasia. Cell. 2001;104:195–203.
87. Makitie O, Marttinen E, Kaitila I. Skeletal growth in cartilage-hair hypoplasia. A radiological study of 82 patients. Pediatr Radiol. 1992;22:434–9.
88. Rider NL, Morton DH, Puffenberger E, et al. Immunologic and clinical features of 25 Amish patients with RMRP 70A-G cartilage-hair hypoplasia. Clin Immunol. 2009;131:119–28.
89. Kavadas FD, Giliani S, Gu Y, et al. Variability of clinical and laboratory features among patients with ribonuclease mitochondrial RNA processing endoribonuclease gene mutations. J Allergy Clin Immunol. 2008;122:1178–84.
90. Makitie O, Kaitila I. Cartilage-hair hypoplasia - clinical manifestations in 108 Finnish patients. Eur J Pediatr. 1993;152:211–7.
91. McCann LJ, McPartland J, Barge D, et al. Phenotypic variations of cartilage hair hypoplasia: granulomatous skin inflammation and severe T cell immunodeficiency as initial clinical presentation in otherwise well child with short stature. J Clin Immunol. 2014;34:42–8.
92. Mäkitie O, Vakkilainen S. Cartilage-hair hypoplasia_anauxetic dysplasia spectrum disorders. In: Pagon RA, Bird TD, Dolan CR, Stephens K, Adam MP, editors. GeneReviews. Seattle, WA: University of Washington; 2018.
93. Toiviainen-Salo S, Kajosaari M, Piilonen A, et al. Patients with cartilage-hair hypoplasia have an increased risk for bronchiectasis. J Pediatr. 2008;152:422–8.
94. Roifman CM, Gu Y, Cohen A. Mutations in the RNA component of RNase mitochondrial RNA processing might cause Omenn syndrome. J Allergy Clin Immunol. 2006;117:897–903.
95. Ip W, Gaspar H, Kleta R, et al. Variable phenotype of severe immunodeficiencies associated with *RMRP* gene mutations. J Clin Immunol. 2015;35:147–57.
96. Makitie O, Pukkala E, Teppo L, et al. Increased incidence of cancer in patients with cartilage-hair hypoplasia. J Pediatr. 1999;134:315–8.
97. Bordon V, Gennery AR, Slatter MA, et al. Clinical and immunologic outcome of patients with cartilage hair hypoplasia after hematopoietic stem cell transplantation. Blood. 2010;116:27–35.
98. Merico D, Roifman M, Braunschweig U, et al. Compound heterozygous mutations in the noncoding RNU4ATAC cause Roifman syndrome by disrupting minor intron splicing. Nat Commun. 2015;6:8718.
99. Dinur Schejter Y, Ovadia A, Alexandrova R, et al. A homozygous mutation in the stem II domain of *RNU4ATAC* causes typical Roifman syndrome. NPJ Genom Med. 2017;2:23.
100. Roifman CM. Antibody deficiency, growth retardation, spondyloepiphyseal dysplasia and retinal dystrophy: a novel syndrome. Clin Genet. 1999;55:103–099.
101. Heremans J, Garcie-Perez JE, Turro E, et al. Abnormal differentiation of B cells and megakaryocytes in patients with Roifman syndrome. J Allergy Clin Immunol. 2018. (in press;142:630–46.
102. Briggs TA, Rice GI, Adib N, et al. Spondyloenchondrodysplasia due to mutations in ACP5: a comprehensive survey. J Clin Immun. 2016;36:220–34.

103. Renella R, Schaefer E, LeMerrer M, et al. Spondyloenchondrodysplasia with spasticity, cerebral calcifications, and immune dysregulation: clinical and radiologic delineation of a pleiotropic disorder. Am J Med Genet. 2006;140A:541–50.
104. Roifman CM, Melamed I. A novel syndrome of combined immunodeficiency, autoimmunity and spondylometaphyseal dysplasia. Clin Genet. 2003;63:522–9.
105. Alsultan A, Shamseldin HE, Osman ME, et al. MYSM1 is mutated in a family with transient transfusion-dependent anemia, mild thrombocytopenia, and low NK- and B-cell counts. Blood. 2013;122:3844–5.
106. Le Guen T, Touzot F, André-Schmutz I, et al. An in vivo genetic reversion highlights the crucial role of Myb-like, SWIRM, and MPN domains 1 (MYSM1) in human hematopoiesis and lymphocyte differentiation. J Allergy Clin Immunol. 2015;136:1619–26. e5
107. Volpi S, Yamazaki Y, Brauer PM, et al. *EXTL3* mutations cause skeletal dysplasia, immune deficiency, and developmental delay. J Exp Med. 2017;214:623–37.
108. Guo L, Elcioglu NH, Mizumoto S, et al. Identification of biallelic *EXTL3* mutations in a novel type of spondylo-epi-metaphyseal dysplasia. J Hum Genet. 2017;62:797–801.
109. Oud MM, Tuijnenburg P, Hempel M, et al. Mutations in EXTL3 cause neuro-immuno-skeletal dysplasia syndrome. Am J Hum Genet. 2017;100:281–96.
110. Samuels ME, Majewski J, Alirezaie N, et al. Exome sequencing identifies mutations in the gene TTC7A in French-Canadian cases with hereditary multiple intestinal atresia. J Med Genet. 2013;50:324–9.
111. Bigorgne AE, Farin HF, Lemoine R, et al. TTC7A mutations disrupt intestinal epithelial apicobasal polarity. J Clin Invest. 2014;124:328–37.
112. Chen R, Giliani S, Lanzi G, et al. Whole-exome sequencing identifies tetratricopeptide repeat domain 7A (TTC7A) mutations for combined immunodeficiency with intestinal atresias. J Allergy Clin Immunol. 2013;132:656–664.e17.
113. Lemoine R, Pachlopnik-Schmid J, Farin HF, et al. Immune deficiency-related enteropathy-lymphocytopenia-alopecia syndrome results from tetratricopeptide repeat domain 7A deficiency. J Allergy Clin Immunol. 2014;134:1354–1364.e6.
114. Kammermeier J, Lucchini G, Pai SY, et al. Stem cell transplantation for tetratricopeptide repeat domain 7A deficiency: long-term follow-up. Blood. 2016;128:1306–8.
115. Kaur M, Singh M, Silakari O. Insight into the therapeutic aspects of 'zeta-chain associated protein kinase 70 kDa' inhibitors: a review. Cell Signal. 2014;26:2481–92.
116. Elder ME, Lin D, Clever J, et al. Human severe combined immunodeficiency due to a defect in ZAP-70, a T cell tyrosine kinase. Science. 1994;264:1596–9.
117. Turul T, Tezcan I, Artac H, et al. Clinical heterogeneity can hamper the diagnosis of patients with ZAP70 deficiency. Eur J Pediatr. 2009;168:87–93.
118. Picard C, Dogniaux S, Chemin K, et al. Hypomorphic mutation of ZAP70 in human results in a late onset immunodeficiency and no autoimmunity. Eur J Immunol. 2009;39:1966–76.
119. Chan AY, Punwani D, Kadlecek TA, et al. A novel human autoimmune syndrome caused by combined hypomorphic and activating mutations in ZAP-70. J Exp Med. 2016;213:155–65.
120. Roifman CM, Dadi H, Somech R, et al. Characterization of zeta-associated protein, 70 kd (ZAP70)-defi- cient human lymphocytes. J Allergy Clin Immunol. 2010;126:1226–1233.e1.
121. Cuvelier GD, Rubin TS, Wall DA, et al. Long-term outcomes of hematopoietic stem cell transplantation for ZAP70 deficiency. J Clin Immunol. 2016;36:713–24.
122. de la Calle-Martin O, Hernandez M, Ordi J, et al. Familial CD8 deficiency due to a mutation in the CD8 alpha gene. J Clin Invest. 2001;108:117–23.
123. Mancebo E, Moreno-Pelayo MA, Mencía A, et al. Gly111Ser mutation in CD8A gene causing CD8 immunodeficiency is found in Spanish gypsies. Mol Immunol. 2008;45:479–84.
124. Dumontet E, Osman J, Guillemont-Lambert N, et al. Recurrent respiratory infections revealing CD8α deficiency. J Clin Immunol. 2015;35:692–5.
125. Smith DK, Neal JJ, Holmberg SD. Unexplained opportunistic infections and CD4+ T-lymphocytopenia without HIV infection. An investigation of cases in the United States. The centers for disease control idiopathic CD4 1 T-lymphocytopenia task force. N Engl J Med. 1993;328:373–9.

126. Spira TJ, Jones BM, Nicholson JK, et al. Idiopathic CD4+ T-lymphocytopenia _ an analysis of five patients with unexplained opportunistic infections. N Engl J Med. 1993;328:386–92.
127. Busch MP, Valinsky JE, Paglieroni T, et al. Screening of blood donors for idiopathic CD4+ T-lymphocytopenia. Transfusion. 1994;34:192–7.
128. Kuijpers TW, Ijspeert H, van Leeuwen EM, et al. Idiopathic CD4+ T lymphopenia without autoimmunity or granulomatous disease in the slipstream of RAG mutations. Blood. 2011;117:5892–6.
129. Albin-Leeds S, Ochoa J, Mehta H, et al. Idiopathic T cell lymphopenia identified in New York state new- born screening. Clin Immunol. 2017;183:36–40.
130. Jyonouchi S, Jongco AM, Puck J, et al. Immunodeficiencies associated with abnormal newborn screening for T cell and B cell lymphopenia. J Clin Immunol. 2017;37:363–74.
131. Thakar MS, Hintermeyer MK, Gries MG, et al. A practical approach to newborn screening for severe combined immunodeficiency using the T cell receptor excision circle assay. Front Immunol. 2017;8:1470.
132. Gorska MM, Alam R. A mutation in the human uncoordinated 119 gene impairs TCR signaling and is associated with CD4 lymphopenia. Blood. 2012;119:1399–406.
133. Gorska MM, Alam R. Consequences of a mutation in the UNC119 gene for T cell function in idiopathic CD4 lymphopenia. Curr Allergy Asthma Rep. 2012;12:396–401.
134. Hauck F, Randriamampita C, Martin E, et al. Primary T-cell immunodeficiency with immunodysregulation caused by autosomal recessive LCK deficiency. J Allergy Clin Immunol. 2012;130:1144–1152.e11.
135. Bader-Meunier B, Rieux-Laucat F, Touzot F, et al. Inherited immunodeficiency: a new association with early-onset childhood panniculitis. Pediatrics. 2018;141(Suppl 5):S496–500.
136. Sawabe T, Horiuchi T, Nakamura M, et al. Defect of lck in a patient with common variable immunodeficiency. Int J Mol Med. 2001;7:609–14.
137. Goldman FD, Ballas ZK, Schutte BC, et al. Defective expression of p56lck in an infant with severe combined immunodeficiency. J Clin Invest. 1998;102:421–9.
138. Salzer E, Cagdas D, Hons M, et al. RASGRP1 deficiency causes immunodeficiency with impaired cytoskeletal dynamics. Nat Immunol. 2016;17:1352–60.
139. Platt CD, Fried AJ, Hoyos-Bachiloglu R, et al. Combined immunodeficiency with EBV positive B cell lymphoma and epidermodysplasia verruciformis due to a novel homozygous mutation in RASGRP1. Clin Immunol. 2017;183:142–4.
140. Mao H, Yang W, Latour S, et al. RASGRP1 mutation in autoimmune lymphoproliferative syndrome-like disease. J Allergy Clin Immunol. 2018;142:595–604.e16.
141. Winter S, Martin E, Boutboul D, et al. Loss of RASGRP1 in humans impairs T-cell expansion leading to Epstein-Barr virus susceptibility. EMBO Mol Med. 2018;10:188–99.
142. Somekh I, Marquardt B, Liu Y, et al. Novel mutations in RASGRP1 are associated with immunodeficiency, immune dysregulation, and EBV-induced lymphoma. J Clin Immunol. 2018;38:699–710.
143. Ghosh S, Drexler I, Bhatia S, et al. Interleukin 2 inducible T-cell kinase deficiency – new patients, new insight? Front Immunol. 2018;9:979.
144. Cagdas D, Erman B, Hanoglu D, et al. Course of IL-2-inducible T-cell kinase deficiency in a family: lymphomatoid granulomatosis, lymphoma and allogeneic bone marrow transplantation in one sibling; and death in the other. Bone Marrow Transplant. 2017;52:126–9.
145. Cipe FE, Aydogmus C, Serwas NK, et al. ITK deficiency: how can EBV be treated before lymphoma? Pediatr Blood Cancer. 2015;62:2247–8.
146. Alme C, Satwani P, Alobeid B, et al. Atypical clinical course in pediatric Hodgkin lymphoma: association with germline mutations in interleukin-2-inducible T-cell kinase. J Pediatr Hematol Oncol. 2015;37:507–8.
147. Bienemann K, Borkhardt A, Klapper W, et al. High incidence of Epstein- Barr virus (EBV)-positive Hodgkin lymphoma and Hodgkin lymphoma-like B-cell lymphoproliferations with EBV latency profile 2 in children with interleukin-2-inducible T-cell kinase deficiency. Histopathology. 2015;67:607–16.

148. Serwas NK, Cagdas D, Ban SA, et al. Identification of ITK deficiency as a novel genetic cause of idiopathic CD4+ T-cell lymphopenia. Blood. 2014;124:655–7.
149. Ghosh S, Bienemann K, Boztug K, et al. Interleukin-2-inducible T-cell kinase (ITK) deficiency – clinical and molecular aspects. J Clin Immunol. 2014;34:892–9.
150. Mansouri D, Mahdaviani SA, Khalilzadeh S, et al. IL-2-inducible T-cell kinase deficiency with pulmonary manifestations due to disseminated Epstein-Barr virus infection. Int Arch Allergy Immunol. 2012;158:418–22.
151. Linka RM, Risse SL, Bienemann K, et al. Loss- of-function mutations within the IL-2 inducible kinase ITK in patients with EBV-associated lymphoproliferative diseases. Leukemia. 2012;26:963–71.
152. Stepensky P, Weintraub M, Yanir A, et al. IL-2-inducible T-cell kinase deficiency: clinical presentation and therapeutic approach. Haematologica. 2011;96:472–6.
153. Huck K, Feyen O, Niehues T, et al. Girls homozygous for an IL-2-inducible T cell kinase mutation that leads to protein deficiency develop fatal EBV-associated lymphoproliferation. J Clin Invest. 2009;119:1350–8.
154. Li FY, Chaigne-Delalande B, Kanellopoulou C, et al. Second messenger role for Mg2+ revealed by human T-cell immunodeficiency. Nature. 2011;475:471–6.
155. Chaigne-Delalande B, Li FY, O'Connor GM, et al. Mg2+ regulates cytotoxic functions of NK and CD8 T cells in chronic EBV infection through NKG2D. Science. 2013;341:186–91.
156. Morgan NV, Goddard S, Cardno TS, et al. Mutation in the TCRα subunit constant gene (TRAC) leads to a human immunodeficiency disorder characterized by a lack of TCRαβ+ T cells. J Clin Invest. 2011;121:695–702.
157. Chou J, Badran YR, Yee CSK, et al. A novel mutation in ORAI1 presenting with combined immunodeficiency and residual T-cell function. J Allergy Clin Immunol. 2015;136:479–482.e1.
158. Maul-Pavicic A, Chiang SC, Rensing-Ehl A, et al. ORAI1-mediated calcium influx is required for human cytotoxic lymphocyte degranulation and target cell lysis. Proc Natl Acad Sci U S A. 2011;108:3324–9.
159. McCarl CA, Picard C, Khalil S, et al. ORAI1 deficiency and lack of store-operated Ca2+ entry cause immunodeficiency, myopathy, and ectodermal dysplasia. J Allergy Clin Immunol. 2009;124:1311–1318.e7.
160. Feske S, Gwack Y, Prakriya M, et al. A mutation in Orai1 causes immune deficiency by abrogating CRAC channel function. Nature. 2006;441:179–85.
161. Schaballie H, Rodriguez R, Martin E, et al. A novel hypomorphic mutation in STIM1 results in a late-onset immunodeficiency. J Allergy Clin Immunol. 2015;136:816–819.e4.
162. Fuchs S, Rensing-Ehl A, Speckmann C, et al. Antiviral and regulatory T cell immunity in a patient with stromal interaction molecule 1 deficiency. J Immunol. 2012;188:1523–33.
163. Byun M, Abhyankar A, Lelarge V, et al. Whole-exome sequencing-based discovery of STIM1 deficiency in a child with fatal classic Kaposi sarcoma. J Exp Med. 2010;207:2307–12.
164. Picard C, McCarl CA, Papolos A, et al. STIM1 mutation associated with a syndrome of immunodeficiency and autoimmunity. N Engl J Med. 2009;360:1971–80.
165. Sherkat R, Sabri MR, Dehghan B, et al. EBV lymphoproliferative-associated disease and primary cardiac T-cell lymphoma in a STK4 deficient patient: a case report. Medicine (Baltimore). 2017;96:e8852.
166. Dang TS, Willet JD, Griffin HR, et al. Defective leukocyte adhesion and chemotaxis contributes to combined immunodeficiency in humans with autosomal recessive MST1 deficiency. J Clin Immunol. 2016;36:117–22.
167. Crequer A, Picard C, Patin E, et al. Inherited MST1 deficiency underlies susceptibility to EV-HPV infections. PLoS One. 2012;7:e44010.
168. Abdollahpour H, Appaswamy G, Kotlarz D, et al. The phenotype of human STK4 deficiency. Blood. 2012;119:3450–7.
169. Nehme NT, Schmid JP, Debeurme F, et al. MST1 mutations in autosomal recessive primary immunodeficiency characterized by defective naive T-cell survival. Blood. 2012;119:3458–68.
170. Charbit-Henrion F, Jeverica AK, Bègue B, et al. GENIUS group. Deficiency in mucosa-associated lymphoid tissue lymphoma translocation 1: a novel cause of IPEX-like syndrome. J Pediatr Gastroenterol Nutr. 2017;64:378–84.

171. Rozmus J, McDonald R, Fung SY, et al. Successful clinical treatment and functional immunological normalization of human MALT1 deficiency following hematopoietic stem cell transplantation. Clin Immunol. 2016;168:1–5.
172. Punwani D, Wang H, Chan AY, et al. Combined immunodeficiency due to MALT1 mutations, treated by hematopoietic cell transplantation. J Clin Immunol. 2015;35:135–46.
173. Torres JM, Martinez-Barricarte R, García-Gómez S, et al. Inherited BCL10 deficiency impairs hematopoietic and nonhematopoietic immunity. J Clin Invest. 2014;124:5239–48.
174. Pérez de Diego R, Sánchez-Ramón S, López-Collazo E, et al. Genetic errors of the human caspase recruitment domain-B-cell lymphoma 10-mucosa-associated lymphoid tissue lymphoma-translocation gene 1 (CBM) complex: molecular, immunologic, and clinical heterogeneity. J Allergy Clin Immunol. 2015;136:1139–49.
175. Turvey SE, Durandy A, Fischer A, et al. The CARD11-BCL10-MALT1 (CBM) signalosome complex: stepping into the limelight of human primary immunodeficiency. J Allergy Clin Immunol. 2014;134:276–84.
176. Jabara HH, Ohsumi T, Chou J, et al. A homozygous mucosa-associated lymphoid tissue 1 (MALT1) mutation in a family with combined immunodeficiency. J Allergy Clin Immunol. 2013;132:151–8.
177. McKinnon ML, Rozmus J, Fung SY, et al. Combined immunodeficiency associated with homozygous MALT1 mutations. J Allergy Clin Immunol. 2014;133:1458–62. e1-7
178. Stepensky P, Keller B, Buchta M, et al. Deficiency of caspase recruitment domain family, member 11 (CARD11), causes profound combined immunodeficiency in human subjects. J Allergy Clin Immunol. 2013;131:477–845. e1
179. Greil J, Rausch T, Giese T, et al. Whole-exome sequencing links caspase recruitment domain 11 (CARD11) inactivation to severe combined immunodeficiency. J Allergy Clin Immunol. 2013;131:1376–1383.e3.
180. Snow AL, Xiao W, Stinson JR, et al. Congenital B cell lymphocytosis explained by novel germline CARD11 mutations. J Exp Med. 2012;209:2247–61.
181. Crequer A, Troeger A, Patin E, et al. Human RHOH deficiency causes T cell defects and susceptibility to EV-HPV infections. J Clin Invest. 2012;122:3239–47.
182. Erman B, Bilic I, Hirschmugl T, et al. Combined immunodeficiency with CD4 lymphopenia and sclerosing cholangitis caused by a novel loss-of-function mutation affecting IL21R. Haematologica. 2015;100:e216–9.
183. Stepensky P, Keller B, Abuzaitoun O, et al. Extending the clinical and immunological phenotype of human interleukin-21 receptor deficiency. Haematologica. 2015;100:e72–6.
184. Kotlarz D, Ziętara N, Uzel G, et al. Loss-of-function mutations in the IL-21 receptor gene cause a primary immunodeficiency syndrome. J Exp Med. 2013;210:433–43.
185. Watkins D, Schwartzentruber JA, Ganesh J, et al. Novel inborn error of folate metabolism: identification by exome capture and sequencing of mutations in the MTHFD1 gene in a single proband. J Med Genet. 2011;48:590–2.
186. Keller MD, Ganesh J, Heltzer M, et al. Severe combined immunodeficiency resulting from mutations in MTHFD1. Pediatrics. 2013;131:e629–34.
187. Alazami AM, Al-Helale M, Alhissi S, et al. Novel CARMIL2 mutations in patients with variable clinical dermatitis, infections, and combined immunodeficiency. Front Immunol. 2018;9:203.
188. Schober T, Magg T, Laschinger M, et al. A human immunodeficiency syndrome caused by mutations in CARMIL2. Nat Commun. 2017;8:14209.
189. Sorte HS, Osnes LT, Fevang B, et al. A potential founder variant in CARMIL2/RLTPR in three Norwegian families with warts, molluscum contagiosum, and T-cell dysfunction. Mol Genet Genomic Med. 2016;4:604–16.
190. Wang Y, Ma CS, Ling Y, et al. Dual T cell- and B cell-intrinsic deficiency in humans with biallelic RLTPR mutations. J Exp Med. 2016;213:2413–35.

Chapter 3
Pulmonary Manifestations of Predominantly Antibody Deficiencies

Amene Saghazadeh and Nima Rezaei

3.1 Introduction

Predominantly antibody deficiencies (PADs) are the most frequent forms of primary immunodeficiency diseases (PIDs). These conditions are resulted from a primary defect in B-cells. Though to a lesser extent, they are caused by a defect in T-cells or other immune cell populations known to contribute to B-cell or plasma cell development and function. Overall, PADs are characterized by a malfunctioned antibody response which is reflected in low or undetectable levels of immunoglobulin(s). As a result, recurrent infection is the most common presentation leading to diagnosis of PADs. It would also remain the cause of most complications during the course of disease. Overall, physicians who are the most likely to encounter patients with PADs are those of infectious disease specialists [1].

Patients with chronic and recurrent respiratory infections are prone to develop severe respiratory conditions such as bronchiectasis and obliterative bronchiolitis. Therefore, patients with respiratory infections need particular attention. They should be prescribed an appropriate therapy as soon as possible and have to be adhering to

A. Saghazadeh
Research Center for Immunodeficiencies, Children's Medical Center, Tehran University of Medical Sciences (TUMS), Tehran, Iran

Systematic Review and Meta-analysis Expert Group (SRMEG), Universal Scientific Education and Research Network (USERN), Tehran, Iran

N. Rezaei (✉)
Research Center for Immunodeficiencies, Children's Medical Center, Tehran University of Medical Sciences (TUMS), Tehran, Iran

Department of Immunology, School of Medicine, Tehran University of Medical Sciences (TUMS), Tehran, Iran

Network of Immunity in Infection, Malignancy and Autoimmunity (NIIMA), Universal Scientific Education and Research Network (USERN), Tehran, Iran
e-mail: rezaei_nima@tums.ac.ir

S. A. Mahdaviani, N. Rezaei (eds.), *Pulmonary Manifestations of Primary Immunodeficiency Diseases*, https://doi.org/10.1007/978-3-030-00880-2_3

more and longer medical therapies. Immunoglobulin substitution therapy along with prophylactic antibiotics remained the cornerstone of treatment for PADs and related complications [2]. Generally, immunoglobulin replacement therapy can effectively reduce both incidence and severity of infections [2]. However, immunoglobulin products contain only purified IgG antibodies and lack other antibody isotypes. It is thus expected that pulmonary infections may persist and even flourish under regular immunoglobulin replacement therapy. Thereby, the patient will be more predisposed to chronic lung diseases and related severe sequels such as respiratory failure [3]. Recent studies have identified a gap for screening protocols to monitor respiratory manifestations in patients with PADs [4].

(For further information you may see Aghamohammadi A, Plebani A, Lougaris V, Durandy A, Condino-Neto A, Kanegane H, Hammarström L. Predominantly antibody deficiencies. In: Rezaei N, Aghamohammadi A, Notarangelo LD, editors. *Primary immunodeficiency diseases: definition, diagnosis, and management*. 2nd ed. p. 183–244.)

3.2 X-Linked Agammaglobulinemia (Bruton's Disease or BTK Deficiency)

Among the most severe types of PADs is X-linked agammaglobulinemia (XLA), the first PID described by Ogden Bruton in 1952. XLA is the most common monogenic immunodeficiency [5] resulting from mutations on the X chromosome in the gene encoding a tyrosine kinase, the so-called Bruton's tyrosine kinase (Btk). These mutations are of loss-of-function type, making an arrest in the early stages of B-cell development [5]. XLA is therefore a humoral immunodeficiency characterized by depletion of B-cells and low levels of all immunoglobulins (IgG, IgA, IgM, IgD, and IgE) [6]. While the number of T-cells and NK cells varies within normal range, it is however realized that lack of B-cells might lower the optimal function of T-cells, as reflected in the diminished T-cell memory to specific antigens. For example, patients with XLA show a defect in T-cell memory to *N. meningitidis* but not influenza [7]. The presentation of this antibody immunodeficiency is expected to occur (a) earlier than other types of PADs, (b) after maternal antibodies waned, and (c) during the first 2 years of life with recurrent and severe sinopulmonary infections [8–11]. However, there are reports, for example, from China, where the mean age at diagnosis was more than 6 years. Even, there have been reports of late-onset XLA (up to the fourth decade of life) [12]. Overall, the mean age at diagnosis falls within the range 3.2–7.7 years, whereas the mean age at onset of symptoms happens within the range 1.8–4.2 years [13–17, 10, 18]. This reflects the delay in diagnosis ranging from 1.4 to 3.6 years.

In conjunction with its expression on different cells such as B-cells, monocytes, macrophages, granulocytes, dendritic cells, and osteoclasts, BTK serves as a potential contributor to various intracellular functions, essentially B-cell development [19] and differentiation [20], natural killer (NK) cell activation [21], and T-cell memory [22]. While BTK deficiency can leave the body in a state of immunodeficiency (e.g., XLA), its upregulation may lead to autoimmune states, such as rheumatoid arthritis and systemic lupus erythematosus [19], as well as malignant states, notably B-cell malignancies [23], squamous cell carcinoma, and pancreatic cancer [24]. Hundreds of variants have been identified in the gene BTK from patients with XLA [25–29, 18] which may explain phenotypic divergence in XLA [30]. Therefore, data are integrated to investigate genotype-phenotype interactions [31]. Overall, the most common complications of XLA are pulmonary infections and bronchiectasis.

3.2.1 Pulmonary Infections

Generally, infections account for the highest proportion of presenting manifestations of XLA [9, 10, 16, 29]. In particular, a prospective study of 101 individuals with XLA reported the presence of at least one of these three infectious complications: pneumonia, sinusitis, and chronic lung disease with bronchiectasis in 76% of patients with XLA [14]. Moreover, the majority of infections affect the upper and lower respiratory tracts [16, 10, 18, 32] and are of bacterial origin, among which bronchitis, pneumonia, chronic sinusitis, otitis, and conjunctivitis are the most common complications of XLA [33]. Infections occur not only before diagnosis but remain a major cause of complications during the course of disease, immunoglobulin substitution, and death in patients with XLA [32, 10]. The most common infections prior to and after diagnosis include otitis media, pneumonia, and sinusitis [9, 29].

Pneumonia is the most common acute infection associated with XLA [14]. Recurrent pneumonia should be, therefore, regarded as an alarm sign for PIDs including XLA [34, 35]. Before the diagnosis is made, between 60% and 83% of patients with XLA have a history of at least one episode of pneumonia [36], and approximately 30% of patients have a history of hospitalization due to pneumonia [16]. With an adequate immunoglobulin therapy, the rate of pneumonias is reduced by more than 10% [14] and lies within the range of 0.00–0.10 pneumonias per treatment year [13, 37]. However, approximately 50% of patients might experience deterioration in their respiratory status while receiving immunoglobulin therapy [38]. The rate of infectious episodes during immunoglobulin therapy seems to be age-related, since there is a threefold increased risk for infections in adult patients compared with pediatric patients (2.12 vs. 0.74 infections/patient/year) [38]. More important is that pneumonias after initiation of immunoglobulin therapy might be severe as many as half of episodes might require hospitalization for intravenous antibiotic treatment [13]. In multivariate analysis, patients with bronchiectasis had a > 3-fold increased risk of pneumonia during the 5-year immunoglobulin therapy [14]. Its source remained unknown in almost 80% of cases. However, sputum cultures could reveal the following as bacterial pathogens underlying pneumonia in patients with XLA: *Haemophilus influenzae*, *Streptococcus pneumoniae*, *Staphylococcus aureus*, and *Mycoplasma pneumonia* [13, 33]. Analysis of bronchoalveolar lavage (BAL) in patients with XLA without acute pulmonary function identified bacterial pathogens such as *Haemophilus influenzae* and *Veillonella* [39]. Also, bacteria that were observed through protected specimen brush samples included *Haemophilus influenzae*, *β-hemolytic streptococci*, and *Porphyromonas* [39]. Other bacterial pathogens found in association with pneumonia among patients with XLA are *Pseudomonas* species and *M. tuberculosis* [16]. Looking at chest X-ray, pneumonia in patients with XLA can cause peribronchial thickening and then segmental atelectasis [13]. Antigen-specific immunological responses might predict the risk of respiratory tract infections in patients with XLA. More precisely, individuals who developed IgG and IgM responses specific to bacteriophage phi-X 174 were less likely to be affected by respiratory tract infections (RTI) compared with those who developed only IgM responses [22]. Although very rare, there are reports of pulmonary infections with fungal (aspergillosis and *Pneumocystis jiroveci*) [40] and viral pathogens (respiratory syncytial virus) [41–43] in patients with XLA even despite regular immunoglobulin substitution therapy. Chronic sinusitis seems to predispose individuals with XLA to pulmonary aspergillosis [40].

3.2.2 Bronchiectasis

There are individuals with impaired pulmonary function, as revealed through pulmonary function test, that show a normal chest X-ray [13]. However, an abnormal chest X-ray clearly warrants that pulmonary function is impaired [13]. Patients with XLA show changes in pulmonary function test (PFT) that favor obstructive lung disease. These include a reduction in forced expiratory volume in the first second (FEV1) as well as a reduction in forced expiratory flow (FEF) [13]. Pulmonary function abnormalities appear not to be age-related [13]. The delay in diagnosis has shown an inverse association with the risk of chronic lung disease. Supporting this, lung function decreases with aging in patients with XLA and is worsened by smoking and bronchiectasis. A longitudinal study of patients with XLA ($n = 8$) over an average period of 7.6 years calculated an average annual decline of 65 ± 11 mL/year and 58 ± 20 mL/year for FEV1 and FVC, respectively [15]. Immunoglobulin therapy dose demonstrated a negative association with lung function decline. This reflects the protective effect of immunoglobulin therapy [15].

Evidence of chronic lung disease (CLD) before diagnosis is present in nearly one-third of patients with XLA [16]. Factors known to increase the risk of CLD before diagnosis of XLA include higher age at diagnosis and the presence of a lower respiratory tract infection (LRTI) [16]. This may indicate that delayed diagnosis might leave patients facing higher risk of CLD [18]. CLD is observed in 40% of patients with XLA who had a history of LRTI. Approximately, 30% of patients develop CLD later in the course of disease [16]. CLD risk after diagnosis of XLA is predicted by pneumonia and inappropriate immunoglobulin substitution therapy [16]. Study of 201 US patients with XLA identified CLD as the cause of death in 25% of cases [9]. CLD also has been shown to have a negative impact on the life quality of patients with XLA [44].

Keeping in mind the high incidence of pulmonary infections, bronchiectasis is considered a common complication of XLA. A study of Australian adults estimated a twofold incidence of infection with bronchiectasis compared to infection without bronchiectasis among patients with XLA (67% vs. 33%) [45]. In a multicenter study of 199 patients with XLA, the use of high-resolution chest CT imaging indicated a prevalence of bronchiectasis as high as 56% [33]. The prevalence of bronchiectasis increases with age [14] and that turning 18 years old was the most important factor predictive of bronchiectasis [33]. However, other factors associated with an increased risk of bronchiectasis included a history of pneumonia and treatment with IVIG compared with subcutaneous IG [33]. In addition, patients with chronic sinusitis were four times more likely to have bronchiectasis [14]. It is important that almost half of patients with XLA suffer from chronic sinusitis [14], whereas no effect of IgG levels on the risk of bronchiectasis was found [14]. The age range for development of bronchiectasis was 7–45 years [33]. Regardless of age, bronchiectasis lowers lung function as reflected in reduced FEV1 [33]. Bronchiectasis is, therefore, the real cause of diminished life quality among patients with XLA [38]. CXR findings are often evident in the middle and lower lobes of the lung(s) [11]. HRCT appears to be more sensitive than CXR for evaluation of pulmonary abnormalities in patients with primary hypogammaglobulinemia including XLA [46].

3.2.3 *Chronic Pleurisy*

There is report of recurrent chronic pleurisy presented with thickened pleura and calcification in CT imaging and intraluminal fibrosis, foamy alveolar macrophages, and chronic inflammation in histopathological examination of the pleural tissue [47]. Broad-range bacterial polymerase chain reaction (PCR) identified *H. equorum*-like bacterium as the underlying pathogen of these abnormalities. Taking high-dose panipenem/betamipron (PAPM/BP) and clarithromycin significantly improved the patients' situation.

3.2.4 *Potential Mechanisms of Respiratory Manifestations in XLA*

Both lipopolysaccharide (LPS) and anti-IL-8/IL-8 immune complexes act as stimulus to neutrophils [48]. Upon stimulation, FcγRIIa is recruited from intracellular compartments to the cell surface. FcγRIIa recruitment is accompanied with activation of Btk, which in turn induces the expression of adaptor molecule MyD88. In this manner, Btk act to direct cross talk between FcγRIIa and toll-like receptor 4 (TLR4) [49]. It is followed by engagement of MyD88 adapter-like (Mal)/TIRAP interaction which plays a crucial role in TLR-dependent NF-kappaB (NF-κB) proinflammatory responses [50]. Matrix metalloproteinases (MMP) mainly MMP9 induced by NF-κB contribute to tissue remodeling in acute lung injury. As expected, Btk inhibitors could abrogate the expression of both Btk and MyD88 in human neutrophils activated with anti-IL-8/IL-8 immune complexes [48]. Additionally, treatments blocking either Btk or MMP9 diminished the expression of MMP9 in neutrophils from mice exposed to secondhand smoke [51]. Altogether, it is plausible to think of Btk-targeted neutrophil-specific therapy in conditions associated with acute lung injury (ALI)/acute respiratory distress syndrome (ARDS) [48] and chronic obstructive pulmonary disease (COPD) [51].

Ibrutinib is used in targeted therapy of malignancies and autoimmune diseases to inhibit BTK. It has been shown to prevent influenza-induced acute lung injury through reduction of pro-inflammatory mediators [52]. Btk inhibitor RN983 showed much more anti-inflammatory potency than corticosteroid budesonide in mouse lung in form of inhalation [53]. This makes it effective in the treatment of allergic asthma. RNA interference (RNAi) of Btk has been demonstrated to decrease protein levels of Btk and phosphorylated Btk (p-Btk) and diminish the expression and activation of Btk in alveolar macrophages [54]. In a mouse model of cecal ligation and puncture (CLP)-induced sepsis, pretreatment with Btk RNAi was able to prevent epithelial cell apoptosis, pulmonary edema, vascular permeability, the expression of inflammatory cytokines (TNF-α, IL-1β, and IL-6) and signaling (NF-κB), and neutrophil lung infiltration.

On the contrary, there is evidence that the over-suppression of innate immunity by ibrutinib might cause toxic events. Ibrutinib can lead to epithelial cell apoptosis and inflammation that promote pulmonary infections [55] and fibrosis [56]. Even, there is report of invasive aspergillus infection in association with ibrutinib in patients with chronic lymphocytic leukemia [57]. These toxic effects induced by ibrutinib draw a picture of what happens in patients with XLA, where loss-of-function mutations lead to downregulation of Btk.

Study of XLA mice suggest that IgM contributes to alveolar macrophage phagocytosis and thereby confining the fungal infection to limited areas [58]. In this manner, low IgM levels in patients with XLA make them prone to develop more severe infections with fungal pathogens such as *Cryptococcus neoformans*.

B-cells act as the regulator of neutrophil migration to the site of stimulus. Depletion of B-cells in XLA dictates the rapid migration of neutrophils to the site of stimulus whereby the opportunity of macrophages to attract to the site of stimulus is captured, while macrophage activation is required for engagement of interferon gamma (IFNy)-producing T-cells, which in turn elicit an effective response to bacillus Calmette-Guérin (BCG) vaccination [59]. In this manner, impairment in antituberculosis immunity exists as a result of disrupted IFNy-producing T-cell-macrophage axis in XLA.

TLR signaling pathways as well as TLR effector function are maintained despite loss of Btk function [60]. Neutrophils from patients with XLA upon stimulation with LPS revealed activation of MAPK cascades, production of reactive oxygen species (ROSs), and reduction of neutrophil apoptosis. All these events occurred in a comparable fashion in neutrophils from controls. Particularly, ROSs are required for phagocytosis of pathogens [61].

Impairment in B-cell development causes airway inflammation [62], and therefore allergic symptoms might be present in patients with XLA [63]. Compared with wild-type mice, X-linked immunodeficiency (Xid) mice exhibited an increase in production of cytokines (IL-4, IL-5, IL-10, IL-13, CCL5, and IFNγ), lung inflammation, interstitial eosinophilia, and mucus production in response to challenge with cockroach antigen.

3.2.5 Management of Respiratory Manifestations in XLA

Immunoglobulin therapy helps to restore IgG levels to protective levels [13]. Patients on high-dose intravenous immunoglobulin therapy rather than low-dose or intramuscular immunoglobulin therapy are more likely to achieve recommended levels of IgG [64]. Analysis of serial determination of IgG levels in patients with XLA receiving IVIG therapy indicated that a median IgG level of 354 mg/dl predicts that individual immunity against infections is acceptable [65]. The annual incidence of bacterial infections (pneumonia) was estimated to be 0.16 (0.12), 0.05 (0.05), and 0.00 (0.00) when IgG levels are below 500 mg/dL, between 500 and 800 mg/dL, and above 800 mg/dL [37]. Of note, a 5-year prospective study of 101 individuals with XLA identified only one episode of pneumonia in cases with IgG levels >1000 mg/dL [14]. Individuals taking a high dose of IVIG (397 mg/kg) are expected to be infection-free [65].

Lung transplantation (LTx) is the option available for patients with bronchiectasis and end-stage respiratory failure caused by XLA. Even after LTx, regular immunoglobulin substitution is still required for prevention of infections [66]. Although it is promising that the lungs often reach an acceptable or predicted functional level, post-lung transplant infection and respiratory failure remain life-threatening [45]. The authors in [67] reported the long-term outcome of six patients with XLA who underwent LTx. All patients but one died within the first 3 years after LTx. The pulmonary infection (bronchiolitis and pulmonary sepsis) was the cause of death for all but one case who died from progressive multifocal leukoencephalopathy.

3.3 Autosomal Recessive Agammaglobulinemia (μ Heavy Chain Deficiency, λ5 Deficiency, Igα Deficiency, Igβ Deficiency, BLNK Deficiency)

When we have a male child with congenital hypogammaglobulinemia and absent B-cells, the first differential diagnosis to consider is XLA, which is resulted from mutant BTK. When we have a female child with similar clinical and immunological presentation, the first differential diagnosis to consider is autosomal recessive (AR) agammaglobulinemia (ARA). Mutations identified as the cause of autosomal recessive forms of agammaglobulinemia occur in the genes encoding molecules that contribute to the structure and function of pre-B-cell receptor (BCR) or its downstream pathways such as the μ heavy chain (IGHM), B-cell linker adaptor protein (BLNK), the immunoglobulin λ-like polypeptide1 (IGLL1), leucine-rich repeat-containing 8 (LRRC8A), Igα (CD79A), and Igβ (CD79B) [31].

As pre-B-cells are known as precursors of B-cells, the pre-B-cell receptor (BCR) is considered as precursor of B-cell receptor. As a result, pre-BCR is an essential to B-cell development. It is composed of the μ heavy chain (μHC) and the surrogate light chain (SLC). The SLC, in turn, includes invariant Vpre-B and λ5 polypeptides. Also, transmembrane protein Igα in association with Igβ serves as the signal transduction component for the pre-BCR complex. Abnormalities in pre-BCR structure and function hinder the transition from pro-B- to pre-B-cell stage [68], predisposing individuals to immunodeficiency, malignancy, and autoimmunity (for review see [69]).

3.3.1 μ Heavy Chain Deficiency

Yel et al. 1996 [70] were the first group to identify mutations in the IGHM gene as a cause of agammaglobulinemia. They reported seven patients from two families with AR B-cell defects. Patients presented between 1 and 15 months of age. Clinical manifestations included fever, weakness, rashes, chronic enteroviral encephalitis, recurrent infections (pneumonia, bronchopneumonia, and otitis), failure to thrive, gastrointestinal disorders, septic shock (due to *Pseudomonas aeruginosa*), arthritis, and perirectal abscesses.

Thereafter, more studies have investigated the IGHM as a potential candidate gene for AR B-cell defects [31, 71–74]. These studies indicate that (a) the IGHM gene is very polymorphic [72], (b) the presence of large deletions rather than point mutations is more likely in patients with agammaglobulinemia [74], and (c) mutant IGHM accounts for about 20–30% of patients who have AR B-cell defects [71] and as well for about 5% of all patients with agammaglobulinemia [74]. Also, it is concluded that patients carrying mutant IGHM experience an earlier onset and more difficult course of agammaglobulinemia compared to patients carrying mutant BTK [71]. Overall, mutant IGHM may cause respiratory manifestations such as recurrent upper respiratory tract infections (viral rhinitis, sinusitis, otitis, pharyngitis, and rhinopharyngitis), recurrent pneumonia, bronchopneumonia, bronchiectasis, and asthma.

3.3.2 λ5 Deficiency

Studies show that despite allelic exclusion of Ig μ heavy chain would remain normal, B-cell development is, however, not completely [75] ablated in mice deficient in λ5 [76]. Minegishi et al. 1998 [77] reported a case with hypogammaglobulinemia, less than 1% of normal number of B-cells, and undetectable levels of CD19. He presented with recurrent otitis at 2 months of age.

3.3.3 Igα Deficiency

Minegishi et al. 1999 [78] published the first case of defect in Igα (CD79a) with agammaglobulinemia. The patient presented with recurrent diarrhea, failure to thrive, bronchitis, and neutropenia. The age at onset of disease was before 1 month of age. The authors demonstrated that defect in the Igα gene results in complete blocking of B-cell development as defect in the IGHM. This study proved that the functional role of Igα as a component of signal transduction molecule is not less than the role that the mu heavy chain plays as a structural component of pre-BCR. The second one was reported by Wang et al. 2002 [79]. Clinical and immunologic features consisted recurrent upper and lower respiratory tract infections, otitis media, weakness, almost complete absence of B-cells but not T-cells, hypogammaglobulinemia, dermatomyositis, and diarrhea.

3.3.4 Igβ Deficiency

Study in *Drosophila melanogaster* [80] showed that mutant Igβ is a contributing factor to the dissociation of Igα/Igβ, whereby the pre-BCR complex cannot be assembled and B-cell development is blocked. Moreover, deletion of Igβ dictated death in murine developing B-cells including pre-B-cells and immature B-cells [81]. The first patient carrying mutant Igβ (CD79b) was described by Dobbs et al. 2007 [82]. She presented with recurrent bronchitis, persistent cough, pneumonia, and hypogammaglobulinemia. The age at onset of symptoms was about 5 months. Ferrari et al. 2007 [80] were the second group who found mutant Igβ in a patient presented with less than 1% of normal CD19 levels, hypogammaglobulinemia, but normal counts of T and NK cells. His symptoms began to appear at 8 months of age and included recurrent pneumonia, conjunctivitis, otitis media, sinusitis, and bronchitis. At the time of evaluation, he was 20 and demonstrated chronic sinusitis at his CT scan. The third case was recently introduced by Lougaris et al. 2014 [83]. The patient was a female child, whose symptoms started at 14 months of age. She presented with recurrent upper respiratory tract infections, fever, neutropenia, profound hypogammaglobulinemia, and complete absence of B-cells but normal numbers of T and NK cells.

3.3.5 BLNK Deficiency

BLNK is essential for B-cell development and function. Mice deficient in BLNK failed to generate B220 + CD43− precursor B-cells and lacked mature B-cells in the periphery [84]. BLNK deficiency also led to reduce IL-10 production in mice [85]. Mutant BLNK in a patient lacking pre-B-cells or mature B-cells was first reported in 1999 [86]. The patient presented with recurrent otitis, pneumonia, and hypogammaglobulinemia. His symptoms commenced at 8 months of age. Other studies that have found mutant BLNK in association with agammaglobulinemia can be found here [87–89]. They confirm recurrent otitis and sinopulmonary infections as the most common initial presentation of BLNK deficiency [88, 89]. However, other clinical manifestations included diarrhea, enteroviral infection, arthritis, dermatitis, and bronchiectasis [89].

3.4 Other Forms of Agammaglobulinemia with Absent B-Cells (TCF3 Deficiency, LRRC8 Deficiency, Thymoma with Immunodeficiency)

3.4.1 TCF3 Deficiency

Studies of mice have shown that the transcription factor 3 (TCF3) gene plays a crucial role in B-cell development [90–92]. This gene which is also known as E22 gene encodes transcription factors E12 and E47. Mutations in TCF3 have been reported in both autosomal recessive [93] and autosomal dominant [94] agammaglobulinemia. The authors in [93] described a patient with B-cell acute lymphoblastic leukemia (B-ALL) presented with profound hypogammaglobulinemia, recurrent pneumonia, meningitis, pancytopenia, and splenomegaly. His immunological findings included less than 1 percent normal number of CD19+ B-cells in the periphery in the presence of normal counts of CD3+, CD4+, and CD8+ T-cells. Boisson et al. 2013 [94] identified the same de novo mutation in the TCF3 gene (within the exon that encodes E47) in four patients with an unusual phenotype characterized by almost complete absence of BCR in the presence of increased expression of CD19 on B-cells [95]. All patients presented severe hypogammaglobulinemia and less than 3 percent CD19+ cells in the periphery. Age at diagnosis ranged from 9 months to 4 years. Clinical presentations included pneumococcal meningitis, recurrent otitis, vaccine-associated polio, and arthritis. Other clinical findings were dermatitis and hepatomegaly.

3.4.2 LRRC8 Deficiency

Sawada et al. 2003 [96] are the first group that isolated the leucine-rich repeat-containing 8 (LRRC8) and showed that B-cell development is impaired in mouse model for a truncated expression of LRRC8. They also provided a report describing a girl patient with agammaglobulinemia, absence of B-cells, epicanthic folds, mild hypertelorism, high-arched palate, and lowered ears. The patient carried mutant LRRC8. To our knowledge, no other report of mutant LRRC8 in association with agammaglobulinemia has been published.

3.4.3 Thymoma with Immunodeficiency (Good's Syndrome)

Good's syndrome (GS) or thymoma with immunodeficiency refers to the combined conditions of thymoma and immunodeficiency. It is mainly characterized by thymoma, hypogammaglobulinemia, and low number of B-cells in the periphery. However, low number of T-cells and an inverted CD4/CD8 ratio are also common.

Tarr et al. 2001 [97] in the study provided a report of 5 patients with GS presented with infection as well as a review of 46 other patients with GS and infections. Infections have a propensity to affect the respiratory and gastrointestinal tract [98, 99]. The following are infectious complications documented in GS: recurrent sinopulmonary infection, CMV disease, bacteremia, oral or esophageal candidiasis, persistent mucocutaneous candidiasis, chronic diarrhea, urinary tract infections, *P. carinii* pneumonia, tuberculosis, Kaposi sarcoma, disseminated varicella, candidemia, wound infection with *Clostridium perfringens*, Mycoplasma arthritis, etc. However, the main clinical findings at presentation appear to be sinopulmonary infections with encapsulated bacteria. When compared to patients with CVID, patients with GS experience a more difficult course of immunodeficiency complicated with opportunistic infections such as *P. carinii* pneumonia, mycobacterium tuberculosis, and mucocutaneous candidiasis, resembling that which occurs in human immunodeficiency virus (HIV) infection [100]. Therefore, if a patient with thymoma or CVID develops refractory infections, then we should consider GS as a differential diagnosis. Particularly, persistent infection (pneumonia) following thymectomy might warrant that your patient is very likely to have GS [101–105]. Overall, respiratory manifestations in association with GS include recurrent sinopulmonary infections (sinusitis, rhinosinusitis, otitis media, and pneumonia) [106–114] with bacterial (especially with encapsulated bacteria including *Haemophilus influenzae*), fungal (aspergillus and *P. carinii*), and viral (CMV and HSV) pathogens [115–121], tracheobronchitis [118], diffuse panbronchiolitis [122–124], granulomatous lung disease [125], and pulmonary nodules [123]. As for patients with other forms of agammaglobulinemia, patients with GS remain dependent on immunoglobulin replacement therapy. A recent study has estimated the median survival of 14 years for 47 patients with GS [111].

3.5 Activated PI3K-δ Syndrome

Activated PI3K-δ syndrome (APDS) is a heterogeneous disorder associated with a spectrum of clinical pictures and immunological findings classified under two types [126]. Autosomal dominant gain-of-function mutations (E1021K and C416R) in the gene PIK3CD (PI3K-δ, phosphoinositide 3-kinase δ) can cause activated PI3K-δ syndrome type 1 (APDS1), while activated PI3K-δ syndrome type 2 (APDS2) is caused by an autosomal dominant gain-of-function mutation in the gene PIK3R1 (phosphoinositide-3-kinase regulatory subunit 1), inducing the skipping of exon 11.

Both types are characterized with similar immunological findings including low levels of IgG2 and lymphocytes and high levels of IgM and B-cells [127]. Overall, patients with APDS are prone to recurrent respiratory infections, airway disease [127], lymphoproliferation, cytopenias, skin diseases, chronic EBV and CMV viremia, and enteropathy [126]. All these major manifestations tend to decrease over time [126]. Of notable importance is that respiratory infections are the most frequent, initial manifestations of APDS [126].

The prospective European Society for Immunodeficiencies (ESID)-APDS registry has recently reported data on 51 patients with APDS1 and 26 patients with APDS2 [126]. Overall, respiratory infections, particularly pneumonia, otitis media, and sinusitis, were observed in nearly all patients and in most patients occurred before 15 years of age. Looking at CT scans, evidences of bronchiectasis were found in 60% of patients with APDS1 and 27% of patients with APDS2. Mean age at diagnosis of bronchiectasis was 11.2 years. Therapeutic options available to patients with APDS include antibiotics, antifungal agents, immunoglobulin replacement therapy, systemic immunosuppressive therapy, and HSCT [126]. Particularly a cohort study of 36 patients with APDS2 revealed that recurrent upper respiratory tract infections were experienced by all patients [128]. Other common respiratory complications in this population included pneumonia and respiratory tract lymphoid hyperplasia, which were found in about 70% and 50% patients.

3.5.1 Potential Mechanisms of Respiratory Manifestations in APDS

PI3K as lipid kinases play role to maintain normal function of airway. Abnormal PI3K signaling can alter airway function, so that inflammatory responses are aggravated [129]. Such a condition is seen in patients with respiratory diseases especially allergic inflammation and asthma. Airway biopsies from 11 patients with atopic asthma provide evidence of increased activation of the PI3K signaling after exposure to allergen [130].

PI3K-δ is a class I PI3K isoform proven to particularly contribute to both innate and adaptive immune responses [129]. Such contribution is resulted from its interaction with Akt, together triggering the PI3K-δ/Akt signaling pathway. Increased activation of this signaling pathway is thought to mediate airway inflammation as seen in obstructive lung diseases [131, 132] and induced by cigarette smoking [133]. Moreover, PI3K-δ is able to reduce glucocorticoid sensitivity of airways ([131, 132]. This explains why some patients are resistant to glucocorticoids. Supporting this, PI3K-δ inhibitor can mitigate allergic inflammation in asthma models [134]. The effect remained true upon exposure to *Aspergillus fumigatus*. At least part of this anti-inflammatory effect of PI3K-δ inhibitor appears to be mediated through reducing endoplasmic reticulum stress [135], hypoxia-inducible factor-1α (HIF-1α), and nucleotide-binding domain, leucine-rich-containing family, and pyrin domain-containing-3 (NLRP3) expression in lung tissue [136, 134]. All these factors are involved in generating inflammatory responses upon stimulation [136]. Additionally, PI3K-δ contributes to virus escape possibly by increasing the expression of B7-H1 (PD-L1) [137]. Therefore, it is well-expected that APDS, a condition associated with PI3K-δ upregulation, should be accompanied with bacterial and viral infections as well as different respiratory manifestations.

The current literature also supports the potential of PI3K-δ to be exploited as a target for treatment of respiratory infections and airway diseases [138, 139]. For example, anti-inflammatory effect of erythromycin and dexamethasone seems to be mediated via suppression of PI3K-δ signaling [140]. Animal models of asthma demonstrate that PI3K-δ blockade hampers infiltration of inflammatory cells by decreasing vascular permeability [141]. Moreover, PI3K-δ inhibition can help to regain glucocorticoid sensitivity and, therefore, enhance anti-inflammatory effects of glucocorticoids [131, 132, 142]. However, attention should be paid that over-suppression of this pathway might cause toxicities. As for APDS, PI3K-δ function is abnormally high in malignant states particularly B-cell malignancies [143]. As a result, PI3K-δ inhibitor (idelalisib) can be used to treat these malignancies [144]. However, it might reduce cellular respiration and so be toxic to lung tissues [145].

3.6 LRBA Deficiency

Lipopolysaccharide (LPS)-responsive and beige-like anchor (LRBA) protein deficiency is a rare PID characterized by hypogammaglobulinemia and CD19+ B-cell deficiency and also to a lesser extent by CD4+ T-cell deficiency and NK-cell deficiency [146]. Patients with LRBA deficiency often present with recurrent infections (pneumonia, urinary tract infections, and otitis media), lymphoproliferative disorders (lymphadenopathy, splenomegaly, hepatomegaly, and granuloma), autoimmune disorders (type 1 diabetes, ulcerative colitis, immune thrombocytopenic purpura, autoimmune hemolytic anemia, and Graves' disease), atopic disorders (food allergy, insect sting allergies, allergic dermatitis, urticaria, and asthma), enteropathy, and failure to thrive [147, 148, 146]. Therefore, LRBA can be appropriately considered as a subgroup of CVID with autoimmune and inflammatory features.

A retrospective cohort of ten patients with LRBA deficiency in Israel highlighted chronic cough as the most common respiratory manifestation in patients with LRBA deficiency [147]. Less frequent respiratory manifestations were dyspnea, perioral cyanosis, and clubbing. Chest X-rays and CT scans in these cases provided evidences of axillary, hilar, and mediastinal lymphadenopathy, consolidation, lobar and sub-lobar atelectasis, bronchiectasis, and interstitial lung disease [147]. Patients with LRBA deficiency demonstrated no serious abnormalities on PFT. They also were likely to have a normal bronchoscopy. Potential findings in bronchoscopy included tracheomalacia and adenoid hypertrophy. The mean age at onset of symptoms was 4.65 [147].

In a longitudinal study of patients with LRBA ($n = 17$) in Iran [146], respiratory tract infections were the most common first presentation of immunodeficiency, seen in more than 40% of patients. Additionally, there were two patients (11.8%) presented with allergy and asthma. The median age at onset of symptoms and diagnosis were 2.0 and 7.0 years, respectively. With a median follow-up of 14 years, all patients (100%) developed infectious complications, which in order of frequency were pneumonia, sinusitis, and otitis media.

There is a case report of bronchiolitis obliterans organizing pneumonia (BOOP) in a 10-year-old boy who presented with recurrent respiratory infections, anemia, and thrombocytopenia [149]. He showed hypogammaglobulinemia of IgA and IgG, while IgM levels were normal. He was refractory to regular IVIG and all antimicrobial agents, and his respiratory condition deteriorated during these treatments. Diffuse lung disease with peripheral nodules was found at CT scans. PCR of BAL fluid was positive for *Pseudomonas aeruginosa*, *Pneumocystis jiroveci*, and CMV. Looking at lung tissue, there were evidences of disseminated infiltration of inflammatory cells and bronchiolitis obliterans organizing pneumonia (BOOP). To establish genetic causality, combined homozygosity mapping and exome sequencing was performed and showed a homozygous mutation (NM_001199282: c.743_744insAAGA: p. Asp248Glufs*2) in the gene LRBA. Each parent carried a copy of this mutation, supporting the autosomal recessive form of disease.

In this manner, different mutations in the gene LRBA are associated with the spectrum of phenotypes [150]. Even two siblings might present with incompatible pictures of LRBA deficiency [151].

Polymorphisms of the gene LRBA known to influence the function of LRBA protein have been associated with risk of pneumoconiosis in coal workers [152].

In conclusion, it is promising that respiratory manifestations of LRBA patients are mostly sensitive to therapy with IVIG, systemic immunosuppression, abatacept (CTLA4-Ig), or hematopoietic stem cell transplantation (HSCT) [147]. Drugs for prophylaxis of recurrent infections include antibiotics, antivirals, and antifungal medicines [146]. Mastoidectomy might be indicated in a severe case with frequent otitis media [146]. Therapeutic options for autoimmune complications vary from individual to individual and include IVIG, systemic immunosuppression, thymectomy, and HSCT [146]. However, respiratory failure remains the leading cause of death in these patients [85].

3.7 CD19 Complex Deficiencies

The CD19 complex is a transmembrane complex comprising CD19, CD21, CD81, and CD225. It can function as a co-receptor for B-cells that promotes B-cell receptor (BCR) signaling. Therefore, it is well-appreciated that defects in the formation of CD19 complex can cause autoimmunity and impairment of humoral immunity [153].

3.7.1 CD19 Deficiency

CD19 includes two extracellular immunoglobulin superfamily (IgSF) constant domains: a transmembrane region and a cytoplasmic region. Its cytoplasmic tail is comprised of nine tyrosine kinase residues that contribute to intracellular signaling. To our knowledge, there have been reported ten cases of CD19 deficiency [154–160]. The genetic defects responsible for CD19 deficiency include mutations resulting in premature termination codons and also missense mutations leading to an amino acid change. Overall, CD19 deficiency is featured by respiratory manifestations such as recurrent respiratory tract infections (pneumonia, bronchiolitis, and otitis media), wheezing, chronic obstructive pulmonary disease, atopy, and asthma [154]. Hypogammaglobulinemia (IgG and IgM) is also commonly found in patients with CD19 deficiency. Infectious pathogens found in these patients are respiratory syncytial virus, *Haemophilus influenzae*, and *Streptococcus pneumoniae*. CXR and CT scans reveal lobar atelectasis, peribronchial thickening, and bronchiectasis. Despite absence of CD19+ B-cells, flow cytometry can be used to confirm presence of CD20+ B-cells. Patients are also likely to have reduced numbers of transitional B-cells, memory B-cells, CD3+ T cells, and CD16+/CD56+ NK cells. Interestingly, studies indicate a delay between Ca2+ influx and stimulation with anti-IgM in B-cells from patients with CD19 deficiency. It should be noted that Ca2+ influx plays a crucial role in BCR signaling.

3.7.2 CD81 Deficiency

CD81 is a 26KDa surface protein also known as TAPA-1 (target of the antiproliferative antibody 1) and Tetraspanin-28 (Tspan-28). CD81 acts as regulator of proliferation of different cells such as glial cells, astrocytes, oocytes, and retinal pigment epithelial cells [161–164]. It is also required for the expression of CD19 on B-cells and thereby contributes to the activation of B-cells and production of antibodies against T-cell-dependent antigens. Its deficiency interferes with the formation of CD19 complex, resulting in the spectrum of respiratory manifestations related to CD19 deficiency.

The authors in the study [165] presented a patient suffering from recurrent respiratory tract infections during the first 2 years of life. She then developed glomerulonephritis, recurrent thrombocytopenia, and hypogammaglobulinemia of IgG. There was no significant change in the numbers of B, T, and NK cells. However, flow cytometry revealed a reduction in the relative number of transitional B-cells and memory B-cells. Additionally, the patient's B-cells showed loss of both CD19 and CD81. Genetic analysis revealed an intact CD19 gene but homozygous splice site mutation (c.561+1G>A) in the CD81 gene. While the patient's family members (her parents and her brother) harboring a single copy of this mutation were immunologically healthy, the patient did not show the expected increase in IgA and IgG levels upon vaccination with tetanus toxoid and pneumococcal antigens. CD81 is thus essential to produce an appropriate antibody response to protein and polysaccharide antigens.

A study of mice links CD9/CD81 double knockout to the spontaneous development of pulmonary emphysema [166]. It is accompanied with an increase in the activity of matrix metalloproteinases MMP-2 and MMP-9 in alveolar macrophages. The role of MMPs is well-appreciated in the degradation of the alveolar matrix as well as in the aggravation of pulmonary inflammatory processes, which both events have been implicated in COPD [167]. It is thus suggested that obstructive lung disease might arise from CD81 deficiency, owing to abnormal activity of MMPs.

Also, allergen-induced airway activity in CD81-deficient mice is decreased compared to wild-type mice [168]. CD81-deficient mice also demonstrated a reduced production of Th2 inflammatory cytokines IL-4, IL-5, and IL-13. It is therefore possible to assume that CD81 plays role in allergen-induced airway hyperactivity by inducing the expression of cytokines.

3.7.3 CD21 Deficiency

CD21 or complement receptor type 2 (CR2) precursor is a 145 KDa protein implicated in EBV entry [169]. It is expressed by mature B-cells and follicular dendritic cells, whereby activation of B-cell responses is enhanced by binding of immune complexes that comprise cleavage products of C3d and antigens [170]. This is beneficial in combating against toxic or infectious agents and on the other hand can cause an imbalance favoring autoimmunity.

The study [171] provides a report of first case of CD21 deficiency. Early childhood respiratory tract infections forced the patient to undergo tonsillectomy at 6 years old. Then, the patient experienced a long remission for about 20 years. At 28 years old, his symptoms including recurrent respiratory tract infections, myalgia, diarrhea, and weight loss began to flare up. The pathogen found in his respiratory secretions was *Haemophilus influenzae*. The patient also showed hypogammaglobulinemia of IgG1 and IgG4 and was thus considered for immunoglobulin replacement therapy. The patient's B-cells completely lacked CD21. Genetic analysis revealed two heterozygous mutations: one resulting in the skipping of exon 6 and the other being a premature stop codon mutation occurring in exon 13.

The patient reported in [172] was a 13-year-old boy who presented with myalgia, rigidity, and hypogammaglobulinemia of IgG1, 2, and 4. Flow cytometry revealed absence of CD21. Sequencing of CD21 gene identified two heterozygous mutations: one nonsense mutation occurring in exon 2 and the other being a frameshift mutation in exon 15. Interestingly, the patient remained free of serious infections until writing the paper.

In the study [173], the authors have described two siblings who carried CD21 deficiency. Symptoms began to manifest at 5 and 7 years of age. Clinical manifestations mainly included recurrent otitis media, rhinopharyngitis, bronchitis, and lobar pneumonia.

3.8 Common Variable Immunodeficiency

Common variable immunodeficiency (CVID) is the most common symptomatic PID estimated to occur in 1/10,000–1/200,000 depending on the study population. It is mainly characterized by a defective B-cell differentiation resulting in hypogammaglobulinemia of IgA, IgG, and IgM with two or more standard deviations below the normal mean. Also, about half of patients manifest characteristics of malfunctioning T-cells and cytokine/chemokine system including a reduction in CD40 ligand expression and IL-2 production [174]. Therefore, CVID covers a spectrum of disease phenotypes, and the diagnosis should only be made after ruling out other potential causes of hypogammaglobulinemia including other PIDs and immunodeficiency diseases due to infectious agents, malignancies, protein-losing agents, and drugs [175]. CVID involves a complex interaction of different disease processes. However, there are a few monogenetic forms of CVID that are caused by defect in a single gene such as ICOS [176, 177], TACI [178, 179], and CD19 [155]. Clinical presentations mainly include recurrent bacterial infections especially affecting upper and lower respiratory tracts, inflammatory diseases, autoimmune disorders, lymphoproliferative disorders, chronic lung diseases, gastrointestinal disorders, malabsorption, hepatitis, and malignancies (especially lymphomas). Clinical symptoms usually peak in the second or third decade of life. Early-onset disease is, however, common, especially in male patients [180]. Recently a multicenter study of 2212 patients with CVID has reported that the median diagnostic delay is around 4–5 years in most populations [181]. Overall, as much as all patients with CVID experience infectious respiratory diseases [182–184] and more than half of patients develop noninfectious respiratory complications as well [185].

3.8.1 Respiratory Tract Infections

The French national study of adults with CVID ($n = 252$) confirmed recurrent respiratory tract infections, e.g., bronchitis, sinusitis, and pneumonia, as the most common initial presentation [181]. In order they were found in about 69%, 63%, and 58% of patients. Lower respiratory tract infections are also found in 84% of patients [182]. In particular, pneumonia is experienced by about 32–77% of patients [180, 182, 184, 186]. Early-onset CVID in male (before 10 years of age) patients is considered a discrete disease entity characterized by a higher risk of infectious complications including pneumonia, but not noninfectious complications [180]. Encapsulated bacteria such as *Streptococcus pneumoniae*, *Staphylococcus aureus*, and *Haemophilus influenzae* are the main pathogens associated with respiratory tract infections in patients with CVID. In particular, *Bordetella pertussis* may contribute to the development of respiratory disease in children with CVID. About 13% of patients reveal a severe defect in switched memory B-cells (IgD-CD27+ cell percentage ≤2% of B-cells), which is related to an increased need for antibiotic therapy. Follow-up studies indicate that the incidence of acute pneumonia and otitis will decrease by time [186]. Other infectious respiratory manifestations that are possible but less frequent than the aforementioned ones include mycoplasma pneumonia, cryptococcal lung abscess, and *Mycobacterium avium* complex pulmonary disease [184].

3.8.2 Chronic Lung Disease

Of note, some patients remain refractory to immunoglobulin therapy and continue to suffer from upper respiratory tract infections [181]. These patients are prone to progress to chronic sinusitis and CLD including bronchiectasis. As expected, longitudinal studies show that the prevalence of chronic sinusitis and CLD will increase by time [186]. Studies estimate the prevalence of CLD to be between 22% and 67.5% in patients with CVID [182–184, 186]. In particular, bronchiectasis is found in 37–58% of patients with CVID [181, 182]. Patients who have a positive sputum culture are more likely to demonstrate evidence of bronchiectasis in HRCT [187]. In addition to the pathogens mostly involved in respiratory tract infections including *Streptococcus pneumoniae* and *Haemophilus influenzae*, bronchiectasis has been associated with *Pseudomonas aeruginosa*, *Staphylococcus aureus*, and *Corynebacterium* spp. [182]. A severe defect in total B-cells (CD19+ cell percentage $\leq$1%) was present in about 40% of patients and was associated with a higher risk of bronchiectasis. In addition, patients with CD4+ cell count below 700 cells/μL, patients with a history of pneumonia, and patients with older age were more prone to bronchiectasis [188].

3.8.3 Lymphocytic Interstitial Lung Disease and Follicular Bronchitis/Bronchiolitis

As reviewed in [189], both profiles of lymphocytic interstitial pneumonia (LIP) and follicular bronchitis/bronchiolitis have been detected in lung tissues from patients with CVID. LIP presents "with a diffuse, interstitial infiltrate of lymphocytes, immunoblasts, plasma cells, fibroblasts, and scattered macrophages that sometimes aggregate into granulomas" [189]. Follicular bronchitis/bronchiolitis is characterized by "reactive lymphoid follicles mainly around airways with minimal interstitial disease" [189]. While LIP has been associated with both hypogammaglobulinemia and hypergammaglobulinemia, follicular bronchitis/bronchiolitis does not appear to have been accompanied by any immunoglobulin abnormalities [189]. Clinical symptoms include cough, dyspnea, fever, and pleuritic chest pain.

The first case of LIP in CVID was described by Levinson et al. [190] and that the first case of nodular lymphoid interstitial pneumonia in CVID was documented by Kohler et al. [191]. Duke et al. also found two other cases with pulmonary infiltration in CXR, which were then histologically diagnosed with LIP [192].

3.8.4 Granulomatous Lung Disease

Generally, granulomatous lesions are found in 5.4–10% of patients with CVID [189]. Noninfectious diffuse lung complications which are collectively referred to granulomatous-lymphocytic interstitial lung disease (GLILD) predict worse survival in patients with CVID [185]. Patients with defects in T-cell function, low CD3+ cell count, and low CD8+ cell count are more likely to develop GLILD. The presence of GLILD has been linked to dyspnea, splenomegaly, restrictive pattern of pulmonary function (a low DL_{CO}), consolidation, ground-glass opacity, interstitial infiltrates, and reticular pulmonary opacification. GLILD in CVID has been associated with a higher prevalence of HHV8 infection, leading to an increased risk of lymphoproliferative disorders [193]. It is promising that monoclonal antibodies and immunosuppressive agents can effectively assist with resolution of granulomas and restoration of lung structure [194]. FDG PET-CT imaging can be used to monitor therapeutic response [194].

3.8.5 Pulmonary Function

The majority of patients in spirometry are normal. About 25% of patients show abnormal features favoring an airflow obstruction and to a lesser extent a restrictive pattern [187]. When compared to patients without bronchiectasis, the spirometry test revealed reduced values of FEV_1, $FEF_{25-75\%}$, and FVC in patients with bronchiectasis [182].

On the contrary, more than 60% of patients have abnormal MMEF. Therefore, there is a large subgroup of patients who are abnormal in MMEF and normal in spirometry [187].

3.8.6 Imaging Findings

HRCT in patients with CVID may provide evidence of granulomatous lung disease, hilar and mediastinal lymphadenopathy, pulmonary nodules, ground-glass opacity, bronchiectasis, and reduced peribronchiectatic shadowing [187, 188]. In particular, patients with bronchiectasis may demonstrate parenchymal scarring, pleural thickening, and atelectasis [182]. Bronchiectasis in patients with CVID has been shown to occur with the involvement of left lower lobe; lingual, right lower lobe; right middle lobe; right upper lobe; multiple lobes; and both lungs [182]. Patients with LIP demonstrate pulmonary infiltration especially basilar, coarse interstitial-alveolar infiltrations in CXR [189]. Patients with ground-glass appearance are more likely to have a high monocyte count, reduced number of CD19 + IgM-IgD-CD27+ isotype-switched memory B-cells, a history of lung disease, and pulmonary nodule(s) and be younger than those with bronchiectasis without interstitial lung disease [188]. Patients who exhibit evidence of bronchiectasis on their CT scan are more likely to have lower CD4+ T-cell counts [188]. Patients with five or more pulmonary nodules have lower CD8+ T-cell counts [188].

3.8.7 *Morbidity and Mortality*

Immunoglobulin dose required for prevention of bacterial infections is between 0.2 and 1.2 g/kg/months [195]. A higher dose of replacement immunoglobulin is, however, required to benefit cases with CLD including bronchiectasis [196]. Regular immunoglobulin therapy has shown to be effective in reducing the incidence of acute infections. A study of 50 patients with CVID with pneumonia demonstrated that the prevalence of pneumonia was reduced from 84% to 22% following immunoglobulin therapy [197]. Additionally, immunoglobulin therapy can effectively improve pulmonary function test results and HRCT scores in patients with CVID with CLD [196]. Such improvement does not appear to reach significance in cases with CVID without CLD [196]. Given that the mortality of CVID increases with age, it is not clear whether it can be effective in long term as well as short term. Lung transplant is the option available to patients with respiratory failure. Altogether, acute or chronic respiratory tract infections and associated respiratory failure are a leading cause of morbidity and mortality in patients with CVID [187, 186], especially in cases below 40 years of age [183].

3.9 CD20 Deficiency

It is a humoral immunodeficiency resulting from a homozygous mutation (MS4A1) in a splice junction of the CD20 gene, leading to the production of nonfunctional mRNA species [198]. Despite normal development of antigen-independent B-cells, CD20-deficient mice fail to generate normal antibody response to T-cell-independent antigens. Also, T-cell-dependent humoral immunity is impaired in CD20 deficiency [199]. This is thought to be a secondary effect of the impairment in B-cell function [199].

3.9.1 *Potential Mechanisms of Respiratory Manifestations in CD20 Deficiency*

CD20 acts as a regulator of B-cell development. It is thus well-understood that chronic administration of anti-CD20 antibodies can lead to B-cell depletion [200]. The effects that CD20 deficiency might have on lung tissues can be tackled in those who received anti-CD20 treatments. As reviewed by [201], anti-CD20 treatments predispose patients to severe and refractory respiratory infections with bacteria, fungi, and viruses, while, anti-CD20 antibodies are being increasingly used to treat autoimmune diseases and non-Hodgkin lymphoma [202]. This has been parallel by increasing the number of cases of pneumocystis pneumonia [203]. This increased susceptibility might be due to suppressive effect of anti-CD20 antibodies on type 2 helper T (Th2) responses, e.g., production of cytokines interleukin (IL)-4, IL-5, and IL-13 [202]. Moreover, there is a report of antisynthetase syndrome after treatment with rituximab, a CD20 monoclonal antibody [204]. The patient was presented with recurrent respiratory infections, arthropathy, and interstitial pneumonitis. Immunoglobulin replacement therapy was shown to improve immunodeficiency and pneumonitis. It is also interesting that treatment with 25-OH vitamin D3 has been shown to enhance CD20 levels [205].

3.10 Other Monogenic Defects Associated with Hypogammaglobulinemia (ICOS Deficiency, TACI Deficiency, BAFF Receptor Deficiency, TWEAK Deficiency, and NFKB2 Deficiency)

As above explained, CVID is not usually a single-gene disorder but rather is a complex disorder resulting from the combined effect of several genes. Overall, monogenic defects account for just 2–10% of cases with CVID [206].

3.10.1 ICOS Deficiency

The inducible T-cell co-stimulator (ICOS) is shown to stimulate differentiation of T follicular helper (TFH) cells and development of Treg, Th17, and Th2 cells that can promote autoimmunity and local inflammation [207]. In this manner, myeloid cells (CD11+ cells) expressing this co-stimulator can contribute to the generation of inflammatory processes in lung tissues [207]. What more supports this is increased expression of ICOS in autoimmune conditions (acute graft-versus-host disease) and allergic airway diseases [208]. Also, its ligand ICOS-L display by dendritic cells is capable to improve Treg or Th17 responses [209], whose pathogenic roles in autoimmunity and organ rejection have been well-described [210]. ICOS deficiency in mice could diminish lung tissue fibrosis [211] and delay rejection of the transplanted bronchus by reduction of relative numbers of Th17, Th2, and Treg cells [54]. By contrast, lung fibrosis was exacerbated in isolated ICOS-L deficiency and in double ICOS/ICOS-L deficiency [211].

Loss-of-function mutations in the ICOS gene as seen in patients with ICOS deficiency lead to reduce the numbers of TFH cells [212]. It has been demonstrated that intranasal application of Protollin, a TLR4 ligand adjuvant, can play a protective role against allergic lower airway disease upon stimulation with pollen allergen. This TLR4-dependent protection was accompanied by engagement of

CD4+ T-cells expressing ICOS [213]. Additionally, adoptive transfer of CD4+ T-cells expressing ICOS could reverse allergen-induced airway hyper-responsiveness [213]. Whereas, inhibition of TLR4 signaling (TLR4-TRIF pathway) exacerbating allergen-induced airway hyper-responsiveness resulted in a reduction of CD4+ T-cells expressing ICOS [214]. Therefore, ICOS deficiency is expected to increase the risk of allergic airway diseases. As for B-cells expressing CD40, all CVID patients show diminished number of CD4+ T-cells expressing ICOS [215].

As above mentioned, ICOS is also implicated in development of Th2 immunity. Th2 cytokines (IL-5) are essential to the recruitment of eosinophils into the airway [216]. Therefore, it is expected that ICOS-deficient mice exhibit impairment in the generation of antigen-induced airway eosinophilia and inflammation [217]. It should be noted that CD28 also plays a crucial role in this context.

3.10.2 TACI Deficiency

Antiviral antibodies are essential to the generation of antiviral immunity. Animals deficient in transmembrane activator and calcium-modulator and cyclophilin ligand interactor (TACI) were not able to achieve protective titers of antibodies against influenza virus [218]. Even, mice that carried only a single copy of mutation in the TACI gene showed reduction of TACI expression on B-cells and were more susceptible to pneumococcal infections [219]. In this manner, TACI deficiency would predispose the lungs to viral and bacterial infections. TACI deficiency has been observed among patients with PADs who had hypogammaglobulinemia of IgG [220] and IgA [221]. It can cause phenotypes in the spectrum of clinical presentations correlated to CVID or even beyond them, for example, lymphoproliferation and IgG subclass deficiencies [222]. Later in life, it might lead to autoimmune disorders [221, 223].

3.10.3 NFKB2 Deficiency

Germline heterozygous mutations in NFKB2 are known to cause an early-onset type of CVID characterized by B-cell deficiency, T-cell deficiency, hypogammaglobulinemia, central adrenal insufficiency, alopecia totalis or areata, and trachyonychia [224–230]. They can contribute to changes in NK-cell count or function as well. Autoimmunity is present in the majority of patients with NFKB2 deficiency. Other presentations of this immunodeficiency include recurrent respiratory tract infections [228, 231].

Animal studies provide evidence that NFKB2 deficiency can cause serious lung inflammation by inducing the expression IFN-γ and thereby Th1 cytokines. Due to extensive infiltration of lymphocytes, this long inflammation is considered an autoimmune condition that can be potentially fatal [232, 233].

3.10.4 BAFF Receptor Deficiency

B-cell-activating factor of the TNF family (BAFF) emerged as an innate mediator that is involved in antiviral immunity. Upon exposure to viral dsRNA, Ig class switching is induced by TLR3-expressing B-cells of the upper respiratory tract. NFKB activation and TLR3 signaling are central to Ig class switching, which are in turn required for production of IgA and IgG antibodies in response to viral antigens [234]. Patients in intensive care unit (ICU) show increased susceptibility to hospital-acquired pneumonia. This is suggested to be caused by pulmonary IgA deficiency secondary to antibiotic therapy. Patients in this condition often reveal low expression of BAFF [235]. BAFF neutralization in mice has been associated with reduction in the number of antibody-secreting cells (ASC) that contribute to antiviral immunity [218]. Interestingly, immunoglobulin D has been shown to improve immunity in basophils of the upper respiratory tract. Its role is mediated by increasing the expression of pro-inflammatory in addition to B-cell stimulating factors, for example, BAFF [236].

On the other hand, BAFF acts to facilitate the cross talk between IL-1β and Th17 cell development, whereby Th1 and Th17 responses which mainly contribute to inflammatory and autoimmune processes are augmented [237]. Overexpression of BAFF is implicated in lung fibrosis [238], and therefore its inhibition is proposed as a targeted therapy for conditions associated with long fibrosis such as scleroderma [239].

3.10.5 TWEAK Deficiency

Tumor necrosis factor-like weak inducer of apoptosis (TWEAK) binding to fibroblast growth factor-inducible 14 (Fn14) leads to activation of intracellular signaling cascades that are likely to contribute to progression of a variety of tumors favorably non-small cell lung cancer (NSCLC) [240].

To the knowledge of the authors, there are not any respiratory manifestations documented as complications of other monogenic defects associated with hypogammaglobulinemia such as MOGS deficiency, TRNT1 deficiency, and TTC37 deficiency.

3.11 Immunoglobulin Class Switch Recombination Deficiencies Affecting B-Cells (AICDA Deficiency, UNG Deficiency, MMR Deficiency, and INO80 Deficiency)

3.11.1 AICDA Deficiency

The activation-induced cytidine deaminase (AICDA) gene encodes the enzyme activation-induced cytidine deaminase (AID) required to CSR in addition to Ig gene somatic hypermutation (SHM) [241]. More importantly, AID plays a crucial role in DNA methylation and reprogramming of somatic cells into induced pluripotent stem cells (iPSC) [242]. Besides the role of activated B-cell CD40 signaling, bacterial and viral antigens can lead to the expression of AID by engaging IL-4-secreting CD4+ T cells or TLR signaling [241].

Patients with AICDA deficiency often present with lymphoid hyperplasia [243]. Also, they frequently develop sinopulmonary infections (sinusitis and pneumonia), and finally their CT scan may reveal evidences of bronchiectasis [244]. Immunological findings include hypogammaglobulinemia of IgA, IgG, and IgE in addition to hypergammaglobulinemia of IgM [244].

The early clearance is an important component in engendering protective immunity against pneumococci [245]. Mice deficient in AID failed to effectively clear pneumococcal bacteria from pulmonary tissues at early time points [246]. The issue was resolved by adoptive transfer of AID+ B1a cells.

3.11.2 UNG Deficiency

The uracil-DNA glycosylase (UNG) gene encodes a base excision repair (BER) enzyme that functions to exclude misincorporated uracil. Cancerous cells deficient in UNG will develop hypersensitivity to pemetrexed (a chemotherapy drug). On the contrary, lung cancer cells carrying high expression of UNG reveal resistance to pemetrexed [247]. Moreover, it has been shown that viral UNG aids replication and dissemination of murine gammaherpesvirus 68 [248]. It seems that viral UNG expression is induced as a compensatory mechanism to increase UNG activity in host lung cells, which typically express low values of UNG [248]. As for AICDA deficiency, UNG deficiency is characterized with hypergammaglobulinemia of IgM along with hypogammaglobulinemia of other immunoglobulins. Also, lymphoid hyperplasia is commonly seen in patients with this immunodeficiency.

3.11.3 MMR Deficiency

DNA mismatch repair (MMR) is a mechanism of DNA repair conserved during evolution from bacteria to humans. It provides a compensatory pathway for correcting mismatched bases during DNA replication. Therefore, patients with MMR deficiency are prone to genomic instability and ultimately malignant transformation. MMR defects have been discovered in cancers of different primary sites such as the colon, rectum [249, 250], stomach [251], prostate, esophagus, endometrium, oral cavity [252], skin, head and neck, and brain [253]. Due to their role in class switch DNA recombination (CSR) and somatic hypermutation (SHM), MMR components are required for the regulation of antibody response as well [254]. Mice deficient in MMR components exhibit spontaneous development of premalignant and malignant lung lesions [255]. It is consistent with some observations of MMR defects in human lung cancers [256–258]. Moreover, defective mismatch repair system can contribute to chronic lung infection with *Pseudomonas aeruginosa* [259].

3.11.4 INO80 Deficiency

The INO80 ATPase takes part in formation of the ATP-dependent chromatin remodeling complex, which is involved in nuclear transactions, e.g., DNA replication, DNA repair, and transcription [260]. Energy-dependent metabolic pathways are accompanied by increased expression of the INO80 complex. While, defective INO80 complex correlates to decreased glycolysis, increased oxidative stress, and increased oxygen consumption. In this manner, the INO80 complex acts as a regulator of respiratory capacity [261]. On the other hand, INO80 is also generated as a nuclear protein to assist with genome replication of herpes simplex virus [262] and with oncogenic transcription and tumorigenesis of non-small cell lung cancer (NSCLC) [263]. However, study of NSCLC cells has recently revealed that the increased activity of chemotherapeutic agents (cisplatin) is underpinned by increased expression of more than 100 genes among which is INO80 [264].

Two patients with nonsynonymous, compound heterozygous single-nucleotide variants in INO80 have been described in [143]. The first one presented with recurrent bacterial infections at 5 years of age and the second with severe and recurrent respiratory infections at 18 years of age. The second also progressed to chronic obstructive pulmonary disease (of course with a history of 35 years of smoking).

3.12 Transient Hypogammaglobulinemia of Infancy

The physiologic hypogammaglobulinemia is what is typically happening in the first 3–6 months of life. Along with IgG subclass deficiency, partial antibody deficiency with impaired polysaccharide responsiveness, and selective IgA deficiency, transient hypogammaglobulinemia of infancy (THI) is one of the common immune-deficiency conditions of children [265], where the certain period of the physiologic hypogammaglobulinemia is extended. The way to diagnose THI is not straightforward; but its diagnosis requires a retrospective look of the patient characteristics: early hypogammaglobulinemia of at least one immunoglobulin isotype, later achieving normal levels for all immunoglobulin isotypes, and no diagnosis more likely than THI is suspected [266]. Overall, recurrent respiratory tract (pneumonia) infections, ENT (otitis media) infections, bronchitis, and asthma are the most common presentations of THI [267–269]. However, other infectious complications that may affect patients with THI include sinusitis, enteritis, lymphadenitis, meningitis, mastoiditis, impetigo [267], urinary tract infections, and sepsis [266]. Moreover, atopic reactions in THI are common and mainly include bronchial hyperreactivity, food allergy, and atopic dermatitis [266]. Study of a single center in Jordan estimated that the average age of onset and diagnosis for THI ($n = 10$) are 1 and 1.6 years [267]. So the diagnostic delay was less than 1 year [267]. In other studies from Turkey and the United States, the mean age of onset was less than 1 year of age [266, 270]. Often it is spontaneously resolved by 3–5 years of age [270], and more than 90% of patients achieve normal immunoglobulin levels by 10 years of age. However, some patients continue to have hypogammaglobulinemia, the so-called undefined/unclassified hypogammaglobulinemia. Of note is that both conditions, i.e., THI and undefined/unclassified hypogammaglobulinemia, share common clinical characteristics [268]. However, patients with persistent antibody deficiency are less able to produce IgA responses against pneumococcal polysaccharide (PnPS) vaccine compared to patients with transient antibody deficiency [271].

3.12.1 Respiratory Tract Infections

Infections affecting the upper and lower respiratory tract are commonly seen among patients with THI. Overall patients with THI have a benign clinical outcome [272]. They usually do not develop life-threatening infections [269] requiring long-term immunoglobulin replacement therapy [267]. Immediate treatment is, however, indicated in severe respiratory tract infections. Also, additional treatments may be warranted according to the type and severity of infection. For example, extracorporeal membrane oxygenation (ECMO), ribavirin, and steroid (albeit along with immunoglobulin replacement therapy) benefited a THI case with severe human parainfluenza viruses (HPIVs) [273]. Moreover there are reports of *Pneumocystis carinii* pneumonia in patients with THI [274–276]. It is a life-threatening infection [277], and despite high rates of drug adverse reactions, drug therapy should be started once the diagnosis of *Pneumocystis carinii* pneumonia is suspected.

3.12.2 Asthma

Studies estimate that about 27–55% of patients with THI suffer from asthma [268, 269]. The history of recurrent upper respiratory tract infections showed a negative association to asthma. Whereas, patients with THI who had history of recurrent lower respiratory tract infections were more likely to suffer from asthma [268].

3.12.3 Potential Mechanisms of Respiratory Manifestations in Transient Hypogammaglobulinemia of Infancy

Patients with THI are categorized into three according to their initial immunoglobulin levels: isolated IgG deficiency, isolated IgA deficiency, isolated IgM deficiency, IgG and IgA deficiency, IgG and IgM deficiency, and IgG, IgA, and IgM deficiency. The majority of patients show IgG and IgA deficiency [266], whereas isolated deficiency of IgA or IgM are relatively rare in patients with THI [269]. It has been well-appreciated that hypogammaglobulinemia either in primary immunodeficiency disorders or secondary to other conditions (malignancies and immunosuppressive drugs) increases the risk of infections.

It has been shown that antibody response to specific respiratory viral antigens (influenzas A and B, adenovirus, mycoplasma, respiratory syncytial virus, and para-influenzas 1, 2, and 3) is more likely to be impaired in patients with THI than in age-matched controls without THI [270]. This is reflected in increased risk of viral infections in these patients.

3.13 Selective IgA Deficiency

Selective IgA deficiency (SIgAD) is the most common PID where B-cell switching to IgA-producing cells is impaired [278]. For children aged 1–18 years with recurrent infections and warning signs of immunodeficiency, it is the most commonly diagnosed disease [279]. Compared to other PIDs, patients with SIgAD appear to less prone to lower respiratory tract infection, sepsis, skin infections, mucocutaneous candidiasis, dental alterations, cardiovascular malformations, angioedema, hospitalizations, and death [280]. The world's epidemiology data indicate that the incidence of SIgAD varies by a family history of SIgAD and ethnicity ranging from 1:18,500 in Japan to 1:143 in the Arabian Peninsula [278, 281]. Intrinsic factors causing IgA deficiency include both monogenic mutations (TNFRSF13B/TACI) [282, 283, 220] and chromosomal abnormalities mainly involving chromosome 18 [278, 1]. SIgAD is indicated by low levels of serum IgA (below 7 mg/dl) in presence of normal levels of IgG and IgM after the age of 4 years in whom other causes of hypogammaglobulinemia have not been identified. Clinical presentations may range from asymptomatic to clinically overt complications including recurrent sinopulmonary infections [284], autoimmune diseases [285], allergies, atopic disorders [286], gastrointestinal disorders, and malignancies [278]. Fortunately, about 65–90% of patients with SIgAD are asymptomatic [1, 287]. Only the minority of patients suffer from severe disease. They are those who may progress to CVID at later time points [278]. Follow-up study reveals that unlike patients with partial IgA deficiency and patients with partial IgA + IgG subclass deficiency, patients with selective IgA deficiency never can achieve normal levels of IgA during study [288]. This indicates the importance of periodic monitoring in these patients.

After IgG, IgA is the second most abundant immunoglobulin in the blood circulation [281]. It is secreted into the circulation and mucosal secretions. Two subclasses of IgA are present in humans: IgA1 and IgA2. Circulating IgA which is mainly comprised of IgA1 (80–90%) may help to regulate immune response via activation of the phagocyte system and inhibition of neutrophil chemotaxis. Mucosal secretions mainly include IgA2, which is more resistant to bacterial proteases present in the respiratory and gastrointestinal tract than IgA1. Secretory IgA contributes to the coating of mucosa-associated bacteria and therefore plays an important role to prevent penetration of bacteria into the mucosa. In addition, patients with SIgAD demonstrated altered cytokine/chemokine system in terms of increased levels of CXCL10/IP-10, IL-10, and G-CSF and decreased levels of IL-9 and IL-12 (p70) [289]. In this manner, SIgAD is regarded as a risk factor of recurrent respiratory infections and bronchial hyper-responsiveness [290].

About 40–90% of patients with symptomatic SIgAD report recurrent sinopulmonary infections as the most important manifestations leading to diagnosis of SIgAD. In particular, adults with SIgAD are more prone to upper respiratory tract infections (e.g., infectious conjunctivitis, common viral cold, pharyngitis, and laryngitis) and lower respiratory tract infections (e.g., bronchitis and pneumonia) [287]. Overall, the main pathogens involved are encapsulated bacteria including *Haemophilus influenzae* and *Streptococcus pneumoniae*. Bronchiectasis and obliterative bronchiolitis represent the most severe respiratory conditions experienced by patients with SIgAD. Studies demonstrate that deficiency of any of IgG subclasses is also present in about 20% of patients with SIgAD [291], rendering them more susceptible to sinopulmonary infections and respiratory insufficiency [292]. Moreover, patients with a low percentage of switched memory B-cells have a higher incidence of pneumonia and bronchiectasis compared to patients with a high percentage of switched memory B-cells [293]. On the contrary, an increased number of IgM-producing B-cells as a compensatory mechanism are commonly found in SIgAD. Because of the functional overlap between IgA and IgM, high levels of secretory IgM may protect patients against infections and help to maintain them asymptomatic [281]. When compared to controls without SIgAD, adults with SIgAD are more likely to be diagnosed with allergic rhinoconjunctivitis, but not asthma [287].

Rarely, SIgAD has been observed concurrent with other respiratory conditions including severe asthma, chronic granulomatous disease [294–296], chronic pulmonary aspergillosis [297], tracheobronchopathia osteochondroplastica [298], pulmonary nodules, disseminated cat-scratch disease [299], pleuropulmonary blastoma [300, 301], eosinophilic pneumonia [302], cryptococcal pneumonia [303], and idiopathic pulmonary hemosiderosis [304]. Also, SIgAD can mimic Churg-Strauss syndrome and hypereosinophilic syndrome [302].

As reviewed in [278], the management of patients with SIgAD includes education and periodic monitoring (every 4–6 months), treatment of allergic and autoimmune disorders, prophylactic antibiotics (especially for patients with chronic and recurrent sinopulmonary infections), pneumococcal vaccine (especially for patients with IgG subclass deficiency), and intravenous or subcutaneous immunoglobulin replacement therapy (especially for patients with recurrent infections). Immunoglobulin products low in IgA that can be administered to those patients include lyophilized Gammagard, Gammaplex, Vigam, Iveegam, Polygam, and Nanogam with IgA <10 mg/ml. Also lobectomy can be considered in cases of bronchiectasis [305]. Monoclonal antibodies such as rituximab (anti-CD20) might be effective in treating autoimmune disorders associated with SIgAD such as autoimmune thrombocytopenia [296].

References

1. Fried AJ, Bonilla FA. Pathogenesis, diagnosis, and management of primary antibody deficiencies and infections. Clin Microbiol Rev. 2009;22(3):396–414.
2. Maarschalk-Ellerbroek LJ, Hoepelman IM, Ellerbroek PM. Immunoglobulin treatment in primary antibody deficiency. Int J Antimicrob Agents. 2011;37(5):396–404.
3. Shillitoe B, Gennery A. X-linked agammaglobulinaemia: outcomes in the modern era. Clin Immunol (Orlando, Fla). 2017;183:54–62.
4. Jolles S, Sanchez-Ramon S, Quinti I, Soler-Palacin P, Agostini C, Florkin B, et al. Screening protocols to monitor respiratory status in primary immunodeficiency disease: findings from a European survey and subclinical infection working group. Clin Exp Immunol. 2017;190(2):226–34.
5. Hendriks RW, Bredius RGM, Pike-Overzet K, Staal FJT. Biology and novel treatment options for XLA, the most common monogenetic immunodeficiency in man. Expert Opin Ther Targets. 2011;15(8):1003–21.
6. Justiz Vaillant AA, Qurie A. Immunodeficiency. StatPearls. Treasure Island: StatPearls Publishing LLC; 2018.
7. Morales-Aza B, Glennie SJ, Garcez TP, Davenport V, Johnston SL, Williams NA, et al. Impaired maintenance of naturally acquired T-cell memory to the meningococcus in patients with B-cell immunodeficiency. Blood. 2009;113(18):4206–12.
8. Smith CIE, Berglof A. X-Linked Agammaglobulinemia. In: Adam MP, Ardinger HH, Pagon RA, Wallace SE, LJH B, Stephens K, et al., editors. GeneReviews((R)). Seattle: University of Washington, Seattle; 1993. GeneReviews is a registered trademark of the University of Washington, Seattle. All rights reserved.
9. Winkelstein JA, Marino MC, Lederman HM, Jones SM, Sullivan K, Burks AW, et al. X-linked agammaglobulinemia: report on a United States registry of 201 patients. Medicine. 2006;85(4):193–202.
10. Moin M, Aghamohammadi A, Farhoudi A, Pourpak Z, Rezaei N, Movahedi M, et al. X-linked agammaglobulinemia: a survey of 33 Iranian patients. Immunol Investig. 2004;33(1):81–93.
11. Buckley RH. Pulmonary complications of primary immunodeficiencies. Paediatr Respir Rev. 2004;5:S225–S33.
12. Ishida F, Kobayashi H, Saito H, Futatani T, Miyawaki T, Kiyosawa K. The oldest case with X-linked agammaglobulinemia in Japan lacking Bruton-type tyrosine kinase protein detected by flow cytometry. [Rinsho ketsueki]. Jpn J Clin Hematol. 1998;39(1):44–7.
13. Sweinberg SK, Wodell RA, Grodofsky MP, Greene JM, Conley ME. Retrospective analysis of the incidence of pulmonary disease in hypogammaglobulinemia. J Allergy Clin Immunol. 1991;88(1):96–104.
14. Quinti I, Soresina A, Guerra A, Rondelli R, Spadaro G, Agostini C, et al. Effectiveness of immunoglobulin replacement therapy on clinical outcome in patients with primary antibody deficiencies: results from a multicenter prospective cohort study. J Clin Immunol. 2011;31(3):315–22.
15. Chen Y, Stirling RG, Paul E, Hore-Lacy F, Thompson BR, Douglass JA. Longitudinal decline in lung function in patients with primary immunoglobulin deficiencies. J Allergy Clin Immunol. 2011;127(6):1414.
16. Basile N, Danielian S, Oleastro M, Rosenzweig S, Prieto E, Rossi J, et al. Clinical and molecular analysis of 49 patients with X-linked agammaglobulinemia from a single center in Argentina. J Clin Immunol. 2009;29(1):123–9.
17. He JX, Zhao SY, Jiang ZF. Clinical features of 17 cases of X-linked agammaglobulinemia. Zhongguo dang dai er ke za zhi= Chinese Journal of Contemporary Pediatrics. 2008;10(2):139–42.
18. Plebani A, Soresina A, Rondelli R, Amato GM, Azzari C, Cardinale F, et al. Clinical, immunological, and molecular analysis in a large cohort of patients with X-linked agammaglobulinemia: an Italian multicenter study. Clin Immunol. 2002;104(3):221–30.

19. Rip J, Van Der Ploeg EK, Hendriks RW, Corneth OBJ. The role of Bruton's tyrosine kinase in immune cell signaling and systemic autoimmunity. Crit Rev Immunol. 2018;38(1):17–62.
20. Pal Singh S, Dammeijer F, Hendriks RW. Role of Bruton's tyrosine kinase in B cells and malignancies. Mol Cancer. 2018;17(1):57.
21. Bao Y, Zheng J, Han C, Jin J, Han H, Liu Y, et al. Tyrosine kinase Btk is required for NK cell activation. J Biol Chem. 2012;287:23769–78. https://doi.org/10.1074/jbc.M112.372425.
22. Ochs HD, Davis SD, Wedgwood RJ. Immunologic responses to bacteriophage ϕX 174 in immunodeficiency diseases. J Clin Invest. 1971;50(12):2559–68.
23. Hendriks RW, Yuvaraj S, Kil LP. Targeting Bruton's tyrosine kinase in B cell malignancies. Nat Rev Cancer. 2014;14(4):219–32.
24. Burger JA, Wiestner A. Targeting B cell receptor signalling in cancer: preclinical and clinical advances. Nat Rev Cancer. 2018;18(3):148–67.
25. Lee J, Rhee M, Min TK, Bang HI, Jang MA, Kang ES, et al. A novel BTK gene mutation, c.82delC (p.Arg28 Alafs(*)5), in a Korean family with X-linked agammaglobulinemia. Korean J Pediatr. 2016;59(Suppl 1):S49–s52.
26. Xu Y, Qing Q, Liu X, Chen S, Chen Z, Niu X, et al. Bruton's agammaglobulinemia in an adult male due to a novel mutation: a case report. J Thorac Dis. 2016;8(10):E1207–e12.
27. Wang S, Lu Y, Li H, Wang Z, Mo X, Chai Z, et al. A novel deletion mutation and structural abnormality in the Bruton's tyrosine kinase gene identified in a Chinese patient with X-linked agammaglobulinemia. Clin Lab. 2014;60(5):859–62.
28. Graziani S, Di Matteo G, Benini L, Di Cesare S, Chiriaco M, Chini L, et al. Identification of a Btk mutation in a dysgammaglobulinemic patient with reduced B cells: XLA diagnosis or not? Clin Immunol. 2008;128(3):322–8.
29. Aghamohammadi A, Fiorini M, Moin M, Parvaneh N, Teimourian S, Yeganeh M, et al. Clinical, immunological and molecular characteristics of 37 Iranian patients with X-linked agammaglobulinemia. Int Arch Allergy Immunol. 2006;141(4):408–14.
30. Jansen AG, Noordzij JG, Bröcker-Vriends AH, Bredius RG. Widely divergent clinical phenotype of X-linked agammaglobulinemia in two cousins. Ned Tijdschr Geneeskd. 2004;148(21):1053–6.
31. Abolhassani H, Vitali M, Lougaris V, Giliani S, Parvaneh N, Parvaneh L, et al. Cohort of Iranian patients with congenital agammaglobulinemia: mutation analysis and novel gene defects. Expert Rev Clin Immunol. 2016;12(4):479–86.
32. Lederman HM, Winkelstein JA. X-linked agammaglobulinemia: an analysis of 96 patients. Medicine. 1985;64(3):145–56.
33. Stubbs A, Bangs C, Shillitoe B, Edgar JD, Burns SO, Thomas M, et al. Bronchiectasis and deteriorating lung function in agammaglobulinaemia despite immunoglobulin replacement therapy. Clin Exp Immunol. 2018;191(2):212–9.
34. Quezada A, Norambuena X, Bravo A, Castro-Rodriguez JA. Recurrent pneumonia as warning manifestation for suspecting primary immunodeficiencies in children. J Investig Allergol Clin Immunol. 2001;11(4):295–9.
35. Usui K, Sasahara Y, Tazawa R, Hagiwara K, Tsukada S, Miyawaki T, et al. Recurrent pneumonia with mild hypogammaglobulinemia diagnosed as X-linked agammaglobulinemia in adults. Respir Res. 2001;2(3):188.
36. Schussler E, Beasley MB, Maglione PJ. Lung disease in primary antibody deficiencies. J Allergy Clin Immunol Pract. 2016;4(6):1039–52.
37. Quartier P, Debré M, De Blic J, de Sauverzac R, Sayegh N, Jabado N, et al. Early and prolonged intravenous immunoglobulin replacement therapy in childhood agammaglobulinemia: a retrospective survey of 31 patients. J Pediatr. 1999;134(5):589–96.
38. Bryan BA, Battersby A, Shillitoe BM, Barge D, Bourne H, Flood T, et al. Respiratory health and related quality of life in patients with congenital agammaglobulinemia in the northern region of the UK. J Clin Immunol. 2016;36(5):472–9.
39. Kainulainen L, Nikoskelainen J, Vuorinen T, Tevola K, Liippo K, Ruuskanen O. Viruses and bacteria in bronchial samples from patients with primary hypogammaglobulinemia. Am J Respir Crit Care Med. 1999;159(4):1199–204.

40. Nishi K, Kawai T, Kubota M, Ishiguro A, Onodera M. X-linked agammaglobulinemia complicated with pulmonary aspergillosis. Pediatr Int Off J Jpn Pediatr Soc. 2018;60(1):90–2.
41. Kawakami C, Inoue A, Takitani K, Kanegane H, Miyawaki T, Tamai H. X-linked agammaglobulinemia complicated with endobronchial tuberculosis. Acta Paediatr. 2011;100(3):466–8.
42. Dogru D, Kiper N, Ozcelik U, Yalcin E, Tezcan I. Tuberculosis in children with congenital immunodeficiency syndromes. Tuberkuloz ve toraks. 2010;58(1):59–63.
43. Alibrahim A, Lepore M, Lierl M, Filipovich A, Assa'ad A. Pneumocystis carinii pneumonia in an infant with X-linked agammaglobulinemia. J Allergy Clin Immunol. 1998;101(4):552–3.
44. Howard V, Greene JM, Pahwa S, Winkelstein JA, Boyle JM, Kocak M, et al. The health status and quality of life of adults with X-linked agammaglobulinemia. Clin Immunol. 2006;118(2–3):201–8.
45. Slade CA, Bosco JJ, Binh Giang T, Kruse E, Stirling RG, Cameron PU, et al. Delayed diagnosis and complications of predominantly antibody deficiencies in a cohort of Australian adults. Front Immunol. 2018;9:694.
46. Kainulainen L, Varpula M, Liippo K, Svedström E, Nikoskelainen J, Ruuskanen O. Pulmonary abnormalities in patients with primary hypogammaglobulinemia. J Allergy Clin Immunol. 1999;104(5):1031–6.
47. Funato M, Kaneko H, Ohkusu K, Sasai H, Kubota K, Ohnishi H, et al. Refractory chronic pleurisy caused by helicobacter equorum-like bacterium in a patient with X-linked agammaglobulinemia. J Clin Microbiol. 2011;49(9):3432–5.
48. Krupa A, Fol M, Rahman M, Stokes KY, Florence JM, Leskov IL, et al. Silencing Bruton's tyrosine kinase in alveolar neutrophils protects mice from LPS/immune complex-induced acute lung injury. Am J Physiol Lung Cell Mol Physiol. 2014;307(6):L435–48.
49. Krupa A, Fudala R, Florence JM, Tucker T, Allen TC, Standiford TJ, et al. Bruton's tyrosine kinase mediates FcgammaRIIa/toll-like receptor-4 receptor crosstalk in human neutrophils. Am J Respir Cell Mol Biol. 2013;48(2):240–9.
50. Verstak B, Nagpal K, Bottomley SP, Golenbock DT, Hertzog PJ, Mansell A. MyD88 adapter-like (Mal)/TIRAP interaction with TRAF6 is critical for TLR2- and TLR4-mediated NF-kappaB proinflammatory responses. J Biol Chem. 2009;284(36):24192–203.
51. Florence JM, Krupa A, Booshehri LM, Gajewski AL, Kurdowska AK. Disrupting the Btk pathway suppresses COPD-like lung alterations in Atherosclerosis Prone ApoE /− mice following regular exposure to cigarette smoke. Int J Mol Sci. 2018;19(2):343.
52. Florence JM, Krupa A, Booshehri LM, Davis SA, Matthay MA, Kurdowska AK. Inhibiting Bruton's tyrosine kinase rescues mice from lethal influenza-induced acute lung injury. Am J Physiol Lung Cell Mol Physiol. 2018;315(1):L52–l8.
53. Phillips JE, Renteria L, Burns L, Harris P, Peng R, Bauer CM, et al. Btk inhibitor RN983 delivered by dry powder nose-only aerosol inhalation inhibits bronchoconstriction and pulmonary inflammation in the ovalbumin allergic mouse model of asthma. J Aerosol Med Pulm Drug Deliv. 2016;29(3):233–41.
54. Zhou P, Ma B, Xu S, Zhang S, Tang H, Zhu S, et al. Knockdown of Burton's tyrosine kinase confers potent protection against sepsis-induced acute lung injury. Cell Biochem Biophys. 2014;70(2):1265–75.
55. Grommes C, Younes A. Ibrutinib in PCNSL: the curious cases of clinical responses and aspergillosis. Cancer Cell. 2017;31(6):731–3.
56. Gu Y, Huang B, Yang Y, Qi M, Lu G, Xia D, et al. Ibrutinib exacerbates bleomycin-induced pulmonary fibrosis via promoting inflammation. Inflammation. 2018;41(3):904–13.
57. Arthurs B, Wunderle K, Hsu M, Kim S. Invasive aspergillosis related to ibrutinib therapy for chronic lymphocytic leukemia. Respir Med Case Rep. 2017;21:27–9.
58. Szymczak WA, Davis MJ, Lundy SK, Dufaud C, Olszewski M, Pirofski LA. X-linked immunodeficient mice exhibit enhanced susceptibility to cryptococcus neoformans Infection. MBio. 2013;4(4):e00265–13.
59. Kondratieva TK, Rubakova EI, Linge IA, Evstifeev VV, Majorov KB, Apt AS. B cells delay neutrophil migration toward the site of stimulus: tardiness critical for effective bacillus Calmette-Guerin vaccination against tuberculosis infection in mice. J Immunol. 2010;184(3):1227–34.

60. Marron TU, Rohr K, Martinez-Gallo M, Yu J, Cunningham-Rundles C. TLR signaling and effector functions are intact in XLA neutrophils. Clin Immunol. 2010;137(1):74–80.
61. Forman HJ, Torres M. Reactive oxygen species and cell signaling: respiratory burst in macrophage signaling. Am J Respir Crit Care Med. 2002;166(Supplement_1):S4–8.
62. Lundy SK, Berlin AA, Martens TF, Lukacs NW. Deficiency of regulatory B cells increases allergic airway inflammation. Inflamm Res. 2005;54(12):514–21.
63. Shabestari MS, Rezaei N. Asthma and allergic rhinitis in a patient with BTK deficiency. J Investig Allergol Clin Immunol. 2008;18(4):300–4.
64. Liese JG, Wintergerst U, Tympner KD, Belohradsky BH. High-vs low-dose immunoglobulin therapy in the long-term treatment of X-linked agammaglobulinemia. Am J Dis Child. 1992;146(3):335–9.
65. Suri D, Bhattad S, Sharma A, Gupta A, Rawat A, Sehgal S, et al. Serial serum immunoglobulin G (IgG) trough levels in patients with X-linked agammaglobulinemia on replacement therapy with intravenous immunoglobulin: its correlation with infections in Indian children. J Clin Immunol. 2017;37(3):311–8.
66. Morales P, Hernandez D, Vicente R, Sole A, Moreno I, Torres JJ, Lanuza A. Lung transplantation in patients with x-linked agammaglobulinemia. In: Transplantation proceedings. Elsevier; 2003. Vol. 35, No. 5, pp. 1942–43.
67. Barnes S, Kotecha S, Douglass JA, Paul E, Hore-Lacy F, Stirling R, et al. Evolving practice: X-linked agammaglobulinemia and lung transplantation. Am J Transpl Off J Am Soc Transpl Am Soc Transpl Surg. 2015;15(4):1110–3.
68. Conley ME, Rohrer J, Rapalus L, Boylin EC, Minegishi Y. Defects in early B-cell development: comparing the consequences of abnormalities in pre-BCR signaling in the human and the mouse. Immunol Rev. 2000;178:75–90.
69. Mårtensson I-L, Almqvist N, Grimsholm O, Bernardi AI. The pre-B cell receptor checkpoint. FEBS Lett. 2010;584(12):2572–9.
70. Yel L, Minegishi Y, Coustan-Smith E, Buckley RH, Trübel H, Pachman LM, et al. Mutations in the mu heavy-chain gene in patients with agammaglobulinemia. N Engl J Med. 1996;335(20):1486–93.
71. Granados EL, Porpiglia AS, Hogan MB, Matamoros N, Krasovec S, Pignata C, et al. Clinical and molecular analysis of patients with defects in μ heavy chain gene. J Clin Invest. 2002;110(7):1029–35.
72. Ferrari S, Zuntini R, Lougaris V, Soresina A, Sourkova V, Fiorini M, et al. Molecular analysis of the pre-BCR complex in a large cohort of patients affected by autosomal-recessive agammaglobulinemia. Genes Immun. 2007;8(4):325–33.
73. Mohammadzadeh I, Yeganeh M, Aghamohammadi A, Parvaneh N, Behniafard N, Abolhassani H, et al. Severe primary antibody deficiency due to a novel mutation of mu heavy chain. J Investig Allergol Clin Immunol. 2012;22(1):78–9.
74. Silva P, Justicia A, Regueiro A, Farina S, Couselo JM, Loidi L. Autosomal recessive agammaglobulinemia due to defect in mu heavy chain caused by a novel mutation in the IGHM gene. Genes Immun. 2017;18(3):197–9.
75. Schuh W, Meister S, Roth E, Jack HM. Cutting edge: signaling and cell surface expression of a mu H chain in the absence of lambda 5: a paradigm revisited. J Immunol. 2003;171(7):3343–7.
76. Karasuyama H, Rolink A, Shinkal Y, Young F, Alt FW, Melchers F. The expression of Vpre-B/λ5 surrogate light chain in early bone marrow precursor B cells of normal and B cell-deficient mutant mice. Cell. 1994;77(1):133–43.
77. Minegishi Y, Coustan-Smith E, Wang YH, Cooper MD, Campana D, Conley ME. Mutations in the human lambda5/14.1 gene result in B cell deficiency and agammaglobulinemia. J Exp Med. 1998;187(1):71–7.
78. Minegishi Y, Coustan-Smith E, Wang Y-H, Cooper MD, Campana D, Conley ME. Mutations in the human λ5/14.1 gene result in B cell deficiency and agammaglobulinemia. J Exp Med. 1998;187(1):71–7.
79. Wang Y, Kanegane H, Sanal O, Tezcan I, Ersoy F, Futatani T, et al. Novel Igalpha (CD79a) gene mutation in a Turkish patient with B cell-deficient agammaglobulinemia. Am J Med Genet. 2002;108(4):333–6.

80. Ferrari S, Lougaris V, Caraffi S, Zuntini R, Yang J, Soresina A, et al. Mutations of the Igβ gene cause agammaglobulinemia in man. J Exp Med. 2007;204(9):2047–51.
81. Meffre E, Nussenzweig MC. Deletion of immunoglobulin beta in developing B cells leads to cell death. Proc Natl Acad Sci U S A. 2002;99(17):11334–9.
82. Dobbs AK, Yang T, Farmer D, Kager L, Parolini O, Conley ME. Cutting edge: a hypomorphic mutation in Igβ (CD79b) in a patient with immunodeficiency and a leaky defect in B cell development. J Immunol. 2007;179(4):2055–9.
83. Lougaris V, Vitali M, Baronio M, Moratto D, Tampella G, Biasini A, et al. Autosomal recessive agammaglobulinemia: the third case of Igbeta deficiency due to a novel non-sense mutation. J Clin Immunol. 2014;34(4):425–7.
84. Pappu R, Cheng AM, Li B, Gong Q, Chiu C, Griffin N, et al. Requirement for B cell linker protein (BLNK) in B cell development. Science. 1999;286(5446):1949–54.
85. Jin G, Hamaguchi Y, Matsushita T, Hasegawa M, Le Huu D, Ishiura N, et al. B-cell linker protein expression contributes to controlling allergic and autoimmune diseases by mediating IL-10 production in regulatory B cells. J Allergy Clin Immunol. 2013;131(6):1674–82.
86. Minegishi Y, Rohrer J, Coustan-Smith E, Lederman HM, Pappu R, Campana D, et al. An essential role for BLNK in human B cell development. Science. 1999;286(5446):1954–7.
87. Van Zelm MC, Geertsema C, Nieuwenhuis N, De Ridder D, Conley ME, Schiff C, et al. Gross deletions involving IGHM, BTK, or Artemis: a model for genomic lesions mediated by transposable elements. Am J Hum Genet. 2008;82(2):320–32.
88. Lagresle-Peyrou C, Millili M, Luce S, Boned A, Sadek H, Rouiller J, et al. The BLNK adaptor protein has a nonredundant role in human B-cell differentiation. J Allergy Clin Immunol. 2014;134(1):145–54.
89. NaserEddin A, Shamriz O, Keller B, Alzyoud RM, Unger S, Fisch P, et al. Enteroviral infection in a patient with BLNK adaptor protein deficiency. J Clin Immunol. 2015;35(4):356–60.
90. Bain G, Maandag ECR, Izon DJ, Amsen D, Kruisbeek AM, Weintraub BC, et al. E2A proteins are required for proper B cell development and initiation of immunoglobulin gene rearrangements. Cell. 1994;79(5):885–92.
91. Zhuang Y, Soriano P, Weintraub H. The helix-loop-helix gene E2A is required for B cell formation. Cell. 1994;79(5):875–84.
92. Sun X-H. Constitutive expression of the Id1 gene impairs mouse B cell development. Cell. 1994;79(5):893–900.
93. Ben-Ali M, Yang J, Chan KW, Ben-Mustapha I, Mekki N, Benabdesselem C, et al. Homozygous transcription factor 3 gene <em>(TCF3)</em> mutation is associated with severe hypogammaglobulinemia and B-cell acute lymphoblastic leukemia. J Allergy Clin Immunol. 2017;140(4):1191–4.e4.
94. Boisson B, Wang Y-D, Bosompem A, Ma CS, Lim A, Kochetkov T, et al. A recurrent dominant negative E47 mutation causes agammaglobulinemia and BCR–B cells. J Clin Invest. 2013;123(11):4781–5.
95. Dobbs AK, Bosompem A, Coustan-Smith E, Tyerman G, Saulsbury FT, Conley ME. Agammaglobulinemia associated with BCR- B cells and enhanced expression of CD19. Blood. 2011;118(7):1828–37.
96. Sawada A, Takihara Y, Kim JY, Matsuda-Hashii Y, Tokimasa S, Fujisaki H, et al. A congenital mutation of the novel gene LRRC8 causes agammaglobulinemia in humans. J Clin Invest. 2003;112(11):1707–13.
97. Tarr PE, Sneller MC, Mechanic LJ, Economides A, Eger CM, Strober W, et al. Infections in patients with immunodeficiency with thymoma (Good syndrome). Report of 5 cases and review of the literature. Medicine. 2001;80(2):123–33.
98. Miyakis S, Pefanis A, Passam FH, Christodulakis GR, Roussou PA, Mountokalakis TD. Thymoma with immunodeficiency (Good's syndrome): review of the literature apropos three cases. Scand J Infect Dis. 2006;38(4):314–20.
99. Miyakis S, Pefanis A, Passam FH, Christodulakis GR, Roussou PA, Mountokalakis TD. Thymoma with immunodeficiency (Good's syndrome): review of the literature apropos three cases. Scand J Infect Dis. 2006;38(4):314–9.

100. Masci AM, Palmieri G, Vitiello L, Montella L, Perna F, Orlandi P, et al. Clonal expansion of CD8+ BV8 T lymphocytes in bone marrow characterizes thymoma-associated B lymphopenia. Blood. 2003;101(8):3106–8.
101. Leibovitz I, Zamir D, Polychuck I, Reitblat T, Gheorghiu D. Recurrent pneumonia post-thymectomy as a manifestation of Good syndrome. Eur J Intern Med. 2003;14(1):60–2.
102. Ohuchi M, Inoue S, Hanaoka J, Igarashi T, Tezuka N, Ozaki Y, et al. Good syndrome coexisting with leukopenia. Ann Thorac Surg. 2007;84(6):2095–7.
103. Ho JK, Wong MM, Tai TK, Tse DM. A rare combination of recurrent pneumonia, diarrhoea, and visual loss in a patient after thymectomy: good syndrome. Hong Kong medical journal = Xianggang yi xue za zhi. 2010;16(6):493–6.
104. Pena C, Intriago M, Munoz P, Gray AM, Cabrera ME. Association of Good syndrome with pure red cell aplasia: report of one case. Revista medica de Chile. 2012;140(8):1050–2.
105. Qu J, Lu X, Gao Q, Zhang Y. Good syndrome, a rare cause of refractory chronic diarrhea and recurrent pneumonia in a Chinese patient after thymectomy. Clin Vaccine Immunol CVI. 2013;20(7):1097–8.
106. Jeandel C, Gastin I, Blain H, Jouanny P, Laurain MC, Penin F, et al. Thymoma with immunodeficiency (Good's syndrome) associated with selective cobalamin malabsorption and benign IgM-kappa gammopathy. J Intern Med. 1994;235(2):179–82.
107. Di Renzo M, Pasqui AL, Voltolini L, Gotti G, Pompella G, Auteri A. Myelodysplasia and Good syndrome. A case report. Clin Exp Med. 2008;8(3):171–3.
108. Jorge LP, Pereira CE, Jorge E. Cytomegalovirus retinitis in good syndrome. Revista Brasileira de Oftalmologia. 2018;77(3):153–5.
109. Numakura T, Matsuura Y, Takiguchi H, Hara Y, Ameku K. A Good syndrome associated with pure red cell aplasia. Nihon Kokyuki Gakkai zasshi = J Jpn Respir Soc. 2011;49(9):647–50.
110. Arnold SJ, Hodgson T, Misbah SA, Patel SY, Cooper SM, Venning VA. Three difficult cases: the challenge of autoimmunity, immunodeficiency and recurrent infections in patients with Good syndrome. Br J Dermatol. 2015;172(3):774–7.
111. Jansen A, van Deuren M, Miller J, Litzman J, de Gracia J, Saenz-Cuesta M, et al. Prognosis of Good syndrome: mortality and morbidity of thymoma associated immunodeficiency in perspective. Clin Immunol (Orlando, Fla). 2016;171:12–7.
112. Takai S, Tagawa A, Ogawa T, Kato H, Saito N, Okada S. Thymoma with immunodeficiency/good syndrome associated with myasthenia gravis. Rinsho shinkeigaku = Clin Neurol. 2017;57(5):208–13.
113. Chen X, Zhang JX, Shang WW, Xie WP, Jin SX, Wang F. Aberrant peripheral immune function in a good syndrome patient. J Immunol Res. 2018;2018:6212410.
114. Aouadi S, Ghrairi N, Braham E, Kaabi M, Maalej S, Elgharbi LD. Acquired hypogammaglobulinemia associated with thymoma: Good syndrome. Pan Afr Med J. 2017;28:253.
115. Makinson A, Corne P, Pelle C, Ben Hadj Salem M, Pouessel D, Landreau L, et al. Good syndrome and cytomegalovirus pneumonia. La Revue de medecine interne. 2003;24(5):330–1.
116. Jian L, Bin D, Haiyun W. Fatal pneumocystis pneumonia with good syndrome and pure red cell aplasia. Clin Infect Dis Off Publ Infect Dis Soc Am. 2004;39(11):1740–1.
117. Katsuki Y, Suzuki S, Takahashi Y, Satoh T, Nogawa S, Tanaka K, et al. A case of good syndrome accompanied by myasthenia gravis: immunological evaluations. Nihon Rinsho Men'eki Gakkai kaishi = Jpn J Clin Immunol. 2006;29(2):102–6.
118. Fernandez-Villar A, Garcia-Tejedor JL, Leiro Fernandez V, Botana Rial M, Mendez Garrido A, Rivo Vazquez E, et al. Tracheobronchial wall thickening secondary to herpesvirus infection in a patient with Goods syndrome. An Med Interna (Madrid, Spain : 1984). 2008;25(5):234–6.
119. Inomata T, Honda M, Murakami A. Atypical VZV retinitis in a patient with Good syndrome. Ocul Immunol Inflamm. 2018;26(2):194–8.
120. Fukushima A, Ichimura Y, Obata S, Kinoshita-Ise M, Fujio Y, Takeno M, et al. Thymoma-associated multi-organ autoimmunity: a case of graft-versus-host disease-like erythro-

derma complicated by good syndrome successfully treated by thymectomy. J Dermatol. 2017;44(7):830–5.
121. Thongngarm T, Boonyasiri A, Pradubpongsa P, Tesavibul N, Anekpuritanang T, Kreetapirom P, Sompornrattanaphan M. Features and outcomes of immunoglobulin therapy in patients with good syndrome at Thailand's largest tertiary referral hospital. Asian Pac J Allergy Immunol. 2018 Jun 1.
122. Chijimatsu Y, Nakazato Y, Homma H, Mizuguchi K. A case report of Good syndrome complicated by diffuse panbronchiolitis. Nihon Kyobu Shikkan Gakkai Zasshi. 1982;20(7):803–8.
123. Tsuburai T, Ikehara K, Suzuki S, Shinohara T, Mishima W, Tagawa A, et al. Hypogammaglobulinemia associated with thymoma (Good syndrome) similar to diffuse panbronchiolitis. Nihon Kokyuki Gakkai zasshi = J Jpn Respir Soc. 2003;41(6):421–5.
124. Ogoshi T, Ishimoto H, Yatera K, Oda K, Akata K, Yamasaki K, et al. A case of good syndrome with pulmonary lesions similar to diffuse panbronchiolitis. Intern Med (Tokyo, Japan). 2012;51(9):1087–91.
125. Lee SH, Lee SM, Yang SC, Yoo CG, Kim YW, Shim YS, et al. A case of granulomatous lung disease in a patient with Good's syndrome. Korean J Intern Med. 2008;23(4):219–22.
126. Maccari ME, Abolhassani H, Aghamohammadi A, Aiuti A, Aleinikova O, Bangs C, Baris S, Barzaghi F, Baxendale H, Buckland M, Burns SO. Disease evolution and response to rapamycin in activated phosphoinositide 3-kinase δ syndrome: the European Society for Immunodeficiencies-activated phosphoinositide 3-kinase δ syndrome registry. Front Immunol. 2018;9:543.
127. Angulo I, Vadas O, Garcon F, Banham-Hall E, Plagnol V, Leahy TR, et al. Phosphoinositide 3-kinase delta gene mutation predisposes to respiratory infection and airway damage. Science. 2013;342(6160):866–71.
128. Elkaim E, Neven B, Bruneau J, Mitsui-Sekinaka K, Stanislas A, Heurtier L, et al. Clinical and immunologic phenotype associated with activated phosphoinositide 3-kinase delta syndrome 2: a cohort study. J Allergy Clin Immunol. 2016;138(1):210–8.e9.
129. Stokes CA, Condliffe AM. Phosphoinositide 3-kinase delta (PI3Kdelta) in respiratory disease. Biochem Soc Trans. 2018;46(2):361–9.
130. Southworth T, Mason S, Bell A, Ramis I, Calbet M, Domenech A, et al. PI3K, p38 and JAK/STAT signalling in bronchial tissue from patients with asthma following allergen challenge. Biomark Res. 2018;6(14):018–0128.
131. Marwick JA, Adcock IM, Chung KF. Overcoming reduced glucocorticoid sensitivity in airway disease: molecular mechanisms and therapeutic approaches. Drugs. 2010;70(8):929–48.
132. Marwick JA, Caramori G, Casolari P, Mazzoni F, Kirkham PA, Adcock IM, et al. A role for phosphoinositol 3-kinase delta in the impairment of glucocorticoid responsiveness in patients with chronic obstructive pulmonary disease. J Allergy Clin Immunol. 2010;125(5):1146–53.
133. Xia M, Xu H, Dai W, Zhu C, Wu L, Yan S, et al. The role of HDAC2 in cigarette smoke-induced airway inflammation in a murine model of asthma and the effect of intervention with roxithromycin. J Asthma. 2018;55(4):337–44.
134. Kim SR, Lee KS, Park HS, Park SJ, Min KH, Moon H, et al. HIF-1alpha inhibition ameliorates an allergic airway disease via VEGF suppression in bronchial epithelium. Eur J Immunol. 2010;40(10):2858–69.
135. Lee KS, Jeong JS, Kim SR, Cho SH, Kolliputi N, Ko YH, et al. Phosphoinositide 3-kinase-delta regulates fungus-induced allergic lung inflammation through endoplasmic reticulum stress. Thorax. 2016;71(1):52–63.
136. Jeong JS, Lee KB, Kim SR, Kim DI, Park HJ, Lee HK, et al. Airway epithelial phosphoinositide 3-kinase-delta contributes to the modulation of fungi-induced innate immune response. Thorax. 2018;73(8):758–68.
137. Kan-o K, Matsumoto K, Asai-Tajiri Y, Fukuyama S, Hamano S, Seki N, et al. PI3K-delta mediates double-stranded RNA-induced upregulation of B7-H1 in BEAS-2B airway epithelial cells. Biochem Biophys Res Commun. 2013;435(2):195–201.

138. Dinavahi SS, Nyayapathy S, Perumal Y, Dharmarajan S, Viswanadha S. Combined inhibition of PDE4 and PI3Kdelta modulates the inflammatory component involved in the progression of chronic obstructive pulmonary disease. Drug Res. 2014;64(4):214–9.
139. Doukas J, Eide L, Stebbins K, Racanelli-Layton A, Dellamary L, Martin M, et al. Aerosolized phosphoinositide 3-kinase gamma/delta inhibitor TG100-115 [3-[2,4-diamino-6-(3-hydroxyphenyl)pteridin-7-yl]phenol] as a therapeutic candidate for asthma and chronic obstructive pulmonary disease. J Pharmacol Exp Ther. 2009;328(3):758–65.
140. Sun XJ, Li ZH, Zhang Y, Zhou G, Zhang JQ, Deng JM, et al. Combination of erythromycin and dexamethasone improves corticosteroid sensitivity induced by CSE through inhibiting PI3K-delta/Akt pathway and increasing GR expression. Am J Physiol Lung Cell Mol Physiol. 2015;309(2):8.
141. Lee KS, Park SJ, Kim SR, Min KH, Jin SM, Puri KD, et al. Phosphoinositide 3-kinase-delta inhibitor reduces vascular permeability in a murine model of asthma. J Allergy Clin Immunol. 2006;118(2):403–9.
142. To Y, Ito K, Kizawa Y, Failla M, Ito M, Kusama T, et al. Targeting phosphoinositide-3-kinase-delta with theophylline reverses corticosteroid insensitivity in chronic obstructive pulmonary disease. Am J Respir Crit Care Med. 2010;182(7):897–904.
143. Kracker S, Di Virgilio M, Schwartzentruber J, Cuenin C, Forveille M, Deau MC, et al. An inherited immunoglobulin class-switch recombination deficiency associated with a defect in the INO80 chromatin remodeling complex. J Allergy Clin Immunol. 2015;135(4):998–1007. e6.
144. Wiestner A. The role of B-cell receptor inhibitors in the treatment of patients with chronic lymphocytic leukemia. Haematologica. 2015;100(12):1495–507.
145. Hammadi SA, Almarzooqi S, Abdul-Kader HM, Saraswathiamma D, Souid AK. The PI3Kdelta inhibitor idelalisib suppresses liver and lung cellular respiration. Int J Physiol Pathophysiol Pharmacol. 2015;7(3):115–25.
146. Azizi G, Abolhassani H, Mahdaviani SA, Chavoshzadeh Z, Eshghi P, Yazdani R, et al. Clinical, immunologic, molecular analyses and outcomes of iranian patients with LRBA deficiency: a longitudinal study. Pediatr Allergy Immunol. 2017;28(5):478–84.
147. Shamriz O, Shadur B, NaserEddin A, Zaidman I, Simanovsky N, Elpeleg O, et al. Respiratory manifestations in LPS-responsive beige-like anchor (LRBA) protein-deficient patients. Eur J Pediatr. 2018;177(8):1163–72.
148. Al Sukaiti N, AbdelRahman K, AlShekaili J, Al Oraimi S, Al Sinani A, Al Rahbi N, Cho V, Field M, Cook MC. Agammaglobulinaemia despite terminal B-cell differentiation in a patient with a novel LRBA mutation. Clin Transl Immunology. 2017;6(5):e144.
149. Shokri S, Nabavi M, Hirschmugl T, Aghamohammadi A, Arshi S, Bemanian MH, et al. LPS-responsive beige-like anchor gene mutation associated with possible bronchiolitis obliterans organizing pneumonia associated with hypogammaglobulinemia and normal IgM phenotype and low number of B cells. Acta Med Iran. 2016;54(10):620–3.
150. Alkhairy OK, Abolhassani H, Rezaei N, Fang M, Andersen KK, Chavoshzadeh Z, et al. Spectrum of phenotypes associated with mutations in LRBA. J Clin Immunol. 2016;36(1):33–45.
151. Schreiner F, Plamper M, Dueker G, Schoenberger S, Gamez-Diaz L, Grimbacher B, et al. Infancy-onset T1DM, short stature, and severe immunodysregulation in two siblings with a homozygous LRBA mutation. J Clin Endocrinol Metab. 2016;101(3):898–904.
152. Liu Y, Yang J, Wu Q, Han R, Yan W, Yuan J, Ji X, Li Y, Yao W, Ni C. LRBA gene polymorphisms and risk of coal workers' pneumoconiosis: a case–control study from China. Int J Environ Res Public Health. 2017;14(10):1138.
153. Tedder TF, Inaoki M, Sato S. The CD19–CD21 complex regulates signal transduction thresholds governing humoral immunity and autoimmunity. Immunity. 1997;6(2):107–18.
154. Skendros P, Rondeau S, Chateil JF, Bui S, Bocly V, Moreau JF, et al. Misdiagnosed CD19 deficiency leads to severe lung disease. Pediatr Allergy Immunol Off Publ Eur Soc Pediatr Allergy Immunol. 2014;25(6):603–6.

155. van Zelm MC, Reisli I, van der Burg M, Castaño D, van Noesel CJM, van Tol MJD, et al. An antibody-deficiency syndrome due to mutations in the CD19 gene. N Engl J Med. 2006;354(18):1901–12.
156. Kanegane H, Agematsu K, Futatani T, Sira MM, Suga K, Sekiguchi T, et al. Novel mutations in a Japanese patient with CD19 deficiency. Genes Immun. 2007;8(8):663.
157. Artac H, Reisli I, Kara R, Pico-Knijnenburg I, Adin-Cinar S, Pekcan S, et al. B-cell maturation and antibody responses in individuals carrying a mutated CD19 allele. Genes Immun. 2010;11(7):523.
158. Vince N, Boutboul D, Mouillot G, Just N, Peralta M, Casanova J-L, et al. Defects in the CD19 complex predispose to glomerulonephritis, as well as IgG1 subclass deficiency. J Allergy Clin Immunol. 2011;127(2):538.
159. van Zelm MC, Smet J, van der Burg M, Ferster A, Le PQ, Schandené L, et al. Antibody deficiency due to a missense mutation in CD19 demonstrates the importance of the conserved tryptophan 41 in immunoglobulin superfamily domain formation. Hum Mol Genet. 2011;20(9):1854–63.
160. van Zelm MC, Smet J, van der Burg M, Ferster A, Le PQ, Schandene L, et al. Antibody deficiency due to a missense mutation in CD19 demonstrates the importance of the conserved tryptophan 41 in immunoglobulin superfamily domain formation. Hum Mol Genet. 2011;20(9):1854–63.
161. Kelic S, Levy S, Suarez C, Weinstein DE. CD81 regulates neuron-induced astrocyte cell-cycle exit. Mol Cell Neurosci. 2001;17(3):551–60.
162. Geisert EE Jr, Williams RW, Geisert GR, Fan L, Asbury AM, Maecker HT, et al. Increased brain size and glial cell number in CD81-null mice. J Comp Neurol. 2002;453(1):22–32.
163. Rubinstein E, Ziyyat A, Prenant M, Wrobel E, Wolf JP, Levy S, et al. Reduced fertility of female mice lacking CD81. Dev Biol. 2006;290(2):351–8.
164. Song BK, Levy S, Geisert EE Jr. Increased density of retinal pigment epithelium in cd81−/− mice. J Cell Biochem. 2004;92(6):1160–70.
165. van Zelm MC, Smet J, Adams B, Mascart F, Schandené L, Janssen F, et al. CD81 gene defect in humans disrupts CD19 complex formation and leads to antibody deficiency. J Clin Invest. 2010;120(4):1265–74.
166. Takeda Y, He P, Tachibana I, Zhou B, Miyado K, Kaneko H, et al. Double deficiency of tetraspanins CD9 and CD81 alters cell motility and protease production of macrophages and causes chronic obstructive pulmonary disease-like phenotype in mice. J Biol Chem. 2008;283(38):26089–97.
167. Churg A, Zhou S, Wright JL. Matrix metalloproteinases in COPD. Eur Respir J. 2012;39(1):197.
168. Deng J, Yeung VP, Tsitoura D, DeKruyff RH, Umetsu DT, Levy S. Allergen-induced airway hyperreactivity is diminished in CD81-deficient mice. J Immunol. 2000;165(9):5054–61.
169. Roberts ML, Luxembourg AT, Cooper NR. Epstein-Barr virus binding to CD21, the virus receptor, activates resting B cells via an intracellular pathway that is linked to B cell infection. J Gen Virol. 1996;77(Pt 12):3077–85.
170. Del Nagro CJ, Kolla RV, Rickert RC. A critical role for complement C3d and the B cell coreceptor (CD19/CD21) complex in the initiation of inflammatory arthritis. J Immunol. 2005;175(8):5379–89.
171. Thiel J, Kimmig L, Salzer U, Grudzien M, Lebrecht D, Hagena T, et al. Genetic CD21 deficiency is associated with hypogammaglobulinemia. J Allergy Clin Immunol. 2012;129(3):801–10.e6.
172. Wentink MW, Lambeck AJ, van Zelm MC, Simons E, van Dongen JJ, IJspeert H, et al. CD21 and CD19 deficiency: two defects in the same complex leading to different disease modalities. Clin Immunol (Orlando, Fla). 2015;161(2):120–7.
173. Rosain J, Miot C, Lambert N, Rousselet MC, Pellier I, Picard C. CD21 deficiency in 2 siblings with recurrent respiratory infections and hypogammaglobulinemia. J Allergy Clin Immunol Pract. 2017;5(6):1765–7.

174. Farrington M, Grosmaire LS, Nonoyama S, Fischer SH, Hollenbaugh D, Ledbetter JA, et al. CD40 ligand expression is defective in a subset of patients with common variable immunodeficiency. Proc Natl Acad Sci. 1994;91(3):1099–103.
175. Sneller MC. Common variable immunodeficiency. Am J Med Sci. 2001;321(1):42–8.
176. Grimbacher B, Hutloff A, Schlesier M, Glocker E, Warnatz K, Dräger R, et al. Homozygous loss of ICOS is associated with adult-onset common variable immunodeficiency. Nat Immunol. 2003;4(3):261.
177. Salzer U, Maul-Pavicic A, Cunningham-Rundles C, Urschel S, Belohradsky BH, Litzman J, et al. ICOS deficiency in patients with common variable immunodeficiency. Clin Immunol. 2004;113(3):234–40.
178. Castigli E, Wilson SA, Garibyan L, Rachid R, Bonilla F, Schneider L, et al. TACI is mutant in common variable immunodeficiency and IgA deficiency. Nat Genet. 2005;37(8):829.
179. Salzer U, Chapel HM, Webster ADB, Pan-Hammarström Q, Schmitt-Graeff A, Schlesier M, et al. Mutations in TNFRSF13B encoding TACI are associated with common variable immunodeficiency in humans. Nat Genet. 2005;37(8):820.
180. Gathmann B, Mahlaoui N, Gérard L, Oksenhendler E, Warnatz K, Schulze I, et al. Clinical picture and treatment of 2212 patients with common variable immunodeficiency. J Allergy Clin Immunol. 2014;134(1):116–26.
181. Oksenhendler E, Gérard L, Fieschi C, Malphettes M, Mouillot G, Jaussaud R, et al. Infections in 252 patients with common variable immunodeficiency. Clin Infect Dis. 2008;46(10):1547–54.
182. Garcia MAM, De Rojas MDHF, Manzur MDN, Pamplona MPM, Torrero LC, Macian V, et al. Respiratory disorders in common variable immunodeficiency. Respir Med. 2001;95(3):191–5.
183. Cunningham-Rundles C. Clinical and immunologic analyses of 103 patients with common variable immunodeficiency. J Clin Immunol. 1989;9(1):22–33.
184. Cunningham-Rundles C. Common variable immunodeficiency. Curr Allergy Asthma Rep. 2001;1(5):421–9.
185. Bates CA, Ellison MC, Lynch DA, Cool CD, Brown KK, Routes JM. Granulomatous-lymphocytic lung disease shortens survival in common variable immunodeficiency. J Allergy Clin Immunol. 2004;114(2):415–21.
186. Quinti I, Soresina A, Spadaro G, Martino S, Donnanno S, Agostini C, et al. Long-term follow-up and outcome of a large cohort of patients with common variable immunodeficiency. J Clin Immunol. 2007;27(3):308–16.
187. Thickett KM, Kumararatne DS, Banerjee AK, Dudley R, Stableforth DE. Common variable immune deficiency: respiratory manifestations, pulmonary function and high-resolution CT scan findings. QJM. 2002;95(10):655–62.
188. Maglione PJ, Overbey JR, Radigan L, Bagiella E, Cunningham-Rundles C. Pulmonary radiologic findings in common variable immunodeficiency: clinical and immunological correlations. Ann Allergy Asthma Immunol. 2014;113(4):452–9.
189. Park JH, Levinson AI. Granulomatous-lymphocytic interstitial lung disease (GLILD) in common variable immunodeficiency (CVID). Clin Immunol. 2010;134(2):97–103.
190. Levinson AI, Hopewell PC, Stites DP, Spitler LE, Fudenberg HH. Coexistent lymphoid interstitial pneumonia, pernicious anemia, and agammaglobulinemia: comment on autoimmune pathogenesis. Arch Intern Med. 1976;136(2):213–6.
191. Kohler PF, Cook RD, Brown WR, Manguso RL. Common variable hypogammaglobulinemia with T-cell nodular lymphoid interstitial pneumonitis and B-cell nodular lymphoid hyperplasia: different lymphocyte populations with a similar response to prednisone therapy. J Allergy Clin Immunol. 1982;70(4):299–305.
192. Dukes RJ, Rosenow EC, Hermans PE. Pulmonary manifestations of hypogammaglobulinaemia. Thorax. 1978;33(5):603–7.
193. Wheat WH, Cool CD, Morimoto Y, Rai PR, Kirkpatrick CH, Lindenbaum BA, et al. Possible role of human herpesvirus 8 in the lymphoproliferative disorders in common variable immunodeficiency. J Exp Med. 2005;202(4):479–84.

194. Jolles S, Carne E, Brouns M, El-Shanawany T, Williams P, Marshall C, et al. FDG PET-CT imaging of therapeutic response in granulomatous lymphocytic interstitial lung disease (GLILD) in common variable immunodeficiency (CVID). Clin Exp Immunol. 2017;187(1):138–45.
195. Lucas M, Lee M, Lortan J, Lopez-Granados E, Misbah S, Chapel H. Infection outcomes in patients with common variable immunodeficiency disorders: relationship to immunoglobulin therapy over 22 years. J Allergy Clin Immunol. 2010;125(6):1354–60.
196. de Gracia J, Vendrell M, Álvarez A, Pallisa E, Rodrigo M-J, de la Rosa D, et al. Immunoglobulin therapy to control lung damage in patients with common variable immunodeficiency. Int Immunopharmacol. 2004;4(6):745–53.
197. Busse PJ, Razvi S, Cunningham-Rundles C. Efficacy of intravenous immunoglobulin in the prevention of pneumonia in patients with common variable immunodeficiency. J Allergy Clin Immunol. 2002;109(6):1001–4.
198. Kuijpers TW, Bende RJ, Baars PA, Grummels A, Derks IAM, Dolman KM, et al. CD20 deficiency in humans results in impaired T cell–independent antibody responses. J Clin Invest. 2010;120(1):214–22.
199. Morsy DED, Sanyal R, Zaiss AK, Deo R, Muruve DA, Deans JP. Reduced T-dependent humoral immunity in CD20-deficient mice. J Immunol. 2013;191:3112–8. https://doi.org/10.4049/jimmunol.1202098.
200. Breitling S, Hui Z, Zabini D, Hu Y, Hoffmann J, Goldenberg NM, et al. The mast cell-B cell axis in lung vascular remodeling and pulmonary hypertension. Am J Physiol Lung Cell Mol Physiol. 2017;312(5):L710–L21.
201. Alvarez B, Arcos J, Fernandez-Guerrero ML. Pulmonary infectious diseases in patients with primary immunodeficiency and those treated with biologic immunomodulating agents. Curr Opin Pulm Med. 2011;17(3):172–9.
202. Elsegeiny W, Eddens T, Chen K, Kolls JK. Anti-CD20 antibody therapy and susceptibility to pneumocystis pneumonia. Infect Immun. 2015;83(5):2043–52.
203. Sato M, Ito S, Ogura M, Kamei K, Miyairi I, Miyata I, et al. Atypical pneumocystis jiroveci pneumonia with multiple nodular granulomas after rituximab for refractory nephrotic syndrome. Pediatr Nephrol. 2013;28(1):145–9.
204. Cherin P, de Jaeger C, Crave JC, Delain JC, Tadmouri A, Amoura Z. Subcutaneous immunoglobulins for the treatment of a patient with antisynthetase syndrome and secondary chronic immunodeficiency after anti-CD20 treatment: a case report. J Med Case Rep. 2017;11(1):017–1211.
205. Dogan M, Erol M, Cesur Y, Yuca SA, Doğan Ş. The effect of 25-hydroxyvitamin D3 on the immune system. J Pediatr Endocrinol Metab. 2009;22(10):929–36.
206. Bogaert DJ, Dullaers M, Lambrecht BN, Vermaelen KY, De Baere E, Haerynck F. Genes associated with common variable immunodeficiency: one diagnosis to rule them all? J Med Genet. 2016;53(9):575–90.
207. Teichmann LL, Cullen JL, Kashgarian M, Dong C, Craft J, Shlomchik MJ. Local triggering of the ICOS coreceptor by CD11c(+) myeloid cells drives organ inflammation in lupus. Immunity. 2015;42(3):552–65.
208. Li Z, Lu H, Gu J, Liu J, Zhu Q, Lu Y, et al. Chitinase 3-Like-1-deficient splenocytes deteriorated the pathogenesis of acute graft-versus-host disease via regulating differentiation of Tfh cells. Inflammation. 2017;40(5):1576–88.
209. Gao X, Zhao L, Wang S, Yang J, Yang X. Enhanced inducible costimulator ligand (ICOS-L) expression on dendritic cells in interleukin-10 deficiency and its impact on T-cell subsets in respiratory tract infection. Mol Med. 2013;19:346–56.
210. Afzali B, Lombardi G, Lechler RI, Lord GM. The role of T helper 17 (Th17) and regulatory T cells (Treg) in human organ transplantation and autoimmune disease. Clin Exp Immunol. 2007;148(1):32–46.
211. Tanaka C, Fujimoto M, Hamaguchi Y, Sato S, Takehara K, Hasegawa M. Inducible costimulator ligand regulates bleomycin-induced lung and skin fibrosis in a mouse model indepen-

dently of the inducible costimulator/inducible costimulator ligand pathway. Arthritis Rheum. 2010;62(6):1723–32.
212. Ma CS, Wong N, Rao G, Avery DT, Torpy J, Hambridge T, et al. Monogenic mutations differentially affect the quantity and quality of T follicular helper cells in patients with human primary immunodeficiencies. J Allergy Clin Immunol. 2015;136(4):993–1006.e1.
213. Shalaby KH, Jo T, Nakada E, Allard-Coutu A, Tsuchiya K, Hirota N, et al. ICOS-expressing CD4 T cells induced via TLR4 in the nasal mucosa are capable of inhibiting experimental allergic asthma. J Immunol (Baltimore, Md : 1950). 2012;189(6):2793–804.
214. Shalaby KH, Al Heialy S, Tsuchiya K, Farahnak S, McGovern TK, Risse PA, et al. The TLR4-TRIF pathway can protect against the development of experimental allergic asthma. Immunology. 2017;152(1):138–49.
215. Berron-Ruiz L, Lopez-Herrera G, Vargas-Hernandez A, Mogica-Martinez D, Garcia-Latorre E, Blancas-Galicia L, et al. Lymphocytes and B-cell abnormalities in patients with common variable immunodeficiency (CVID). Allergol Immunopathol. 2014;42(1):35–43.
216. Tamachi T, Watanabe N, Oya Y, Kagami S, Hirose K, Saito Y, et al. B and T lymphocyte attenuator inhibits antigen-induced eosinophil recruitment into the airways. Int Arch Allergy Immunol. 2007;143(Suppl 1):50–5.
217. Shilling RA, Clay BS, Tesciuba AG, Berry EL, Lu T, Moore TV, et al. CD28 and ICOS play complementary non-overlapping roles in the development of Th2 immunity in vivo. Cell Immunol. 2009;259(2):177–84.
218. Wolf AI, Mozdzanowska K, Quinn WJ 3rd, Metzgar M, Williams KL, Caton AJ, et al. Protective antiviral antibody responses in a mouse model of influenza virus infection require TACI. J Clin Invest. 2011;121(10):3954–64.
219. Jabara HH, Lee JJ, Janssen E, Ullas S, Liadaki K, Garibyan L, et al. Heterozygosity for transmembrane activator and calcium modulator ligand interactor A144E causes haploinsufficiency and pneumococcal susceptibility in mice. J Allergy Clin Immunol. 2017;139(4):1293–301.e4.
220. Speletas M, Mamara A, Papadopoulou-Alataki E, Iordanakis G, Liadaki K, Bardaka F, et al. TNFRSF13B/TACI alterations in Greek patients with antibody deficiencies. J Clin Immunol. 2011;31(4):550–9.
221. Ameratunga R, Koopmans W, Woon ST, Leung E, Lehnert K, Slade CA, et al. Epistatic interactions between mutations of TACI (TNFRSF13B) and TCF3 result in a severe primary immunodeficiency disorder and systemic lupus erythematosus. Clin Transl Immunol. 2017;6(10):e159.
222. Speletas M, Salzer U, Florou Z, Petinaki E, Daniil Z, Bardaka F, et al. Heterozygous alterations of TNFRSF13B/TACI in tonsillar hypertrophy and sarcoidosis. Clin Dev Immunol. 2013;2013:532437.
223. Barroeta Seijas AB, Graziani S, Cancrini C, Finocchi A, Ferrari S, Miniero R, et al. The impact of TACI mutations: from hypogammaglobulinemia in infancy to autoimmunity in adulthood. Int J Immunopathol Pharmacol. 2012;25(2):407–14.
224. Chen K, Coonrod EM, Kumanovics A, Franks ZF, Durtschi JD, Margraf RL, et al. Germline mutations in NFKB2 implicate the noncanonical NF-kappaB pathway in the pathogenesis of common variable immunodeficiency. Am J Hum Genet. 2013;93(5):812–24.
225. Lee CE, Fulcher DA, Whittle B, Chand R, Fewings N, Field M, et al. Autosomal-dominant B-cell deficiency with alopecia due to a mutation in NFKB2 that results in nonprocessable p100. Blood. 2014;124(19):2964–72.
226. Lindsley AW, Qian Y, Valencia CA, Shah K, Zhang K, Assa'ad A. Combined immune deficiency in a patient with a novel NFKB2 mutation. J Clin Immunol. 2014;34(8):910–5.
227. Brue T, Quentien MH, Khetchoumian K, Bensa M, Capo-Chichi JM, Delemer B, et al. Mutations in NFKB2 and potential genetic heterogeneity in patients with DAVID syndrome, having variable endocrine and immune deficiencies. BMC Med Genet. 2014;15:139.
228. Lougaris V, Tabellini G, Vitali M, Baronio M, Patrizi O, Tampella G, et al. Defective natural killer-cell cytotoxic activity in NFKB2-mutated CVID-like disease. J Allergy Clin Immunol. 2015;135(6):1641–3.

229. Liu Y, Hanson S, Gurugama P, Jones A, Clark B, Ibrahim MA. Novel NFKB2 mutation in early-onset CVID. J Clin Immunol. 2014;34(6):686–90.
230. Shi C, Wang F, Tong A, Zhang X-Q, Song H-M, Liu Z-Y, et al. NFKB2 mutation in common variable immunodeficiency and isolated adrenocorticotropic hormone deficiency: a case report and review of literature. Medicine. 2016;95(40):e5081.
231. Shi C, Wang F, Tong A, Zhang XQ, Song HM, Liu ZY, et al. NFKB2 mutation in common variable immunodeficiency and isolated adrenocorticotropic hormone deficiency: a case report and review of literature. Medicine. 2016;95(40):e5081.
232. Yang L, Cui H, Wang Z, Zhang B, Ding J, Liu L, et al. Loss of negative feedback control of nuclear factor-kappaB2 activity in lymphocytes leads to fatal lung inflammation. Am J Pathol. 2010;176(6):2646–57.
233. Low JT, Hughes P, Lin A, Siebenlist U, Jain R, Yaprianto K, et al. Impact of loss of NF-kappaB1, NF-kappaB2 or c-REL on SLE-like autoimmune disease and lymphadenopathy in Fas(lpr/lpr) mutant mice. Immunol Cell Biol. 2016;94(1):66–78.
234. Xu W, Santini PA, Matthews AJ, Chiu A, Plebani A, He B, et al. Viral double-stranded RNA triggers Ig class switching by activating upper respiratory mucosa B cells through an innate TLR3 pathway involving BAFF. J Immunol. 2008;181(1):276–87.
235. Lohmeyer J, Morty RE, Herold S. Antibiotic therapy-induced collateral damage: IgA takes center stage in pulmonary host defense. J Clin Invest. 2018;128(8):3234–6.
236. Chen K, Xu W, Wilson M, He B, Miller NW, Bengten E, et al. Immunoglobulin D enhances immune surveillance by activating antimicrobial, proinflammatory and B cell-stimulating programs in basophils. Nat Immunol. 2009;10(8):889–98.
237. Sutherland AP, Ng LG, Fletcher CA, Shum B, Newton RA, Grey ST, et al. BAFF augments certain Th1-associated inflammatory responses. J Immunol. 2005;174(9):5537–44.
238. Francois A, Gombault A, Villeret B, Alsaleh G, Fanny M, Gasse P, et al. B cell activating factor is central to bleomycin- and IL-17-mediated experimental pulmonary fibrosis. J Autoimmun. 2015;56:1–11.
239. Matsushita T, Kobayashi T, Mizumaki K, Kano M, Sawada T, Tennichi M, et al. BAFF inhibition attenuates fibrosis in scleroderma by modulating the regulatory and effector B cell balance. Sci Adv. 2018;4(7):eaas9944.
240. Whitsett TG, Cheng E, Inge L, Asrani K, Jameson NM, Hostetter G, et al. Elevated expression of Fn14 in non-small cell lung cancer correlates with activated EGFR and promotes tumor cell migration and invasion. Am J Pathol. 2012;181(1):111–20.
241. Xu Z, Pone EJ, Al-Qahtani A, Park SR, Zan H, Casali P. Regulation of aicda expression and AID activity: relevance to somatic hypermutation and class switch DNA recombination. Crit Rev Immunol. 2007;27(4):367–97.
242. Bhutani N, Brady JJ, Damian M, Sacco A, Corbel SY, Blau HM. Reprogramming towards pluripotency requires AID-dependent DNA demethylation. Nature. 2010;463(7284):1042–7.
243. Aghamohammadi A, Parvaneh N, Rezaei N, Moazzami K, Kashef S, Abolhassani H, et al. Clinical and laboratory findings in hyper-IgM syndrome with novel CD40L and AICDA mutations. J Clin Immunol. 2009;29(6):769–76.
244. Mahdaviani SA, Hirbod-Mobarakeh A, Wang N, Aghamohammadi A, Hammarstrom L, Masjedi MR, et al. Novel mutation of the activation-induced cytidine deaminase gene in a Tajik family: special review on hyper-immunoglobulin M syndrome. Expert Rev Clin Immunol. 2012;8(6):539–46.
245. Askenase PW, Bryniarski K, Paliwal V, Redegeld F, Groot Kormelink T, Kerfoot S, et al. A subset of AID-dependent B-1a cells initiates hypersensitivity and pneumococcal pneumonia resistance. Ann N Y Acad Sci. 2015;1362:200–14.
246. Yamamoto N, Kerfoot SM, Hutchinson AT, Dela Cruz CS, Nakazawa N, Szczepanik M, et al. Expression of activation-induced cytidine deaminase enhances the clearance of pneumococcal pneumonia: evidence of a subpopulation of protective anti-pneumococcal B1a cells. Immunology. 2016;147(1):97–113.
247. Weeks LD, Fu P, Gerson SL. Uracil-DNA glycosylase expression determines human lung cancer cell sensitivity to pemetrexed. Mol Cancer Ther. 2013;12(10):2248–60.

248. Minkah N, Macaluso M, Oldenburg DG, Paden CR, White DW, McBride KM, et al. Absence of the uracil DNA glycosylase of murine gammaherpesvirus 68 impairs replication and delays the establishment of latency in vivo. J Virol. 2015;89(6):3366–79.
249. Poulogiannis G, Frayling IM, Arends MJ. DNA mismatch repair deficiency in sporadic colorectal cancer and lynch syndrome. Histopathology. 2010;56(2):167–79.
250. Haraldsdottir S, Roth R, Pearlman R, Hampel H, Arnold CA, Frankel WL. Mismatch repair deficiency concordance between primary colorectal cancer and corresponding metastasis. Familial Cancer. 2016;15(2):253–60.
251. Giampieri R, Maccaroni E, Mandolesi A, Del Prete M, Andrikou K, Faloppi L, et al. Mismatch repair deficiency may affect clinical outcome through immune response activation in metastatic gastric cancer patients receiving first-line chemotherapy. Gastric Cancer Off J Int Gastric Cancer Assoc Jpn Gastric Cancer Assoc. 2017;20(1):156–63.
252. Spetsotaki KN, Tsiambas E, Stamatelopoulos A, Fotiades PP, Kastanioudakis I, Tomos P, et al. DNA mismatch repair deficiency in lung and oral cavity carcinomas: the role of histogenetic origin. J BUON Off J Balkan Union Oncol. 2017;22(3):606–9.
253. Bouffet E, Larouche V, Campbell BB, Merico D, de Borja R, Aronson M, et al. Immune checkpoint inhibition for hypermutant glioblastoma multiforme resulting from germline biallelic mismatch repair deficiency. J Clin Oncol Off J Am Soc Clin Oncol. 2016;34(19):2206–11.
254. Wu X, Tsai CY, Patam MB, Zan H, Chen JP, Lipkin SM, et al. A role for the MutL mismatch repair Mlh3 protein in immunoglobulin class switch DNA recombination and somatic hypermutation. J Immunol (Baltimore, Md : 1950). 2006;176(9):5426–37.
255. Downey CM, Jirik FR. DNA mismatch repair deficiency accelerates lung neoplasm development in K-ras(LA1/+) mice: a brief report. Cancer Med. 2015;4(6):897–902.
256. Takamochi K, Takahashi F, Suehara Y, Sato E, Kohsaka S, Hayashi T, et al. DNA mismatch repair deficiency in surgically resected lung adenocarcinoma: microsatellite instability analysis using the Promega panel. Lung Cancer (Amsterdam, Netherlands). 2017;110:26–31.
257. Chung C, Christianson M. Predictive and prognostic biomarkers with therapeutic targets in breast, colorectal, and non-small cell lung cancers: a systemic review of current development, evidence, and recommendation. J Oncol Pharm Pract Off Publ Int Soc Oncol Pharm Pract. 2014;20(1):11–28.
258. Warth A, Korner S, Penzel R, Muley T, Dienemann H, Schirmacher P, et al. Microsatellite instability in pulmonary adenocarcinomas: a comprehensive study of 480 cases. Virchows Archiv Int J Pathol. 2016;468(3):313–9.
259. Moyano AJ, Feliziani S, Di Rienzo JA, Smania AM. Simple sequence repeats together with mismatch repair deficiency can bias mutagenic pathways in Pseudomonas aeruginosa during chronic lung infection. PLoS One. 2013;8(11):e80514.
260. Conaway RC, Conaway JW. The INO80 chromatin remodeling complex in transcription, replication and repair. Trends Biochem Sci. 2009;34(2):71–7.
261. Yao W, King DA, Beckwith SL, Gowans GJ, Yen K, Zhou C, et al. The INO80 complex requires the Arp5-Ies6 subcomplex for chromatin remodeling and metabolic regulation. Mol Cell Biol. 2016;36(6):979–91.
262. Dembowski JA, DeLuca NA. Selective recruitment of nuclear factors to productively replicating herpes simplex virus genomes. PLoS Pathog. 2015;11(5):e1004939.
263. Zhang S, Zhou B, Wang L, Li P, Bennett BD, Snyder R, et al. INO80 is required for oncogenic transcription and tumor growth in non-small cell lung cancer. Oncogene. 2017;36(10):1430–9.
264. Leung AW, Hung SS, Backstrom I, Ricaurte D, Kwok B, Poon S, et al. Combined use of gene expression modeling and siRNA screening identifies genes and pathways which enhance the activity of cisplatin when added at no effect levels to non-small cell lung Cancer cells in vitro. PLoS One. 2016;11(3):e0150675.
265. Stiehm RE. The four most common pediatric immunodeficiencies. Adv Exp Med Biol. 2007;601:15–26.
266. Karaca NE, Aksu G, Gulez N, Yildiz B, Azarsiz E, Kutukculer N. New laboratory findings in Turkish patients with transient hypogammaglobulinemia of infancy. Iran J Allergy Asthma Immunol. 2010;9(4):237–43.

267. Habahbeh ZM, Abu-Shukair ME, Almutereen MA, Alzyoud RM, Wahadneh AM. Primary antibody deficiencies at queen Rania children Hospital in Jordan: single center experience. Iran J Immunol. 2014;11(1):49–58.
268. Keles S, Artac H, Kara R, Gokturk B, Ozen A, Reisli I. Transient hypogammaglobulinemia and unclassified hypogammaglobulinemia: 'similarities and differences'. Pediatr Allergy Immunol. 2010;21(5):843–51.
269. Kilic SS, Tezcan I, Sanal O, Metin A, Ersoy F. Transient hypogammaglobulinemia of infancy: clinical and immunologic features of 40 new cases. Pediatr Int. 2000;42(6):647–50.
270. Cano F, Mayo DR, Ballow M. Absent specific viral antibodies in patients with transient hypogammaglobulinemia of infancy. J Allergy Clin Immunol. 1990;85(2):510–3.
271. Janssen WJ, Nierkens S, Sanders EA, Boes M, van Montfrans JM. Antigen-specific IgA titres after 23-valent pneumococcal vaccine indicate transient antibody deficiency disease in children. Vaccine. 2015;33(46):6320–6.
272. Kidon MI, Handzel ZT, Schwartz R, Altboum I, Stein M, Zan-Bar I. Symptomatic hypogammaglobulinemia in infancy and childhood – clinical outcome and in vitro immune responses. BMC Fam Pract. 2004;5(23):1471–2296.
273. Cotugno N, Manno EC, Stoppa F, Sinibaldi S, Saffirio C, D'Argenio P, et al. Severe parainfluenza pneumonia in a case of transient hypogammalobulinemia of infancy. BMJ Case Rep. 2013. pii: bcr2013009959.
274. Smart JM, Kemp AS, Armstrong DS. Pneumocystis carinii pneumonia in an infant with transient hypogammaglobulinaemia of infancy. Arch Dis Child. 2002;87(5):449–50.
275. Walzer PD, Schultz MG, Western KA, Robbins JB. Pneumocystis carinii pneumonia and primary immune deficiency diseases of infancy and childhood. J Pediatr. 1973;82(3):416–22.
276. Burke EC, Brown AL Jr, Weed LA. Pneumocystis carinii pneumonia: report of case in infant with hypogammaglo-bulinemia. Proc Staff Meet Mayo Clin. 1962;37:129–36.
277. Kramer RI, Cirone VC, Moore H. Interstitial pneumonia due to pneumocystis carinii, cytomegalic inclusion disease and hypogammaglobulinemia occurring simultaneously in an infant. Pediatrics. 1962;29:816–27.
278. Yazdani R, Azizi G, Abolhassani H, Aghamohammadi A. Selective IgA deficiency: epidemiology, pathogenesis, clinical phenotype, diagnosis, prognosis and management. Scand J Immunol. 2017;85(1):3–12.
279. Aldirmaz S, Yucel E, Kiykim A, Cokugras H, Akcakaya N, Camcioglu Y. Profile of the patients who present to immunology outpatient clinics because of frequent infections. Turk pediatri arsivi. 2014;49(3):210–6.
280. Lozano NA, Lozano A, Sasia LV, Saranz RJ, Agresta MF, del Pilar Bovina Martijena M, et al. Clinical comparison between patients with selective immunoglobulin A deficiency and other primary immunodeficiencies. Arch Argent Pediatr. 2015;113(2):141–5.
281. Yel L. Selective IgA deficiency. J Clin Immunol. 2010;30(1):10–6.
282. Karaca NE, Severcan EU, Guven B, Azarsiz E, Aksu G, Kutukculer N. TNFRSF13B/TACI alterations in Turkish patients with common variable immunodeficiency and IgA deficiency. Avicenna J Med Biotechnol. 2018;10(3):192–5.
283. Santos-Valente E, Reisli I, Artac H, Ott R, Sanal O, Boztug K. A novel mutation in the complement component 3 gene in a patient with selective IgA deficiency. J Clin Immunol. 2013;33(1):127–33.
284. Justiz Vaillant AAQA. Immunodeficiency. [Updated 2018 May 2]. In: StatPearls [Internet]. Treasure Island: StatPearls Publishing; 2018.
285. Singh K, Chang C, Gershwin ME. IgA deficiency and autoimmunity. Autoimmun Rev. 2014;13(2):163–77.
286. Azizi G, Bagheri Y, Tavakol M, Askarimoghaddam F, Porrostami K, Rafiemanesh H, et al. The clinical and immunological features of patients with primary antibody deficiencies. Endocr Metab Immune Disord Drug Targets. 2018;18(5):537–45.
287. Jorgensen GH, Gardulf A, Sigurdsson MI, Sigurdardottir ST, Thorsteinsdottir I, Gudmundsson S, et al. Clinical symptoms in adults with selective IgA deficiency: a case-control study. J Clin Immunol. 2013;33(4):742–7.

288. Kutukculer N, Karaca NE, Demircioglu O, Aksu G. Increases in serum immunoglobulins to age-related normal levels in children with IgA and/or IgG subclass deficiency. Pediatr Allergy Immunol Off Publ Eur Soc Pediatr Allergy Immunol. 2007;18(2):167–73.
289. Hel Z, Huijbregts RP, Xu J, Nechvatalova J, Vlkova M, Litzman J. Altered serum cytokine signature in common variable immunodeficiency. J Clin Immunol. 2014;34(8):971–8.
290. Papadopoulou A, Mermiri D, Taousani S, Triga M, Nicolaidou P, Priftis KN. Bronchial hyper-responsiveness in selective IgA deficiency. Pediatr Allergy Immunol Off Publ Eur Soc Pediatr Allergy Immunol. 2005;16(6):495–500.
291. Santaella ML, Peredo R, Disdier OM. IgA deficiency: clinical correlates with IgG subclass and mannan-binding lectin deficiencies. Puerto Rico Health Sci J. 2005;24(2):107–10.
292. Aghamohammadi A, Mohammadi J, Parvaneh N, Rezaei N, Moin M, Espanol T, et al. Progression of selective IgA deficiency to common variable immunodeficiency. Int Arch Allergy Immunol. 2008;147(2):87–92.
293. Aghamohammadi A, Abolhassani H, Biglari M, Abolmaali S, Moazzami K, Tabatabaeiyan M, et al. Analysis of switched memory B cells in patients with IgA deficiency. Int Arch Allergy Immunol. 2011;156(4):462–8.
294. Jindal AK, Rawat A, Suri D, Sharma M, Shandilya JK, Goel S, et al. Severe aspergillus pneumonia and pulmonary artery hypertension in a child with autosomal recessive chronic granulomatous disease and selective IgA deficiency. J Clin Immunol. 2017;37(4):333–5.
295. Patiroglu T, Gungor HE, Lazaroski S, Unal E. Chronic granulomatous disease with markedly elevated IgE levels mimicking hyperimmunoglobulin E syndrome. Acta Microbiol Immunol Hung. 2013;60(2):155–62.
296. Shamsian BS, Mansouri D, Pourpak Z, Rezaei N, Chavoshzadeh Z, Jadali F, et al. Autosomal recessive chronic granulomatous disease, IgA deficiency and refractory autoimmune thrombocytopenia responding to anti-CD20 monoclonal antibody. Iran J Allergy Asthma Immunol. 2008;7(3):181–4.
297. Ragesh R, Ray A, Mian A, Vyas S, Sharma SK. Cavitary lung lesions in a difficult-to-treat asthma patient. J Assoc Physicians India. 2016;64(4):73–6.
298. Dincer HE, Dunitz JM. Tracheobronchopathia osteochondroplastica and selective IgA deficiency. J Bronchol Interv Pulmonol. 2012;19(1):54–6.
299. Rohr A, Ash R, Vadaparampil J, Hill J, Wetzel L. Disseminated cat-scratch disease in an adult with selective IgA deficiency. Radiol Case Rep. 2016;11(2):54–7.
300. Stewart DR, Givens SS, Harris AK, Williams GM, Messinger YH, Schultz KA, et al. Comment on: DICER1-negative pleuropulmonary blastoma in a patient with selective IgA deficiency. Pediatr Blood Cancer. 2016;63(10):1869–70.
301. Chen Y, Jin M, Zhao W, Li S, Wang X, Cai S, et al. DICER1-negative pleuropulmonary blastoma in a patient with selective IgA deficiency. Pediatr Blood Cancer. 2016;63(4):757–8.
302. Takahashi N, Kondo T, Fukuta M, Takemoto A, Takami Y, Sato M, et al. Selective IgA deficiency mimicking Churg-Strauss syndrome and hypereosinophilic syndrome: a case report. Nagoya J Med Sci. 2013;75(1–2):139–46.
303. Hage JE, Wu J, Cunha BA. Cryptococcal pneumonia in a patient with presumptive sarcoidosis and selective immunoglobulin a deficiency. Heart Lung J Crit Care. 2012;41(4):398–400.
304. Erkocoglu M, Civelek E, Kocabas CN. Unusual presentation: concurrent IgA deficiency and idiopathic pulmonary hemosiderosis. Pediatr Pulmonol. 2016;51(10):E34–e6.
305. Dominguez O, Giner MT, Alsina L, Martin MA, Lozano J, Plaza AM. Clinical phenotypes associated with selective IgA deficiency: a review of 330 cases and a proposed follow-up protocol. An Pediatr (Barcelona, Spain: 2003). 2012;76(5):261–7.

Chapter 4
Pulmonary Manifestations of Congenital Defects of Phagocytes

Seyed Amir Mohajerani, Marzieh Tavakol, and Seyed Alireza Mahdaviani

4.1 Introduction

The phagocytic system is an indispensable part of the immune defense mechanism and one of the main components of the innate immune system. Congenital immune defects of phagocytic system could be due to reduced neutrophil numbers or function. Clinically, congenital defects of phagocytes can lead to various specific symptoms such as delayed separation of the umbilical cord, recurrent cutaneous abscesses, periodontitis, liver and lung abscesses, and mucocutaneous aphthous ulcers.

Lung manifestations are one of the unique features of specific congenital defects of phagocytes which will be discussed in this chapter in detail. Infections are significantly the most common complications, but the host reaction to infection often leads to characteristic findings that can be helpful diagnostically.

The prognosis of many congenital defects of phagocytes has been improved dramatically during the last decade. Many patients will survive into their adulthood by applying prophylactic regimen, early diagnosis, and aggressive treatment of infectious and noninfectious complications. Pulmonary involvement in patients

S. A. Mohajerani
Tracheal Diseases Research Center (TDRC) National Research Institute of Tuberculosis and Lung Diseases (NRITLD), Shahid Beheshti University of Medical Sciences, Tehran, Iran

M. Tavakol
Non-communicable Diseases Research Center, Alborz University of Medical Sciences, Karaj, Iran

Department of Allergy and Clinical Immunology, Emam Ali Hospital, Alborz University of Medical Sciences, Karaj, Iran

S. A. Mahdaviani (✉)
Pediatric Respiratory Diseases Research Center, National Research Institute of Tuberculosis and Lung Diseases (NRITLD), Shahid Beheshti University of Medical Sciences, Tehran, Iran

S. A. Mahdaviani, N. Rezaei (eds.), *Pulmonary Manifestations of Primary Immunodeficiency Diseases*, https://doi.org/10.1007/978-3-030-00880-2_4

with chronic granulomatous disease (CGD) is the most important cause of death; it may not necessarily be the initial manifestation, but it grows in severity over time. Longer survival of the patients with congenital defects of phagocytes has indisputably led us to identify cumulative effects of repetitive pulmonary infectious and noninfectious inflammatory disorders. Pulmonary manifestations could be either ambiguous or misleading, particularly if not enough attention and clinical impression are made. In other words, since one of the most common sites of involvement in these defects is the lung, pulmonologists (pediatrics or adult) may be among the first to recognize the pattern of pulmonary manifestation leading to a diagnosis of phagocytic defects.

In this chapter, we will discuss the pulmonary complications of these congenital defects of phagocytes with respect to clinical observations and their management.

(For further information, you may see Wintergerst U, Kuijpers TW, Rosenzweig SD, Holland SM, Abinun M, Malech HL, Rezaei N. Phagocytes defects. In: Rezaei N, Aghamohammadi A, Notarangelo LD, editors. *Primary immunodeficiency diseases: definition, diagnosis, and management*. 2nd ed. p. 245–294).

4.2 Chronic Granulomatous Disease (CGD)

Chronic granulomatous disease (CGD) is an inherited disorder, characterized by defects in superoxide-generating NADPH oxidase of phagocytes. The genetic defects in CGD induce activation failure of the respiratory burst in the phagocytes, that leads to severe recurrent infections and unexplained prolonged inflammatory reactions which produce granulomatous lesions.

4.2.1 Genetics

CGD has five different mutations in genes involved in assembly and activation of the NADPH oxidase [1]. Two-thirds of patients have mutations in gp91phox (CYBB gene, cytochrome b [−245], β subunit, OMIM*300481), on the X chromosome. Other mutations are inherited as autosomal recessive (AR) involving p22phox (CYBA, cytochrome b [−245], β subunit, OMIM*608508), p47phox (NCF1, OMIM*608512), p67phox (NCF2, OMIM*608515), or p40phox (NCF4, neutrophil cytosolic factor 4, p40phox, OMIM*601448). Clinical manifestations are variable in range and severity associated with variation in different involved genes [2]. X-linked forms are more prevalent in the whole world, whereas AR forms are more prevalent in the countries with a high rate of consanguinity [3]. Clinical manifestations could be tremendously diverse in CGD patients even with similar mutations. Overall, X-linked mutations could have more morbidity and less life expectancy among CGD patients [4].

4.2.2 Pulmonary Manifestation

The most common involved organ in CGD is the lung, which manifests with infectious and noninfectious (inflammatory and autoimmune) complications (Box 4.1).

The most frequent pulmonary manifestations are infectious complications, comprising 80% of pulmonary involvements [5]. Infectious involvements are characterized by pneumonia in 40–60% and less frequently abscess in 3–6% of patients [6]. Severe pneumonia in these patients could induce atelectasia, abscess, or extensive reticulonodular infiltration with increased chance of respiratory failure or death [7]. In addition, mediastinal or hilar adenopathy, pulmonary fibrosis, honeycomb lung, pulmonary artery hypertension, and pleural thickening are among complications which may be related to pulmonary infections with prolonged course.

Pulmonary infectious involvement in CGD patients is often caused by uncommon organisms; therefore, a microbiologic smear and culture analysis in all case is necessary before antibiotic therapy [8]. The most common detected causative agent of pneumonia in CGD patients is *Aspergillus*, followed by *Staphylococcus* species, *Burkholderia cepacia*, *Nocardia*, and *Serratia* species [9]. In sporadic cases, causative agents included *Candida*, *Serratia marcescens*, *Burkholderia cepacia*, *Cephalosporium*, and *Staphylococcus epidermidis* [10]. In other words, consensus is made on *Aspergillus* as the most common causative agent in pneumonia, but there is a discrepancy in following commonly detected pathogens responsible for pneumonia between different regions and studies, which may be related to geographical and population variations or diagnostic approaches [9]. CGD is the only phagocytic disorder that is associated with *Aspergillus* infection in the absence of preexisting

Box 4.1 Pulmonary Manifestations of Chronic Granulomatous Disease

- *Infectious manifestations:*
  - Pneumonia
  - Abscesses
  - Pleural effusion
  - Bronchiectasis
  - Bronchitis
  - Atelectasia
  - Respiratory failure
  - Mediastinal or hilar adenopathy
  - Lung tuberculosis
- *Noninfectious manifestations:*
  - Granuloma formations
  - Pneumonitis
  - Extensive fibrosis

lung damage [11]. *Aspergillus* infections have an indolent course unlike bacterial infections [12], and this explains why CGD patients rarely experience pulmonary cavitation or hemoptysis because of *Aspergillus* infection. Contiguous spread of *Aspergillus* infection from the lungs to the vicinity organs such as the pleura or chest wall could occur in CGD patients and lead to osteomyelitis of the ribs or vertebral bodies [13]. Among gram-negative bacteria, *Burkholderia cepacia complex* organisms are commonly found in pneumonia [14]. Interestingly, *Burkholderia* is exclusively detected in pulmonary infection of CGD and cystic fibrosis (CF) patients, which probably indicates a pathophysiologic link between these two diseases [15]. The rarity of *Burkholderia cepacia* isolation in EU papers may not reflect the actual role of this gram-negative organism in pneumonia among CGD patients; hence, more studies are needed to clarify the role of environmental differences.

Uncommon pathogens of pulmonary infection in CGD patients are *Actinomyces* species [16] and a fungus named *Neosartorya udagawae* [17]. *Mycobacterial* workup should be performed in CGD patients [18] that could lead to severe pulmonary (not miliary) tuberculosis [19]. Interestingly, CGD patients are vulnerable to mycobacteria of the tuberculosis complex, such as BCG or *M. tuberculosis*, but not other mycobacteria.

CGD patients experience inflammatory complications, and some might have autoimmune problems [20], which are mainly due to deregulated inflammatory process in CGD in response to a trigger and might be due to either increased proinflammatory or decreased anti-inflammatory mediators [21].

Noncaseating granuloma formations in multiple organs, including the brain, lungs, liver, and spleen, are typically one of the main manifestations of this dysregulation. The granulomas in the lung can manifest themselves as obstructive symptoms in pulmonary branches. Granulomas in CGD are often found to be sterile, possibly underline that granuloma formation does not require the continued presence of microorganism [22].

The pathogenesis of abnormal inflammatory response and granuloma formation is still obscure. Inflammation can occur without infection, possibly due to increase in proinflammatory mediators. In some cases, recurrent infections have been shown to induce chronic inflammatory responses [23]. Although the role of infectious pathogens is not proven in granuloma formation, however, despite negative laboratory tests, it is difficult to exclude the infectious causes [1].

Fungi, alive or dead, could also induce severe inflammatory response in the lungs of CGD patients. Fungi antigens from aerosolized decayed organics, such as mulch, hay, or dead leaves, may induce mulch pneumonitis [21]. Mulch pneumonitis presentation is related to pulmonary hypersensitivity, including fever, dyspnea, and hypoxia; diffuse interstitial infiltrates in CXR and lung biopsy show acute inflammation with necrotizing granulomata and fungi [24].

Pulmonary manifestations in some CGD patients are hypoxia and functional limitation induced by granulomas and extensive fibrosis [25]. The pathogenesis of diffuse pulmonary inflammation is difficult to prove by lab tests. However, empirical treatment with corticosteroids or methotrexate could be helpful. Polymorphism in innate immune system, like mannose-binding lectin and Fc gamma receptors [26], creates autoimmune involvement in CGD patients [27]. Finally, autoimmune lung involvement processes are in association with sarcoidosis, rheumatic diseases, and lupus-like syndrome [23].

4.2.3 Radiologic Findings of Pulmonary Manifestations

Radiologic findings are the mainstay of diagnosis of pulmonary manifestations as the most common findings in CGD. The most common findings in chest radiography include consolidation, reticulonodular opacities, and scarring. And the most common findings in computed tomography (CT) are consolidation, ground-glass opacity, tree-in-bud pattern, centrilobular or random nodules, bronchiectasis, septal thickening, air trapping, or scarring. Infectious complications of the lung could present as focal consolidation or miliary pattern. Lung infections in CGD patients typically have prolonged course and are often complicated by granulomatous formation, persistent hilar or mediastinal lymphadenopathy, pulmonary fibrosis, and honeycomb lung. In addition, pneumonia may be complicated by abscess formation or empyema. Radiographic detection may be delayed if pulmonary infections involve previously scarred areas. Chest wall invasion is not always apparent on routine chest radiograph shadowed by underlying lung parenchymal disease. Technetium-labeled bone scans and CT or MRI can be used to diagnose this complication. Chest CT could reveal osseous erosion with periosteal or endosteal reaction. MRI may demonstrate abnormal bone marrow signal intensity of periosteum, cortical destruction, or surrounding soft tissue.

4.2.4 Treatment

4.2.4.1 Treatment of Infectious Complications

Long-term antibiotics and antifungals are the mainstay of treatment in CGD patients [28]. Bone marrow transplant is the curative treatment for these patients [29]. Acute infections should be treated by early and aggressive antimicrobial agent therapies. All pulmonary infections should be aggressively treated because of the spread risk into the chest wall and osteomyelitis involving the ribs or vertebral bodies which needs surgical resections if it happens [30].

Oral prophylaxis with cotrimoxazole and itraconazole reduces the rate of infection in patients with CGD [31]. CGD patients should be advised to avoid sources of *Aspergillus* spores. Broader-spectrum antimicrobial agents may be needed if *Nocardia* and *Aspergillus* are isolated. If culture results are not available, empiric antibiotic therapy has to cover the most likely involved infectious agents. Antibiotics should be aimed to cover a broad range of bacteria including *S. aureus*, *Burkholderia*,

S. marcescens, and *Nocardia*. Oral ciprofloxacin and intravenous meropenem are mostly first-line agents. If fungal pneumonia is suspected, voriconazole should be started as first choice to cover *Aspergillus*. In CGD, infections often respond slowly, and intravenous treatment must be followed by prolonged oral therapy [32]. Selected CGD patients may benefit from interferon gamma prophylaxis [33].

4.2.4.2 Treatment of Inflammatory Complications

Immunosuppressive therapy by corticosteroids is required for acute granulomatous exacerbation. TNF-α inhibitors (infliximab) are effective anti-inflammatory agents but could increase the risk of severe and fatal infections. CGD patients with invasive lung aspergillosis and nocardiosis should be started by steroids [34]. Patients with "mulch pneumonitis" syndrome may benefit from antifungals and steroids [1].

4.3 Myeloperoxidase Deficiency

Myeloperoxidase deficiency in humans (MPO deficiency) is a rare genetic disease induced by mutations in DNA for MPO in germ-line cells [35]. Secondary form of MPO deficiency has been described in lead poisoning (due to inhibition of heme synthesis), severe infections (due to consumption), neuronal lipofuscinosis, diabetes mellitus, patients treated with cytotoxic drugs and malignant disorders like acute and chronic myeloid leukemia, myelodysplastic syndrome (MDS), and Hodgkin's lymphoma [36].

MPO deficiency is analyzed by using an automated flow analysis of white blood cells. MPO deficiency could be mild, partial (prevalence of 9%), subtotal (prevalence of 0.2%), or total (prevalence of 1 in 2000–4000). However, association of MPO deficiency state with specific pathologies has not been determined yet [35].

Majority of MPO-deficient individuals (>95%) are asymptomatic despite killing defects in neutrophils. However, symptomatic patients could periodically suffer from recurrent *Candida* infections, severe osteomyelitis, meningitis, and sepsis [36].

Invasive fungal infections (IFIs) occur in less than 5% of MPO-deficient patients. Invasive *Candida* (IC) presents as candidemia, disseminated infection, pneumonia, osteomyelitis, meningitis, or liver abscess; however, antifungal prophylaxis is not indicated [37].

Malignant tumors have also been reported in patients with congenital MPO deficiency; however, no solid association has been reported between malignancies and MPO deficiency [35]. Unfortunately, there is no specific treatment for MPO deficiency. In symptomatic patients, long-term antifungal prophylaxis with fluconazole or itraconazole may be beneficial. In diabetic patients, tight control of blood glucose should be achieved [36].

Maintenance or prophylactic antibiotic therapy is not recommended, since most of the MPO-deficient patients are not involved with infections. However, caution is required in patients affected by diabetes mellitus, who suffer from a high tendency to localized and systemic infections, and concomitant complete MPO deficiency. In such cases, aggressive prolonged maintenance antibiotic therapy is crucial to control infections with resistant microorganisms or species of fungi [38].

4.4 Neutrophil-Specific Granule Deficiency

Neutrophil-specific granule deficiency (SGD) is a rare autosomal recessive primary immunodeficiency characterized by either profound reduction or absence of neutrophil-specific granules and bilobed neutrophil nuclei (pseudo-Pelger-Huet anomaly). SGD patients have increased susceptibility to bacterial infections, especially skin, ear, lung, and lymph node infections. The responsible gene for SGD is the CCAAT/enhancer binding protein-ε (C/EBPε) and is a member of the C/EBP transcription factor family that regulates proliferation, differentiation, and apoptosis in various cells. C/EBPε is an essential gene for terminal differentiation of granulocytes [39].

In the blood smear, abnormal segmentations of the granulocytes are pathognomonic. Chemotaxis is significantly reduced, and specific granules are absent from electron microscope images of granulocytes. Definitive diagnosis is made by mutational analysis of the C/EBPε gene [36]. Different clinical symptoms of SGD are not clearly explained due to rarity of this genetic defect [39].

4.4.1 Pulmonary Manifestation

Although these patients mainly suffer from mucocutaneous ulcerative and necrotic lesions, pulmonary manifestation by recurrent pneumonias and lung abscess mostly due to *Staphylococcus aureus* and/or *Pseudomonas aeruginosa* has also been reported [39]. Pus formation is also defective, and patients have ulcerative and necrotic lesions of the skin and mucous membranes as in leukocyte adhesion deficiency (LAD) [36].

4.4.2 Management

Long-term antibiotic prophylaxis is usually necessary in the course of their life span. Antibiotics in acute infections should cover *Staphylococcus aureus*, *Pseudomonas aeruginosa*, and *Klebsiella* spp. [36].

4.5 Leukocyte Adhesion Deficiency I (INTG2 or CD18 Deficiency), Leukocyte Adhesion Deficiency II (SCL35C1 or CDG-IIc Deficiency), and Leukocyte Adhesion Deficiency III (FERMT3 or Kindlin3 Deficiency)

4.5.1 Background

Leukocyte adhesion deficiency (LAD) is an immunodeficiency disease with an estimated frequency of less than 1 case per 106 populations. Three genetic forms of LAD have been described so far. These genetic forms include leukocyte adhesion deficiency I (INTG2 or CD18 deficiency), leukocyte adhesion deficiency II (SCL35C1 or CDG-IIc deficiency), and leukocyte adhesion deficiency III (FERMT3 or kindlin3 deficiency) [40].

4.5.2 Etiology

LAD type 1 (LAD-1) is the most common form of LAD caused by a defect in common chain of the beta 2 integrin family (ITGB2 or CD18). LAD type 2 (LAD-2) is a congenital disorder of glycosylation type IIc caused by mutations in member C1 (SLC35C1) gene from the solute carrier family, which encodes GDP-fucose transporter 1 (FUCT1). This induces absence of fucosylated carbohydrate ligands resulting in defective rolling and impaired transport of fucose via the GDP-fucose transporter into the Golgi apparatus [41].

The third type of LAD (LAD-3) results from failure of cytokine activation of a number of integrins with an abnormality of Rap1 function involved in regulation of integrin signaling [42].

4.5.3 Pulmonary Manifestations

The lung is not the first target in LAD, and involvement of superficial tissues including skin and mucus membranes is a predominant clinical feature in LAD patients [44].

Among upper respiratory tract infections, otitis media frequency is unprecedentedly high (about 16.7%) in LAD patients; however, LAD is rarely accompanied by pneumonia [44]. Pulmonary manifestations of LAD mainly include pneumonia induced by both typical and atypical bacteria.

LAD is characterized by skin ulcers, poor wound healing, and recurrent bacterial infections. It is described in patients with delayed umbilical cord separation and omphalitis, recurrent bacterial infections, periodontitis, defective neutrophil mobility, absence of pus formation, and impaired wound healing. Without appropriate therapy, more than 75% of the patients die before their second birthday [45].

The causative agents are frequently *Staphylococcus aureus* or gram-negative bacilli. In acutely injured lungs, massively recruited polymorphonuclear neutrophils (PMNs) secrete abnormally neutrophil elastase which increases lung injury.

Various types of LAD have variability in severity of manifestation. Infections in patients with LAD-2 are less severe than LAD-1. While there is no delay in the separation of the umbilical cord in LAD-2, skin, lung, or periodontal infections are generally not life-threatening. A hallmark of LAD-2 is severe delay in psychomotor development, microcephaly and cortical atrophy, and short stature [46]. The clinical presentation of LAD-3 is similar to LAD-1, with severe recurrent bacterial infections, delayed separation of the umbilical cord, and bleeding of the skin and mucous membranes [47].

4.5.4 Diagnosis

LAD-1 should be suspected in patients with combination of early bacterial infections, particularly omphalitis, with absent pus formation and marked peripheral blood neutrophilia (up to 50,000–100,000/μl in the presence of infection or in the range of 15,000/μl in the absence of infection). Confirmation of the diagnosis is achieved with flow cytometry analysis of the common beta chain and the alpha subunits using monoclonal antibodies against CD18 and CD11. Severe phenotype is associated with an expression of CD18 of less than 1–2% compared to normal controls, while patients with some surface expression of CD18 (>2–30% of normal) may have a milder to moderate clinical course. However, only 25% of patients with even the "milder" phenotype survive beyond 40 years [40].

These patients with milder phenotype often suffer from large nonhealing infected ulcers of the groin and lower extremities that respond poorly to antibiotics and eventually becoming colonized and infected with unusual organisms that are resistant to most antibiotics.

A diagnosis of LAD-2 should be suspected in a patient with the clinical features of psychomotor delay and with recurrent but mild infections, leukocytosis, and detection of the Bombay blood group (absence of H antigen) [48].

Peripheral blood leukocytes show an absence of Slex expression (CD15A). Confirmation of the diagnosis needs sequence analysis of the GDP-fucose transporter. LAD-3 is a major differential diagnosis of LAD-1 and should be suspected in situations when CD18 expression in an otherwise "typical LAD-1" patient is normal. The confirmation of diagnosis requires the demonstration of impaired integrin activation (e.g., activation of RAP-1) in specialized centers.

4.5.5 *Management*

In all three genetic types of LADs, infections should be treated promptly with appropriate antibiotics. In LAD-1, granulocyte colony-stimulating factor (G-CSF) transfusion stimulates granulocytes in uncontrolled severe infections and large chronic ulcers. The only curative treatment for severe phenotypes is hematopoietic stem cell transplantation (HSCT) [49].

In less severe phenotypes (CD18 > 2–30%), prophylactic antibiotics (e.g., trimethoprim-sulfamethoxazole 5 mg/kg once daily) are sufficient to avoid severe infections, and careful oral hygiene is mandatory to prevent or ameliorate periodontitis in most cases. In LAD-2 patients with recurrent infections, antibiotic prophylaxis with trimethoprim-sulfamethoxazole TMP-SMX is beneficial. Fucose supplementation may achieve a significant clinical improvement in some patients, and therefore, this modality should be tried in these patients [50]. Meanwhile, therapy of LAD-3 is very similar to of LAD-1 patients [36].

4.6 Ras-Related C3 Botulinum Toxin Substrate 2 (RAC-2) Deficiency

Ras-related C3 botulinum toxin substrate 2 (RAC-2) deficiency or neutrophil immunodeficiency syndrome is a severe defect in leukocyte migration manifested by lack of pus formation at the site of infection. RAC-2 (Rho-GTPase) is important for the expression of L-selectin, F-actin assembly, chemotaxis, superoxide generation, and regulation of actin polymerization [51].

Patients with RAC-2 deficiency suffer from delayed separation of the umbilical cord, poor pus formation, nonhealing perirectal or periumbilical abscesses, and leukocytosis similar to LAD-1.

Biopsies from wounds show an appropriate number of neutrophils which differentiate this disease from LAD-1. CD18 expression is also normal, while chemotaxis toward C5a, fMLP, and IL-8 is impaired. Moreover, neutrophil polarization in response to fMLP is also deficient. NADPH oxidase activity is normal after PMA but decreased after fMLP stimulation.

4.6.1 *Pulmonary Manifestations*

In general, pulmonary involvement is uncommon in RAC-2-deficient patients. There are rare cases of recurrent sinopulmonary infections, pneumonia, and bronchiectasis in RAC-2 deficiency, in which majority of them were incorrectly diagnosed [52] as CVID before definitive confirmation of RAC-2 deficiency.

4.6.2 *Management*

Infections should be treated with appropriate antibiotics, while granulocyte transfusions are reserved for patients with critical illnesses and severe infections. Allogenic HSCT is suggested to be a curative treatment [36].

4.7 Congenital Neutropenia (CN)

4.7.1 *Background*

Congenital neutropenia (CN) is a family of genetic diseases associated with three main features of low neutrophil count and susceptibility to infection, various organ dysfunctions, and an extraordinarily high risk of leukemic transformation. Numerous genetic mutations have been identified related to congenital defects in this syndrome.

Neutropenia is defined by a neutrophil count below 1.5 G/l in children over 1 year and below 2 G/l in children aged between 2 and 12 months. Consequently, neutropenia in newborns is defined by a higher threshold as in adult of below 2.5 G/l neutrophils. Severe neutropenia is below 0.5 G/l, and chronic neutropenia lasts more than 3 months. It is important to confirm neutropenia on three samples per week over a 6-week period [53].

Monocytosis, hypereosinophilia, and polyclonal hypergammaglobulinemia appeared to be frequently associated with neutropenia and inversely proportional to its severity. Severe congenital neutropenia is a rare condition, and its prevalence is estimated to be 3–8.5 cases per million individuals [54].

4.7.2 *Pulmonary Manifestations*

Severe infection is the central phenotype of CN in spite of various genotypes of these genetic defects. The most determinant factor linked with infection risk is the residual capacity to mobilize neutrophils from the site of production to the site of infection [55].

The preferential sites of infection are highly variable; frequent sites of infections are the skin and mucosae, ears, nose and throat region, and lungs. During the first weeks of life, the child might begin to have fevers associated with respiratory symptoms, including signs of pneumonia. During the first month of life, skin infections or deep tissue abscesses might be present.

Stomata involvements always manifest after 2 years of age in patients with profound central neutropenia characterized by erosive, hemorrhagic, and painful gingivitis associated with oral furuncles of the tongue and mucosa. Diffuse gastrointestinal lesions could lead to abdominal pain and diarrhea that may resemble Crohn's disease on radiological studies. These lesions may also be associated with bacterial enteritis with atypical symptoms in patients with profound neutropenia, local inflammation, absence of pus and necrosis, and ecthyma gangrenosum. Bacterial infections involved are *Staphylococcus aureus* and *Staphylococcus epidermidis*, *Streptococci*, *Enterococci*, *Pneumococci*, *Pseudomonas aeruginosa*, and gram-negative bacilli. Fungal infections involved are mainly *Candida* or *Aspergillus* species [53].

Thus, patients with severe congenital neutropenia usually present in the first year of life with stomatitis, gingivitis, perirectal inflammation, or cellulitis. Abscesses, pneumonia, and septicemia may also occur. Clinical signs of infections are attenuated by the presence of neutropenia, but fever then serves as a marker of inflammation and regularly develops when infection occurs. These patients are not predisposed to parasitic, viral, or fungal infections. Fungal infections are uncommon except as a complication of prolonged antibiotic therapy [56].

4.8 Severe Congenital Neutropenias (ELANE Deficiency, GFI1 Deficiency, HAX1 Deficiency, G6PC3 Deficiency, VPS45 Deficiency, X-Linked Neutropenia with Myelodysplasia)

4.8.1 ELANE Deficiency

ELANE (neutrophil elastase) mutations are the most frequent congenital form of neutropenia. They are found in about 40% to 55% of patients with congenital neutropenia.

Autosomal-dominant heterozygous mutations of ELANE are the most frequent cause of CN. ELANE deficiency is responsible for cyclic neutropenia (CyN), and severe CN type 1 (SCN1) leads to more severe infections. In CyN, in periods of 21 days, neutrophil counts fluctuate between normal and close to zero, associated with inverse monocyte cycling, sometimes together with variations in reticulocyte, eosinophil, lymphocyte, and platelet counts.

Patients with SCN1 have chronic profound neutropenia characterized by bone marrow maturation suppression at the promyelocyte stage, induced by apoptosis of neutrophil precursors [57].

4.8.1.1 Diagnosis

ELANE-related neutropenia is diagnosed by serial measurements of the absolute neutrophil count (ANC) along with clinical findings. ELANE is the only known gene mutation is known to cause neutropenia. Mutation detection rate is 100% in individuals with documented cyclic neutropenia and known affected family members. However, mutation detection rate is 80% in individuals with congenital neutropenia [58].

4.8.1.2 Pulmonary Manifestation

No specific lung involvement has been reported in ELANE-related neutropenia, same as with other forms of congenital neutropenia. ELANE-related neutropenia is manifested by recurrent fever, skin and oropharyngeal ulcers, gingivitis, sinusitis, pharyngitis, and cervical adenopathy. Infectious complications are basically more severe in congenital neutropenia compared to cyclic neutropenia.

In congenital neutropenia, diarrhea, pneumonia, and deep abscesses in the liver, lung, and subcutaneous tissues are common. Immediate omphalitis after birth may be the first sign. Bacteremia occurs infrequently but has severe consequences in affected individuals [58].

4.8.1.3 Treatment

These patients require large doses of G-CSF, both for the management of active infections and as long-term therapy. There is a high risk of leukemic transformation in this setting. SCN is usually diagnosed before the age of 6 months.

G-CSF treatment increases blood neutrophil levels. Prognosis is generally poor, and many patients expire at young age due to sepsis, colitis, lymphosarcoma, pulmonary complication, and massive gastrointestinal hemorrhage [59].

4.8.2 Neutropenia Associated with G6PC3 Mutations

These mutations induce severe permanent neutropenia associated with granulocyte maturation arrest and susceptibility to infections. Other clinical manifestations are thin skin with a highly visible veins, urogenital malformations, cardiac disorders (in particular arrhythmia due to atrioseptal conduction defect), myopathy (despite a normal histology of muscle), and perception deafness [53].

4.8.2.1 Pulmonary Manifestation

G6PC3 deficiency has highly variable clinical presentations and severity. Majority of patients with G6PC3 deficiency have cardiovascular and urogenital manifestations (so-called classic G6PC3 deficiency). A more severely affected classic disease called Dursun syndrome is manifested with involvement of myeloid cells, primary pulmonary hypertension in the newborn period, and minor dysmorphic features. This syndrome is characterized by a triad of familial primary pulmonary hypertension (PPH), leukopenia, and atrial septal defects [60].

Patients with G6PC3 deficiency usually present in their first 6 months of life with recurrent bacterial infections, recurrent diarrhea, failure to thrive, and sinopulmonary infections. Sinopulmonary infections namely bronchiectasis, and otitis media are the most common pulmonary manifestations. Moreover, urinary tract infections, skin abscesses, and sepsis are also common findings in these patients. Some patients may also suffer from oral ulcers, periodontitis, stomatitis, gingivitis, and fungal infections. G6PC3 deficiency patients remain susceptible to bacterial infections if not treated. Nearly two-thirds of G6PC3 deficiency patients show intermittent thrombocytopenia. Pulmonary hypertension (PHT) has also been described in G6PC3 deficiency patients, and congenital heart defects are also common. In their recent review, Banka and Newman found that more than half of G6PC3 deficiency patients may have congenital cardiac defects, and the most common anomaly is atrial septal defect.

Severe G6PC3 deficiency (Dursun syndrome) has classic finding of G6PC3 deficiency in addition to specific features including primary pulmonary hypertension (PPH) developing in the newborn period, nonmyeloid cell involvement and severe lymphopenia, and thymus hypoplasia.

4.8.2.2 Management

G-CSF has been used for treatment in patients with G6PC3 deficiency; it improves neutrophil count, prevents infections, and increases quality of life. However, in some patients, G-CSF could not control infections [13]. On the other hand, patients with mild disease may not necessarily require G-CSF treatment and can be managed with prophylactic antibiotics [61].

Prognosis of most patients with G6PC3 deficiency is generally good on G-CSF treatment or prophylactic antibiotics in mildly affected individuals. However, untreated G6PC3 deficiency can be fatal.

4.8.3 Neutropenia Associated with GFI1 Mutations

No pulmonary manifestation has been reported for this congenital disease.

4.8.4 HAX1 Deficiency

The only reported form of pulmonary manifestation in HAX1 deficiency of congenital neutropenia is pneumonia. Other manifestations of HAX1 deficiency are recurrent stomatitis, gingivitis, skin abscess, otitis, mastoiditis, and tooth decay [62].

4.8.5 *Mutations in* VPS45

No pulmonary manifestation has been reported.

4.8.6 *X-Linked Neutropenia with Myelodysplasia*

No pulmonary manifestations have been reported.

4.9 Cyclic Neutropenia

Cyclic neutropenia, an autosomal dominant disorder, is a type of SCN in which numbers of blood neutrophils, monocytes, platelets, reticulocytes, and lymphocytes fluctuate within a 21-day period. Mutations in ELANE can induce cyclic neutropenia and some other forms of SCN. Risk of cyclic neutropenia to evolve to MDS and acute myeloid leukemia is low. However, when neutrophil counts are at the lowest count, patients could have painful mouth ulcers, cellulitis, respiratory symptoms, abscesses, and severe infections that could even be fatal [54].

4.9.1 *Pulmonary Manifestation*

Cyclic neutropenia has no specific pulmonary manifestation, the same as other congenital neutropenia; however, upper respiratory infections (sinusitis and/or otitis media), pneumonia, and bronchitis are reported respiratory manifestations of this form of immunodeficiency [63].

Interestingly, patients with cyclic neutropenia are usually asymptomatic. However, they can frequently suffer from severe bacterial infections, oral lesions, and cutaneous manifestations during the episodes of neutropenia. These patients are generally healthy between neutropenic periods but, during the episode of neutropenia, suffer from aphthous stomatitis, oral ulcers, gingivitis, abscesses, and occasionally overwhelming bacterial infections [64].

The symptomatic episodes of fever and infections usually recur approximately every 3–4 weeks. The neutropenic periods are associated with infections especially in oral cavity and mucous membranes, where oral ulcers and periodontitis are common. Cutaneous infections, upper respiratory infections, and skin abscesses are also common. Perirectal and genital areas are susceptible to recurrent infections and abscesses [65].

More than half of patients with cyclic neutropenia experience oral ulcerations, gingivitis, lymphadenopathy, fever, pharyngitis, and skin infections at least five times per year. Adult patients are involved with sinusitis or otitis media, while pediatrics have more than five episodes of bone pain or tooth abscesses per year. More than 10% of individuals report pneumonia and bronchitis. On the other hand, congenital neutropenia is a preleukemic condition of which 20% of patients ultimately develop leukemia after 20 years [66].

4.9.2 Diagnosis

Congenital cyclic neutropenia is diagnosed by periodic oscillations in the circulating neutrophil count from normal to severe neutropenic in at least 3-week period with duration of 3–6 days [67].

In patients with neutropenia, the clinical history and examination of the peripheral blood smear are the most important aspects of diagnostic evaluation. Examination of the oral cavity, perianal region, and skin is necessary in order to assess the clinical impact of neutropenia [68].

In patients not being treated with G-CSF, the cycling period is regularly within 3 month laps. However, the cycling periodicity can vary somewhat from a patient to another patient and can be altered by administration of G-CSF.

Diagnosis is performed by CBC with differential at least twice weekly over 6–9 weeks to determine the typical cyclic pattern of neutropenia. In sporadic cases without a positive family history, cycling pattern from early childhood is absent or is erratically different from 21 days. In such cases, acquired cyclic neutropenia should be considered in the differential diagnosis [36].

4.9.3 Management

The life expectancy and quality of life of patients with congenital cyclic neutropenia are acceptable, if patients are diagnosed and regularly followed up [1].

Although the prognosis is good with a benign course, approximately 10% of patients may experience life-threatening infections. In addition to prophylactic antibiotics, in some patients, treatment with recombinant human G-CSF in anticipation and into the time of "cycling nadir" may be all that is needed only over a period of several days to sufficiently increase blood neutrophil counts to achieve reduction in infection rate and improvement in survival and quality of life. Prophylactic antibiotics and antifungal agents and aggressive therapy during acute infections are keys for long-term survival [65].

4.10 Shwachman-Diamond Syndrome

Shwachman-Diamond syndrome (SDS) is a multi-system AR disease characterized by exocrine pancreatic insufficiency, impaired hematopoiesis, and leukemia predisposition. Other clinical features include skeletal, immunologic, hepatic, and cardiac disorders [69].

Infants with SDS suffer from failure to thrive, foul-smelling stools due to the pancreatic insufficiency, and persistent or intermittent neutropenia with recurrent infections like recurrent otitis media, sepsis, pneumonia, etc. In later stage of their lives, pancreatic insufficiency significantly improves in more than 50% of the patients older than 4 years, while anemia and thrombocytopenia develop in more than 40% of patients. Neutropenia is intermittent in about two-thirds and constant in one-third. Approximately, 10% of patients progress to MDS and acute myelogenous leukemia. Furthermore, patients suffer from skeletal abnormalities (irregularity of metaphyses, osteopenia, short stature), neurodevelopmental delay, dental caries, and hepatic dysfunction [36]. SDS diagnosis is made by association of clinical symptoms of pancreatic exocrine and bone marrow dysfunction [69].

4.10.1 Pulmonary Manifestations

Patients with SDS are susceptible to recurrent bronchopulmonary bacterial, viral, and fungal opportunistic infections [69]. Besides, recurrent otitis media, sinusitis, and mouth sores are seen in these patients as well. Other systemic infections in SDS patients include septicemia, osteomyelitis, and skin infections.

4.10.2 Management

First-line therapy is to ameliorate exocrine pancreatic insufficiency symptoms by pancreatic enzymes substitutes and supplementary fat-soluble vitamins. Blood count monitoring should be performed at least every 6 months and bone marrow once a year. Neutropenia with recurrent bacterial infections could be treated with G-CSF; however, there is increased risk of preleukemic cell stimulation. In patients with symptomatic anemia, leukocyte-depleted and irradiated erythrocyte transfusions are recommended, and in thrombocytopenia and bleeding cases, platelet transfusions are indicated. HSCT could also be offered to patients with pancytopenia, MDS, or leukemia in remission; however, survival is about 60–70% [36].

4.11 Cohen Syndrome

Cohen syndrome (OMIM#216550) is an AR condition with mutations in *COH1* gene manifesting with hypotonia, obesity, microcephaly, mental retardation, short stature, and characteristic faces with short philtrum, prominent upper central incisors, and prominent nasal root. Neutropenia is mild to moderate, intermittent, and not generally associated with severe infection, although gingivitis, periodontitis, and cutaneous infections are common [36].

4.11.1 Pulmonary Manifestations

There is an association between Cohen syndrome and upper respiratory airway problems which may be severe and even life-threatening inducing intrinsic difference in laryngeal function [70]. Stridor is the most common presenting sign in infancy of Cohen patients due to laryngomalacia, laryngeal abnormalities, laryngeal stenosis, and vocal cord paralysis. A high-pitched voice is a consistent finding, even in those patients who have not had previous laryngeal problems.

4.11.2 Treatment of Manifestations

Early intervention including physical, occupational, and speech therapy is appropriate to address gross developmental delay, hypotonia, joint hypermobility, and motor clumsiness. Meanwhile, G-CSF should be considered if neutropenia is documented [71].

4.12 Poikiloderma with Neutropenia (PN)

Poikiloderma is a syndrome of skin atrophy and papular erythematous rash. So far, several subtypes of this genodermatosis have been described. The Clericuzio was first described in Navajo Indians. Onset of this disease is in the first year of life; later on, the rash gradually propagates centripetally from the limbs and forms a papular rash, followed by plaques of hypo- and hyperpigmentation and telangiectasia. The nails could also be affected (pachyonychia), but no hair loss or leukoplasia is observed. More importantly, the skin changes are mostly associated with recurrent infections, especially pneumonia.

The neutropenia in these patients is often severe. Granulocyte maturation arrest at the promyelocyte stage is not observed; however, dysgranulopoiesis with late arrest is often seen [53].

4.12.1 Pulmonary Manifestations

PN patients mostly have recurrent pulmonary infections inducing bronchiectasis, lung abscesses, and lung granulomas. Chronic recurrent otitis media and sinusitis are also common in childhood. The frequency of acute sinopulmonary infections decreases after 5–10 years of age, but most individuals continue to have bronchiectasis, chronic nonproductive cough, and reactive airway disease.

4.12.2 *Management*

Poikiloderma is treated with conservative skin care, applying weak emollients and sun protectives. However, pruritic palmar/plantar hyperkeratosis can be treated with a strong topical steroid or a topical keratolytic after ruling out dermatophyte infection. G-CSF is not clinically effective on PN patients in decreasing frequency of infections, despite increases in absolute neutrophil count. MDS and acute myelogenous leukemia are treated in the usual treatment modalities. Sinopulmonary, middle ear, and skin infections require aggressive treatment with antibiotics. Reactive airway disease and hypogonadotropic hypogonadism are also treated. PN patients with recurrent sinopulmonary infections should be treated with prophylactic antibiotics during the winter to decrease frequency of infections [72].

4.13 Other Phagocytic Deficiencies

In other phagocytic deficiencies, including b-actin, aggressive periodontitis, Papillon-Lefevre syndrome, Barth syndrome, and glycogen storage disease Ib, no pulmonary manifestations have been reported. Although these phagocytic deficiencies present mostly with recurrent infections, however, to the unknown reasons, pulmonary involvement has not been reported so far in reported cases.

References

1. Rezaei N, Pourpak Z, Aghamohammadi A, Farhoudi A, Movahedi M, Gharagozlou M, et al. Consanguinity in primary immunodeficiency disorders; the report from Iranian primary immunodeficiency registry. Am J Reprod Immunol. 2006;56(2):145–51.
2. Matute JD, Arias AA, Wright NA, Wrobel I, Waterhouse CC, Li XJ, et al. A new genetic subgroup of chronic granulomatous disease with autosomal recessive mutations in p40phox and selective defects in neutrophil NADPH oxidase activity. Blood. 2009;114(15):3309–15.
3. Fattahi F, Badalzadeh M, Sedighipour L, Movahedi M, Fazlollahi MR, Mansouri SD, et al. Inheritance pattern and clinical aspects of 93 Iranian patients with chronic granulomatous disease. J Clin Immunol. 2011;31(5):792.
4. Kuhns DB, Alvord WG, Heller T, Feld JJ, Pike KM, Marciano BE, et al. Residual NADPH oxidase and survival in chronic granulomatous disease. N Engl J Med. 2010;363(27):2600–10.
5. Mansouri D, Adimi P, Mirsaedi M, Mansouri N, Tabarsi P, Amiri M, et al. Primary immune deficiencies presenting in adults: seven years of experience from Iran. J Clin Immunol. 2005;25(4):385–91.
6. Van den Berg JM, Van Koppen E, Åhlin A, Belohradsky BH, Bernatowska E, Corbeel L, et al. Chronic granulomatous disease: the European experience. PLoS One. 2009;4(4):e5234.
7. Carnide EG, Jacob CA, Castro AM, Pastorino AC. Clinical and laboratory aspects of chronic granulomatous disease in description of eighteen patients. Pediatr Allergy Immunol. 2005;16(1):5–9.

8. Mahdaviani SA, Mohajerani SA, Rezaei N, Casanova J-L, Mansouri SD, Velayati AA. Pulmonary manifestations of chronic granulomatous disease. Expert Rev Clin Immunol. 2013;9(2):153–60.
9. Johnston RB Jr. Clinical aspects of chronic granulomatous disease. Curr Opin Hematol. 2001;8(1):17–22.
10. Khanna G, Kao SC, Kirby P, Sato Y. Imaging of chronic granulomatous disease in children. Radiographics. 2005;25(5):1183–95.
11. Almyroudis N, Holland S, Segal B. Invasive aspergillosis in primary immunodeficiencies. Med Mycol. 2005;43(sup1):247–59.
12. Dorman SE, Guide SV, Conville PS, DeCarlo ES, Malech HL, Gallin JI, et al. Nocardia infection in chronic granulomatous disease. Clin Infect Dis. 2002;35(4):390–4.
13. Marciano BE, Wesley R, De Carlo ES, Anderson VL, Barnhart LA, Darnell D, et al. Long-term interferon-γ therapy for patients with chronic granulomatous disease. Clin Infect Dis. 2004;39(5):692–9.
14. Lacy D, Spencer D, Goldstein A, Weller P, Darbyshire P. Chronic granulomatous disease presenting in childhood with Pseudomonas cepacia septicaemia. J Infect. 1993;27(3):301–4.
15. Reichenbach J, Lopatin U, Mahlaoui N, Beovic B, Siler U, Zbinden R, et al. Actinomyces in chronic granulomatous disease: an emerging and unanticipated pathogen. Clin Infect Dis. 2009;49(11):1703–10.
16. Vinh DC, Shea YR, Sugui JA, Parrilla-Castellar ER, Freeman AF, Campbell JW, et al. Invasive aspergillosis due to Neosartorya udagawae. Clin Infect Dis. 2009;49(1):102–11.
17. Lee PP, Chan K-W, Jiang L, Chen T, Li C, Lee T-L, et al. Susceptibility to mycobacterial infections in children with X-linked chronic granulomatous disease: a review of 17 patients living in a region endemic for tuberculosis. Pediatr Infect Dis J. 2008;27(3):224–30.
18. Bustamante J, Aksu G, Vogt G, De Beaucoudrey L, Genel F, Chapgier A, et al. BCG-osis and tuberculosis in a child with chronic granulomatous disease. J Allergy Clin Immunol. 2007;120(1):32–8.
19. Kuijpers T, Lutter R. Inflammation and repeated infections in CGD: two sides of a coin. Cell Mol Life Sci. 2012;69(1):7–15.
20. De Ravin SS, Naumann N, Cowen EW, Friend J, Hilligoss D, Marquesen M, et al. Chronic granulomatous disease as a risk factor for autoimmune disease. J Allergy Clin Immunol. 2008;122(6):1097–103.
21. Siddiqui S, Anderson VL, Hilligoss DM, Abinun M, Kuijpers TW, Masur H, et al. Fulminant mulch pneumonitis: an emergency presentation of chronic granulomatous disease. Clin Infect Dis. 2007;45(6):673–81.
22. Morgenstern DE, Gifford MA, Li LL, Doerschuk CM, Dinauer MC. Absence of respiratory burst in X-linked chronic granulomatous disease mice leads to abnormalities in both host defense and inflammatory response to Aspergillus fumigatus. J Exp Med. 1997;185(2):207–18.
23. Segal BH, Leto TL, Gallin JI, Malech HL, Holland SM. Genetic, biochemical, and clinical features of chronic granulomatous disease. Medicine. 2000;79(3):170–200.
24. Brown KL, Bylund J, MacDonald KL, Song-Zhao GX, Elliott MR, Falsafi R, et al. ROS-deficient monocytes have aberrant gene expression that correlates with inflammatory disorders of chronic granulomatous disease. Clin Immunol. 2008;129(1):90–102.
25. Segal BH, Han W, Bushey JJ, Joo M, Bhatti Z, Feminella J, et al. NADPH oxidase limits innate immune responses in the lungs in mice. PLoS One. 2010;5(3):e9631.
26. Foster CB, Lehrnbecher T, Mol F, Steinberg SM, Venzon DJ, Walsh TJ, et al. Host defense molecule polymorphisms influence the risk for immune-mediated complications in chronic granulomatous disease. J Clin Invest. 1998;102(12):2146–55.
27. Khalilzadeh S, Bloorsaz MR, Mansouri D, Baghaie N, Hakimi S, Velayati AA. Clinical and radiological aspects of chronic granulomatous disease in children: a case series from Iran. Iran J Allergy Asthma Immunol. 2006;5(2):85–8.
28. Margolis DM, Melnick DA, Ailing DW, Gallin JI. Trimethoprim-sulfamethoxazole prophylaxis in the management of chronic granulomatous disease. J Infect Dis. 1990;162(3):723–6.

29. Petropoulou T, Liese J, Tintelnot K, Gahr M, Belohradsky B. Long-term treatment of patients with itraconazole for the prevention of Aspergillus infections in patients with chronic granulomatous disease (CGD). Mycoses. 1994;37:64–9.
30. Holland SM. Chronic granulomatous disease. Clin Rev Allergy Immunol. 2010;38(1):3–10.
31. Uzel G, Orange JS, Poliak N, Marciano BE, Heller T, Holland SM. Complications of tumor necrosis factor-±blockade in chronic granulomatous disease—related colitis. Clin Infect Dis. 2010;51(12):1429–34.
32. Grez M, Reichenbach J, Schwäble J, Seger R, Dinauer MC, Thrasher AJ. Gene therapy of chronic granulomatous disease: the engraftment dilemma. Mol Ther. 2011;19(1):28–35.
33. Ott MG, Schmidt M, Schwarzwaelder K, Stein S, Siler U, Koehl U, et al. Correction of X-linked chronic granulomatous disease by gene therapy, augmented by insertional activation of MDS1-EVI1, PRDM16 or SETBP1. Nat Med. 2006;12(4):401.
34. Yamazaki-Nakashimada MA, Stiehm ER, Pietropaolo-Cienfuegos D, Hernandez-Bautista V, Espinosa-Rosales F. Corticosteroid therapy for refractory infections in chronic granulomatous disease: case reports and review of the literature. Ann Allergy Asthma Immunol. 2006;97(2):257–61.
35. Arnhold J, Flemmig J. Human myeloperoxidase in innate and acquired immunity. Arch Biochem Biophys. 2010;500(1):92–106.
36. Rezaei N, Aghamohammadi A, Notarangelo LD. Primary immunodeficiency diseases definition, diagnosis, and management. Berlin/Heidelberg: Springer; 2008.
37. Antachopoulos C. Invasive fungal infections in congenital immunodeficiencies. Clin Microbiol Infect. 2010;16(9):1335–42.
38. Lanza F. Clinical manifestation of myeloperoxidase deficiency. J Mol Med. 1998;76(10): 676–81.
39. Wada T, Akagi T, Muraoka M, Toma T, Kaji K, Agematsu K, et al. A novel in-frame deletion in the leucine zipper domain of C/EBPε leads to neutrophil-specific granule deficiency. J Immunol. 2015;195(1):80–6.
40. Malech HL, Hickstein DD. Genetics, biology and clinical management of myeloid cell primary immune deficiencies: chronic granulomatous disease and leukocyte adhesion deficiency. Curr Opin Hematol. 2007;14(1):29–36.
41. Lübke T, Marquardt T, Etzioni A, Hartmann E, von Figura K, Körner C. Complementation cloning identifies CDG-IIc, a new type of congenital disorders of glycosylation, as a GDP-fucose transporter deficiency. Nat Genet. 2001;28(1):73.
42. Kinashi T, Aker M, Sokolovsky-Eisenberg M, Grabovsky V, Tanaka C, Shamri R, et al. LAD-III, a leukocyte adhesion deficiency syndrome associated with defective Rap1 activation and impaired stabilization of integrin bonds. Blood. 2004;103(3):1033–6.
43. Etzioni A, Tonetti M. Leukocyte adhesion deficiency II–from a to almost Z. Immunol Rev. 2000;178(1):138–47.
44. Bazregari S, Azizi G, Tavakol M, Asgardoon MH, Kiaee F, Tavakolinia N, et al. Evaluation of infectious and non-infectious complications in patients with primary immunodeficiency. Cent Eur J Immunol. 2017;42(4):336.
45. Etzioni A. Novel aspects of phagocytic cell disorders. Curr Opin Allergy Clin Immunol. 2001;1(6):535–40.
46. Etzioni A, Harlan J, Pollack S, Phillips L, Gershoni-Baruch R, Paulson J. Leukocyte adhesion deficiency (LAD) II: a new adhesion defect due to absence of sialyl Lewis X, the ligand for selectins. Immunodeficiency. 1993;4(1–4):307.
47. Etzioni A, Alon R. Leukocyte adhesion deficiency III: a group of integrin activation defects in hematopoietic lineage cells. Curr Opin Allergy Clin Immunol. 2004;4(6):485–90.
48. Frydman M, Etzioni A, Eidlitz-Markus T, Avidor I, Varsano I, Shechter Y, et al. Rambam–Hasharon syndrome of psychomotor retardation, short stature, defective neutrophil motility, and Bombay phenotype. Am J Med Genet. 1992;44(3):297–302.
49. Thomas C, Le Deist F, Cavazzana-Calvo M, Benkerrou M, Haddad E, Blanche S, et al. Results of allogeneic bone marrow transplantation in patients with leukocyte adhesion deficiency. Blood. 1995;86(4):1629–35.

50. Marquardt T, Lühn K, Srikrishna G, Freeze HH, Harms E, Vestweber D. Correction of leukocyte adhesion deficiency type II with oral fucose. Blood. 1999;94(12):3976–85.
51. Bogaert DJ, Dullaers M, Lambrecht BN, Vermaelen KY, De Baere E, Haerynck F. Genes associated with common variable immunodeficiency: one diagnosis to rule them all? J Med Genet. 2016;53(9):575–90.
52. Alkhairy OK, Rezaei N, Graham RR, Abolhassani H, Borte S, Hultenby K, et al. RAC2 loss-of-function mutation in 2 siblings with characteristics of common variable immunodeficiency. J Allergy Clin Immunol. 2015;135(5):1380–4.e5.
53. Donadieu J, Fenneteau O, Beaupain B, Mahlaoui N, Chantelot CB. Congenital neutropenia: diagnosis, molecular bases and patient management. Orphanet J Rare Dis. 2011;6(1):26.
54. Skokowa J, Dale DC, Touw IP, Zeidler C, Welte K. Severe congenital neutropenias. Nat Rev Dis Prim. 2017;3:17032.
55. Donadieu J, Beaupain B, Fenneteau O, Bellanné-Chantelot C. Congenital neutropenia in the era of genomics: classification, diagnosis, and natural history. Br J Haematol. 2017;179(4):557–74.
56. Boxer LA. Severe congenital neutropenia: genetics and pathogenesis. Trans Am Clin Climatol Assoc. 2006;117:13.
57. Lanini LLS, Prader S, Siler U, Reichenbach J. Modern management of phagocyte defects. Pediatr Allergy Immunol. 2017;28(2):124–34.
58. Dale DC. ELANE-related neutropenia. In: Adam MP, Ardinger HH, Pagon RA, Wallace SE, Bean LJH, Stephens K, et al., editors. GeneReviews((R)). Seattle: University of Washington, Seattle. GeneReviews is a registered trademark of the University of Washington, Seattle All rights reserved; 2011.
59. Okolo ON, Katsanis E, Yun S, Reveles CY, Anwer F. Allogeneic transplant in ELANE and MEFV mutation positive severe cyclic neutropenia: review of prognostic factors for secondary severe events. Case Rep Hematol. 2017;2017:1.
60. Banka S. G6PC3 deficiency. In: Adam MP, Ardinger HH, Pagon RA, Wallace SE, Bean LJH, Stephens K, et al., editors. GeneReviews((R)). Seattle: University of Washington, Seattle. GeneReviews is a registered trademark of the University of Washington, Seattle. All rights reserved; 1993.
61. Banka S, Newman WG. A clinical and molecular review of ubiquitous glucose-6-phosphatase deficiency caused by G6PC3 mutations. Orphanet J Rare Dis. 2013;8(1):84.
62. Aydogmus C, Cipe F, Tas M, Akınel A, Öner Ö, Keskindemirci G, et al. HAX-1 deficiency: characteristics of five cases including an asymptomatic patient. Asian Pac J Allergy Immunol. 2016;34(1):73–6.
63. Palmer SE, Stephens K, Dale DC. Genetics, phenotype, and natural history of autosomal dominant cyclic hematopoiesis. Am J Med Genet. 1996;66(4):413–22.
64. Dale DC, Liles WC, Garwicz D, Aprikyan AG. Clinical implications of mutations of neutrophil elastase in congenital and cyclic neutropenia. J Pediatr Hematol Oncol. 2001;23(4):208–10.
65. Dale DC, Bolyard AA, Aprikyan A. Cyclic neutropenia. Semin Hematol. 2002;39(2):89–94.
66. Mansoor MS, Khan MB. A case of cyclic neutropenia in adults. JPMA J Pak Med Assoc. 2012;62(3):289–90.
67. Dale DC, WPt H. Cyclic neutropenia: a clinical review. Blood Rev. 1988;2(3):178–85.
68. Rezaei N, Farhoudi A, Pourpak Z, Aghamohammadi A, Ramyar A, Moin M, et al. Clinical and laboratory findings in Iranian children with cyclic neutropenia. Iran J Allergy Asthma Immunol. 2004;3(1):37–40.
69. Burroughs L, Woolfrey A, Shimamura A. Shwachman-Diamond syndrome: a review of the clinical presentation, molecular pathogenesis, diagnosis, and treatment. Hematol Oncol Clin North Am. 2009;23(2):233–48.
70. Chandler KE, Kidd A, Al-Gazali L, Kolehmainen J, Lehesjoki AE, Black GC, et al. Diagnostic criteria, clinical characteristics, and natural history of Cohen syndrome. J Med Genet. 2003;40(4):233–41.
71. Wang H, Falk MJ, Wensel C, Traboulsi EI. Cohen syndrome. In: Adam MP, Ardinger HH, Pagon RA, Wallace SE, Bean LJH, Stephens K, et al., editors. GeneReviews((R)). Seattle:

University of Washington, Seattle University of Washington, Seattle. GeneReviews is a registered trademark of the University of Washington, Seattle. All rights reserved; 1993.

72. Wang L, Clericuzio C, Larizza L. Poikiloderma with neutropenia. In: Adam MP, Ardinger HH, Pagon RA, Wallace SE, Bean LJH, Stephens K, et al., editors. GeneReviews((R)). Seattle: University of Washington, Seattle University of Washington, Seattle. GeneReviews is a registered trademark of the University of Washington, Seattle. All rights reserved; 1993.

Chapter 5
Pulmonary Manifestations of Genetic Disorders of Immune Regulation

Sebastian F. N. Bode, Ulrich Baumann, and Carsten Speckmann

5.1 Introduction

The immune system has to be tightly balanced between adequate responses against infectious pathogens while maintaining tolerance toward the host. Genetic disorders of immune regulation can lead to both immunodeficiency and autoimmunity/immune dysregulation – sometimes including respiratory manifestations.

Immune dysregulation typically leads to noninfectious pulmonary inflammation ("pneumonitis") localized interstitially but also in the bronchioli and alveolae. This is in stark contrast to respiratory manifestations of antibody deficiencies that typically lead to increased susceptibility to bronchopulmonary infections, often bronchiectasis and chronic cough. Symptoms of pneumonitis are often nonspecific or patients can be even asymptomatic. Pulmonary function tests initially may only show impaired gas exchange that progresses to restrictive lung disease. The lack of clinical symptoms does not prompt pulmonary function tests that are needed for the diagnosis of pulmonary involvement. This might be a reason for the low incidence of respiratory manifestations that are reported in genetic disorders of immune regulation. The following chapter demonstrates available information regarding

S. F. N. Bode (✉)
Center for Pediatrics, Department of General Pediatrics, Adolescent Medicine, and Neonatology, Medical Center, Faculty of Medicine, University of Freiburg, Freiburg, Germany
e-mail: sebastian.bode@uniklinik-freiburg.de

U. Baumann
Department of Paediatric Pulmonology and Neonatalogy, Hanover Medical School, Hannover, Germany

C. Speckmann
Center for Chronic Immunodeficiency and Center for Pediatrics, Department of Pediatric Hematology and Oncology, Medical Center, Faculty of Medicine, University of Freiburg, Freiburg, Germany

S. A. Mahdaviani, N. Rezaei (eds.), *Pulmonary Manifestations of Primary Immunodeficiency Diseases*, https://doi.org/10.1007/978-3-030-00880-2_5

pulmonary pathologies for each genetically defined disease of immune dysregulation. In some cases, animal models can help to better understand the pathophysiology. Some conditions outlined in this chapter only show signs of immune dysregulation, but others share features with antibody deficiencies and combined immunodeficiencies leading to a variable possible respiratory presentation.

Some of the conditions outlined in this chapter lead to the clinical picture of hemophagocytic lymphohistiocytosis (HLH) (Sect. 5.2) which carries a poor prognosis by itself, but an even worse prognosis of pulmonary involvement is present.

Other conditions like LRBA or CTLA-4 deficiency (Sect. 5.3); Hermansky-Pudlak syndrome types 2, 9, and 10 (Sect. 5.7); STAT5b deficiency (Sect. 5.13); or ITCH deficiency (Sect. 5.14) have typical pulmonary manifestations that, in combination with symptoms of autoimmunity or immunodeficiency, can aid the clinical diagnosis of a specific condition.

As some of the conditions outlined in this chapter cause some form of B- or T-cell immunodeficiency, patients with p14 deficiency (Sect. 5.8), SAP/XIAP deficiency (Sect. 5.9), CD27 deficiency (Sect. 5.10), or CD25 deficiency (Sect. 5.12) are at the same risk for infectious pulmonary manifestations as patients with hypogammaglobulinemia or combined immunodeficiency due to other molecular defects.

Evidence-based recommendations on the therapeutic management of these respiratory manifestations or complications are not available in many cases; some suggestions are discussed in the following chapter.

(For further information you may see Speckmann C, Borkhardt A, Gaspar B, Gambineri E, Ehl S. Genetic disorders of immune regulation. In: Rezaei N, Aghamohammadi A, Notarangelo LD, editors. *Primary immunodeficiency diseases: definition, diagnosis, and management*. 2nd ed. p. 295–338)

5.2 Familial Hemophagocytic Lymphohistiocytosis (Perforin Deficiency, UNC13D Deficiency, Syntaxin 11 Deficiency, STXBP2 Deficiency)

5.2.1 Background

Familial hemophagocytic lymphohistiocytosis (FHL) comprises a group of genetically different conditions that lead to the life-threatening clinical picture of hemophagocytic lymphohistiocytosis with uncontrolled proliferation of lymphocytes and the secretion of pro-inflammatory cytokines [1].

Four forms of FHL have been described so far: FHL-2 (OMIN*603553) [2, 3] or perforin deficiency, named after the mutations in the perforin gene (PRF1; OMIN*170280), FHL-3 (OMIN*608898) [4] caused by mutations in MUNC13-4 (UNC13D; OMIN*608897), FHL-4 (OMIN*603552) [5] due to mutations in the gene for syntaxin 11 (STX11; OMIN*605014), and FHL-5 (OMIN*613101)

Table 5.1 Diagnostic criteria for HLH. Modified from histio.org and [10]

A	B (Five out of eight criteria have to be fulfilled)
Molecular diagnosis consistent with HLH	Fever
	Splenomegaly
	Cytopenias in 2/3 cell lines (hemoglobin <9 mg/dl) (<10 mg/dl in infants <4 weeks old), platelets <100.000/µl, neutrophils <1.000/µl
	Hypertriglyceridemia (fasting triglycerides ≥265 mg/dl) and/or hypofibrinogenemia (fibrinogen ≤1.5 g/l)
	Hemophagocytosis in the bone marrow, spleen, lymph nodes, or liquor
	Ferritin >500 ng/ml
	Soluble IL-2 receptor (sCD25) >2.400 U/ml
	Decreased or absent NK cell cytotoxicity

[6, 7] caused by mutations in the gene for STXBP2 (OMIN*601717). All these mutations result in reduced NK cell or T-cell cytotoxicity. While the exact genetic defect of FHL-1 has not been identified yet, it has been linked to chromosome 9q21.3-22 [8].

Ineffective killing of pathogens or infected cells leads to proliferation and hyperstimulation of NK and T-cells causing hypercytokinemia and the clinical picture of HLH [9]. A diagnosis can be established if at least five out of eight diagnostic criteria are fulfilled (see Table 5.1) [10].

5.2.2 Pulmonary Manifestations of HLH

While pulmonary complications in patients with primary or familial hemophagocytic lymphohistiocytosis are rarely reported, there are reports on pulmonary involvement in secondary HLH, for example, caused by infections. In one cohort over 50% of adult patients with HLH showed some form of pulmonary involvement, mostly in the form of dyspnea and cough at onset that quickly led to the need for mechanical ventilation [11]. In a pediatric cohort that might comprise of more cases of FHL (median age 33 months at diagnosis of HLH, at least 3 cases of perforin deficiency), 30% of patients displayed respiratory symptoms including cough, dyspnea, or tachypnea [12].

Patients with HLH and pulmonary involvement were more likely to suffer from a severe episode of HLH and to require intensive care and had a poorer prognosis (<50% survival) than patients without pulmonary involvement and HLH (80% survival).

In pediatric cohorts, bilateral lung infiltrates, pleural effusions, and granulomatous lung disease were most common and in general nonspecific [13–15]. A report on autopsies of 27 children demonstrated signs of hemophagocytosis in the lungs without stating an exact percentage of affected patients [16].

It is worth considering whether the pulmonary involvement in HLH can be directly caused by the underlying disease as suggested by animal models [17, 18] or is secondary due to infections that may be caused by the impaired infection control in HLH. The cytokine storm in HLH or in severe infections can lead to capillary leakage causing acute respiratory distress syndrome with bilateral infiltrates and effusions. Seguin et al. report that 59% of 118 patients with pulmonary symptoms and HLH had an underlying infectious trigger identified underscoring the importance of thorough diagnostics to identify treatable triggers [11].

5.2.3 Management

All patients with HLH should undergo prompt evaluation for underlying causes and promptly receive immunosuppressive therapy according to current protocols [10, 19]. Especially patients with HLH and pulmonary symptoms need to be treated early and aggressively to ameliorate the poor prognosis. The only curative option for patients with FHL is hematopoietic stem cell transplantation (HSCT) [9].

5.3 Autoimmune Lymphoproliferative Syndrome (ALPS) (FAS Defect, FASLG Defect, CASP10 Deficiency, CASP8 Deficiency, RAS-Associated Autoimmune Leukoproliferative Disease, FADD Deficiency)

5.3.1 Background

The autoimmune lymphoproliferative syndromes (ALPS) (OMIN#601859) often present with uncontrolled lymphocyte proliferation leading to lymphadenopathy, splenomegaly, hemolytic anemia, and other symptoms related to a poorly controlled lymphocyte apoptosis [20, 21]. Mutations in the Fas (CD95)-mediated death receptor pathway (FAS, FAS-ligand (FAS-L)) are most common. Mutations affecting the intrinsic apoptotic pathway, namely, in NRAS and KRAS, have been described as RAS-associated autoimmune lymphoproliferative disease (RALD) (OMIN#614470).

Other primary immunodeficiency diseases (PIDs) can lead to lymphoproliferation and cytopenia, including *XLP*, *LRBA*, *STAT3* gain-of-function, *CTLA-4*, and APDS types 1 and 2, but the genetic basis for some patients still remains to be elucidated (unclassified ALPS/ALPS-like syndrome).

Patients with ALPS, especially ALPS-FAS, show an enlarged population of "double-negative T-cells" that express an α/β T-cell receptor [22]. Upregulation of the mTOR pathway and secretion of IL-10 and other cytokines favoring the production of autoantibodies contribute to the clinical picture of ALPS [23–25].

The clinical manifestation and course of ALPS is mainly benign and includes lymphadenopathy, hepatosplenomegaly, and autoimmune cytopenias as well as other autoimmune phenomena. Around 10–15% of ALPS-FAS patients develop B-cell lymphomas [26].

5.3.2 Pulmonary Manifestations of ALPS

Pulmonary symptoms in general are infrequent in the ALPS population. In the largest ALPS cohort reported, 8% (18/255) of patients showed abnormal lung findings on radiographic, especially chest CT, imaging [27].

These abnormalities included mainly ground-glass opacities (alveolar and/or interstitial infiltration) in 16 patients, tree-in-bud nodules (bronchiolitis with impaction and wall thickening) in 15 patients, bronchiectasis in 14 patients, and septal thickening (thickening of the interstitial septa by effusion of fibrous tissue) in 13 patients. Other changes were observed less frequently.

Of those 18 patients, only 2 had clinical symptoms (dyspnea/desaturation on room air). This is unsurprising as the changes mentioned above can be local only or scar tissue in the case of septal thickening. None had a concomitant viral, bacterial, or fungal infection. Over time patients showed fluctuation of CT patterns with no clear influence of treatment choices nor any continuous worsening. Pulmonary function tests were available for 15/18 patients: 6 had a restrictive pattern and 2 had an obstructive pattern. DLCO was pathological in 12/15 (67%).

Interestingly 78% (14) of patients with pulmonary abnormalities had an unclassified ALPS, 3 patients had ALPS-FAS, and 1 had ALPS-FASLG [27].

In conclusion patients with ALPS-FAS or ALPS-FASLG seem to have only rarely pulmonary manifestations. On the other hand, patients with unclassified/undetermined ALPS should be followed up more closely with yearly pulmonary function tests including spirometry, body plethysmography, and CO diffusion as they might develop pulmonary manifestations more frequently. Additionally, patients with unclassified ALPS warrant further immunological investigations as they might have another underlying disease, e.g., STAT3 and STAT1 gain-of-function mutations, APDS mutations, LRBA, or CTLA-4 deficiencies, all known for severe pulmonary involvement (see Sect. 5.3) [27].

5.3.3 Management

Treatment with the mTOR inhibitor, sirolimus, is becoming the first-line therapy for ALPS patients [28]. Its effects on the lymphoproliferation are indisputable – possible positive effects on pulmonary involvement might be secondary in nature. Especially patients with unclassified ALPS might benefit from repeated and invasive pulmonary investigations (histology and microbiology). Treatment should be carried according to the identified obstructive or restrictive lung disease and/or identified microbial agent.

5.3.4 Pulmonary Manifestations of Other Autoimmune Lymphoproliferative Diseases

Caspase-8 deficiency does show a more severe clinical phenotype than ALPS due to activation defect in both B-cells and T-cells. It has been termed caspase-8 deficiency state (CEDS) and is no longer part of the ALPS classification [21]. Niemela et al. described two patients with caspase-8 deficiency: one with pulmonary hypertension and interstitial lung disease that deteriorated quickly leading to lung transplant and the other one with recurrent pulmonary infections leading to bronchiectasis [29]. These two patients showed recurrent sinusitis, bronchitis, and pneumonia [30]. These manifestations are similar to those in combined immunodeficiencies.

Fas-associated via death domain (FADD) deficiency is characterized by ALPS-like features plus severe bacterial and viral infections. Two patients manifested invasive pneumococcal infection due to functional hyposplenism. No further data are available on pulmonary manifestations [31].

Patients with activating *NRAS* (OMIM*164790) or *KRAS* (OMIM*190070) mutations, described as RAS-associated autoimmune leukoproliferative disease (RALD), so far have not been reported to suffer from pulmonary manifestations [32, 33].

5.4 Autoimmune Lymphoproliferative Syndromes with Primary Immunodeficiency (ALPID) (STAT1 and STAT3 Gain-of-Function, APDS1 and APDS2, CTLA-4 Deficiency, LRBA Deficiency)

5.4.1 Background

Conditions caused by *STAT1* and *STAT3* gain-of-function mutations, activated phosphoinositide 3-kinase-δ syndrome (APDS) 1 (caused by mutations in *PIK3CD*) and 2 (mutations in *PIK3R1*) deficiency, CTLA-4 deficiency, and LRBA deficiency traditionally were counted among antibody deficiencies, combined immunodeficiencies, or autoimmune lymphoproliferative syndromes. They all show features of autoimmunity and lymphoproliferation as well as primary immunodeficiency, therefore, termed ALPID to differentiate them from ALPS. Patients with ALPID disease often present with a more severe clinical course with hypogammaglobulinemia and susceptibility to infections than ALPDS patients.

5.4.2 STAT1 and STAT3 Gain-of-Function

The signal transducer and activator of transcription 1 (*STAT1*, OMIN*600555) play a crucial role in different interferon and interleukin pathways impairing, among others, Th17 cell responses [34].

Different types of loss-of-function mutations in *STAT1*, both autosomal-dominant and recessive, are described elsewhere. *STAT1* gain-of-function (GOF) mutations (OMIN*614162) were first described in patients with chronic mucocutaneous candidiasis, but patients with a heterogeneous clinical and immunological phenotype are increasingly recognized [34, 35].

Clinical presentation includes early childhood onset chronic mucocutaneous candidiasis, bacterial infections affecting the respiratory tract in almost half of the patients, as well as viral infections. Additionally, autoimmune features including hypothyroidism, autoimmune hepatitis, diabetes, autoimmune cytopenias, and others were described [35, 36]. In some patients the course of disease is intense and resembles a combined immunodeficiency. Interestingly, nonimmune manifestations such as aneurysms, neurological abnormalities, and carcinomas are not uncommon in patients with *STAT1* GOF [36].

Lower respiratory tract infections occur early. Chronic or frequent infections as well as a noninfectious inflammatory component that is incompletely understood as of yet lead to chronic pulmonary changes with bronchiectasis and obstructive airway disease and are a major mortality factor in *STAT1* GOF-affected individuals [35–37]. HLH has been reported in at least one patient with *STAT1* GOF, and the same implications for pulmonary manifestations apply as laid out in Sect. 5.2.2 [38].

Early detection and treatment of infection are paramount to prevent permanent lung damage, and some patients will need long-term antibiotic prophylaxis [35, 39]. HSCT is a treatment option in *STAT1* GOF, but outcome needs to be improved with an overall survival of 40% in a cohort of 15 patients [38]. First reports are emerging that specific *STAT1*-directed therapy with ruxolitinib, a Janus kinase inhibitor, might be a therapeutic option for patients who are not eligible for HSCT. It might improve susceptibility to infections and autoimmune manifestations, but therapy needs to be closely monitored for potential opportunistic infections including JC virus-induced progressive multifocal leukoencephalopathy [39–41].

STAT3 (OMIM*102582) GOF mutations lead via impaired T-cell signaling pathways to a variable phenotype termed ADMIO1 (autoimmune disease, multisystem, infantile-onset 1) (OMIM*615952).

Patients with *STAT3*-GOF mutations are prone to autoimmune conditions including enteropathy, type 1 diabetes mellitus, cytopenias, lymphoid interstitial lung disease, as well as lymphoproliferation, large granular lymphocytic (LGL) leukemia, and short stature [39]. Some patients present with a combination of clinical features as seen in IPEX syndrome (Sect. 5.11), but especially patients affected by the lymphoid interstitial lung disease share clinical features with patients with STAT5b deficiency (Sect. 5.13) [42].

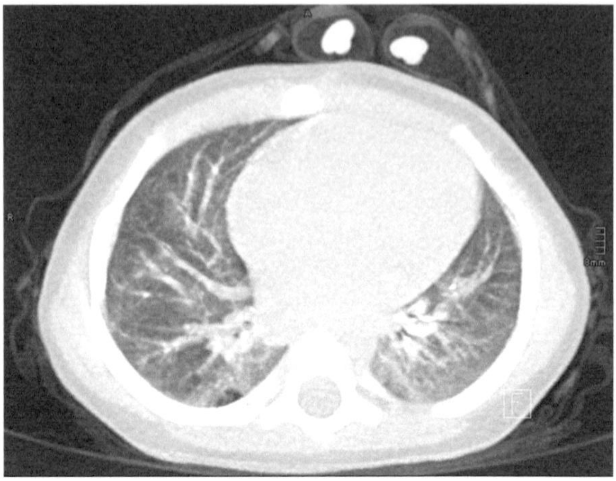

Fig. 5.1 Chest CT of a 5-year-old boy with STAT1 gain-of-function mutation. Chronic parenchymal lung changes with ground-glass opacities

Patients require immunosuppressive treatment to control autoimmunity and lymphoproliferation [43]. The anti-IL-6 antibody, tocilizumab, has been administered to some few patients with success [42]. If ruxolitinib also possesses therapeutic potential in *STAT3*-GOF, patients still need prospective evaluation. Other therapeutic agents that target the *STAT3* signaling pathway are being developed and hold promise for individuals with *STAT3*-GOF mutations [44]. Regarding pulmonary manifestations, no specific therapeutic regimen has been established, and patients should be monitored regularly to identify possible deterioration early on (Fig. 5.1).

5.4.3 Activated Phosphoinositide 3-Kinase-δ Syndrome 1 and 2 (APDS1 and APDS2)

Activated phosphoinositide 3-kinase-δ syndrome (APDS) is a clinically heterogeneous syndrome consisting of two entities caused by either mutation in the *PIK3CD* gene (OMIM*602839) leading to APDS1 (OMIM#615513) or mutation in *PIK3R1* (OMIM*171833) leading to APDS2 (OMIM#616005). PI3Kδ is a heterodimeric enzyme consisting of p85α regulatory subunit (PIK3CD) and a p110δ subunit (PIK3R1). Both gain-of-function and loss-of-function mutations have been described highlighting the importance of this enzyme's regulation for both correct T- and B-cell functioning, thus leading to a combined immunodeficiency [45].

Loss-of-function mutations only have been described in few patients who presented with recurrent sinopulmonary infections, severe B-cell lymphopenia resulting in hypo-/agammaglobulinemia, and autoimmune conditions including inflammatory bowel disease, hepatitis, and lymphoproliferation [46, 47].

GOF mutations lead to increased T-cell senescence and death and increased number of Tregs and transitional B-cells but reduced class-switch recombination and somatic hypermutation leading to immunodeficiency and B-cell lymphoma. Loss-of-function mutations present with reduced T-cell responses and less T-cell

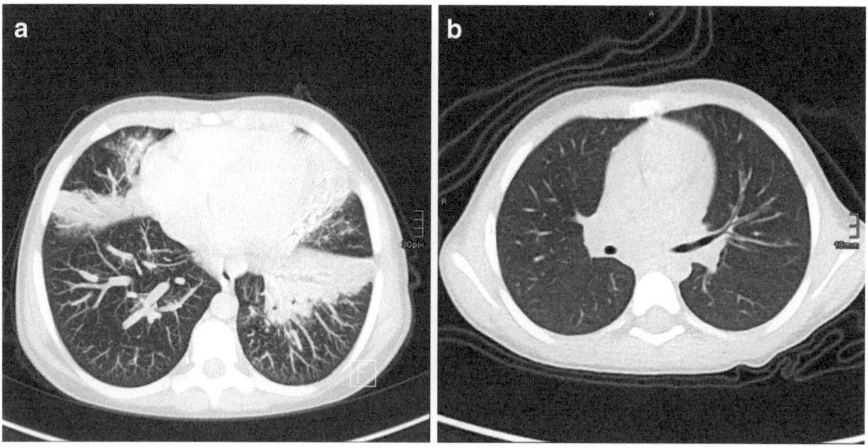

Fig. 5.2 (**a**) Chest CT of a 9-year-old boy with APDS1. Areal hyperintensities in the right middle lobe and the left lower lobe with positive bronchoaerogram and signs of bronchiectasis. Several small speckled consolidations (see red circle). (**b**) Chest CT of a 6-year-old girl with APDS2 and bronchiectasis

cytokine production as well as reduced Tregs and B-cells [45]. Especially the affected regulatory T-cells inflict autoimmune complications.

Activating mutations in *PIK3CD* and *PIK3R1* show a similar clinical phenotype [48]. Patients present with B-cell dysfunction (e.g., impaired vaccine responses) and susceptibility to respiratory infections with encapsulated bacteria such as *Haemophilus influenzae* and *Streptococcus pneumoniae* which are not alleviated by immunoglobulin replacement therapy [45, 49–52].

The two largest cohorts published so far describe respiratory infections in 98–100% of patients with APDS1 [48] and APDS2 [53], pneumonitis in 71%, and bronchiectasis in 18–60%. On CT scan, patients presented with air-space opacities, tree-in-bud opacities, bronchial wall thickening, mosaic attenuation, and bronchiectasis [48]. Abnormal T-cell function leads to recurrent viral infection mostly by EBV or CMV [48, 51, 52].

Treatment consists of immunoglobulin replacement therapy, rapamycin, and HSCT [48, 50]. The PI3Kδ inhibitor, idelalisib, administered orally showed very promising results regarding the lymphoproliferation of affected patients in a clinical trial [54]. Meanwhile, another trial for an inhaled form with a better safety profile is under way (NCT02593539) (Fig. 5.2).

5.4.4 CTLA-4 Deficiency

The protein cytotoxic T-lymphocyte-associated-4 (*CTLA-4*) (OMIM*123890) is essential for inhibitory regulation of immune responses. Mutations in *CTLA-4* cause the autosomal-dominant CTLA-4 deficiency (OMIM#616100) [55] with

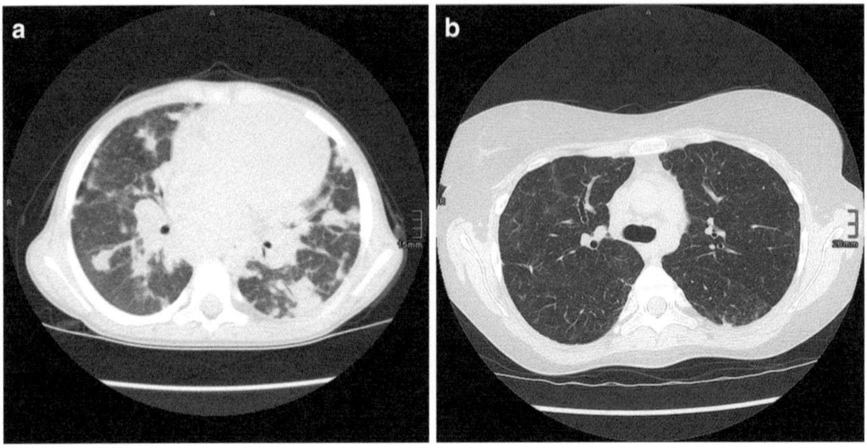

Fig. 5.3 (**a**) Chest CT of a 6-year-old boy with CTLA-4 deficiency. Multiple round infiltrates resembling reversed halo (or atoll) signs as evidence of granulomatous-lymphocytic lung disease. (**b**) Chest CT of a 23-year-old woman with CTLA-4 deficiency. Mosaic attenuation and bronchiectasis

dysregulation of regulatory T-cells, increased activation of T effector cells, and lymphocytic organ infiltration [56].

Patients typically present with features of immune dysregulation, e.g., cytopenias, enteropathy, diabetes, and hepatosplenomegaly [55, 57]. Even though CTLA-4 is essentially a disorder with hyperactive, poorly controlled, T lymphocytes, no episodes of HLH have been reported so far in CTLA-4 deficiency.

Pulmonary manifestations of CTLA-4 deficiency include recurrent bronchopulmonary infections, bronchiectasis, pulmonary fibrosis, and granulomatous-lymphocytic lung disease (GLILD) in up to 2/3 of patients [55, 56].

Treatment needs to be directed both at the immunodeficient and the immune dysregulatory aspects of CTLA-4 deficiency. Immunoglobulins and steroids, sometimes in combination or with additional steroid-sparing agents like sirolimus, rituximab, and others, have been administered to CTLA-4-deficient patients [57]. With abatacept, there is a CTLA-4 fusion protein available that can possibly present a targeted approach for affected patients. The few existing reports so far show a positive response [58, 59]. HSCT was performed in eight patients with CTLA-4 deficiency. Six patients are alive and well, but especially the persisting diabetes in some patients urges at early diagnosis and treatment [60] (Fig. 5.3).

5.4.5 LRBA Deficiency

The autosomal-recessive LRBA deficiency (OMIM#614700) is caused by mutations in the lipopolysaccharide-responsive, beige-like anchor protein gene *LRBA* (OMIM*606453). *LRBA* plays an important role in intracellular trafficking and degradation of *CTLA-4* (see above), and LRBA deficiency leads to increased turnover and, therefore, lower level of CTLA-4. Clinical manifestations include early-onset hypogammaglobulinemia due to impaired B-cell development causing recurrent infections, particularly affecting the respiratory tract, as well as autoimmune manifestations as autoimmune hemolytic anemia, idiopathic thrombocytopenic purpura, and inflammatory bowel disease [61–63].

Apart from recurrent bronchopulmonary infections, patients can develop bronchiectasis often following granulomatous-lymphocytic interstitial lung disease. In a cohort of 21 patients, 11 (52%) had abnormal pulmonary findings, and 8 (38%) had granulomatous-lymphocytic pulmonary disease [62]. Diagnosis of GLILD has to be established by HRCT. Treatment includes supportive care, ventilation, and immunosuppression [64].

As the clinical manifestation can be variable, treatment has to be adapted accordingly from immunoglobulin substitution to immunosuppression, control lymphoproliferation, and HSCT in severe cases. The CTLA-4 fusion protein, abatacept, has been used with excellent results improving both symptoms of autoimmunity and lung function tests and pulmonary changes evident of CT in patients with LRBA deficiency [65] (Fig. 5.4).

5.5 Chédiak-Higashi Syndrome (CHS)

The clinical manifestations of the autosomal-recessive Chédiak-Higashi syndrome (OMIM#214500) are variable. As patients with CHS suffer from a lack of natural killer cell function, they are at risk for infections, including pulmonary infections. Patients show variable oculocutaneous albinism, a bleeding tendency, and a progressive neurological involvement.

Mutations in the *LYST* gene (OMIM*606897) lead to incorrect formation of intracellular granula. Most patients progress to the "accelerated phase" of the disease, which can be clinically indistinguishable from the full picture of HLH and should be treated as such [66]. The pulmonary manifestations in the accelerated phase can be similar to those of HLH (see above). HSCT is the only therapeutic option, and patients' outcome is better if they are transplanted before the accelerated stage [67].

Mouse models for CHS do show pulmonary abnormalities even in the absence of HLH, especially lymphocytic infiltration and fibrosis, even in the absence of an infectious trigger [68]. Details on human lung samples or clinical signs of pulmonary involvement have not been reported.

5.6 Griscelli Syndrome, Type 2

Patients with Griscelli syndrome type 2 (OMIM#607624) have a pronounced form of albinism, hypogammaglobulinemia, and sometimes severe neurological impairment and are at high risk for HLH. Therefore, they are at the same risk for

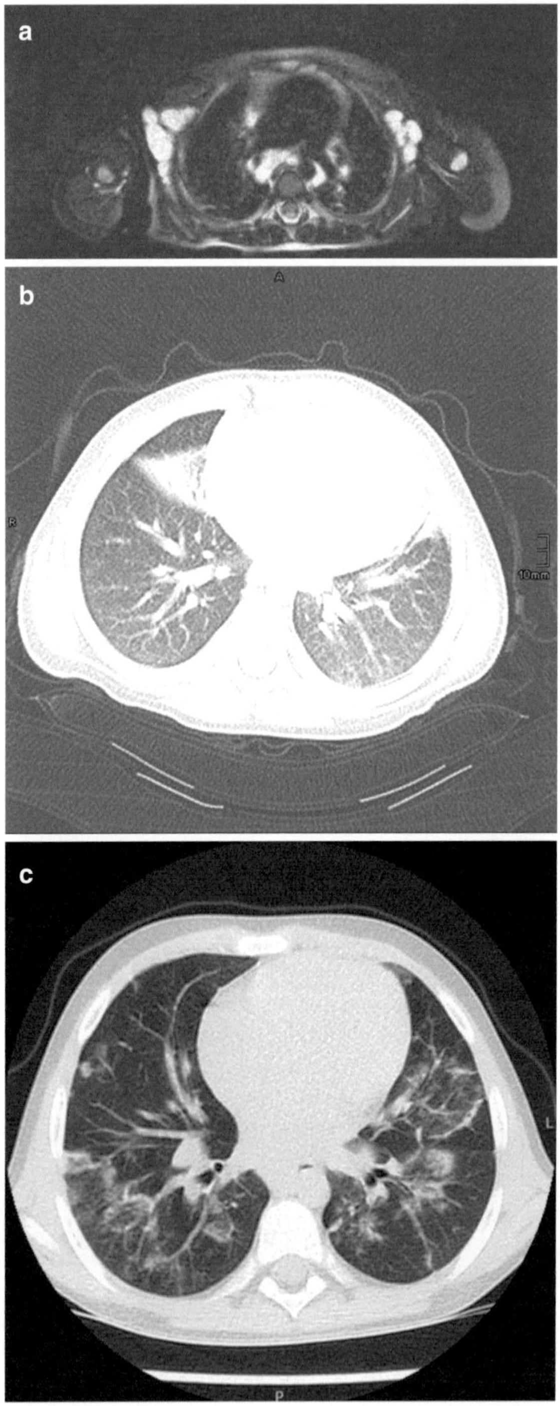

Fig. 5.4 (**a**) Chest MRI of a 1-year-old girl with LRBA deficiency. Enlargement of axillary and mediastinal lymph nodes. (**b**) Chest CT of the same patient with areal infiltrates and bronchoaerogram. (**c**) Chest CT of a 9-year-old girl with LRBA deficiency. Atypical and confluent, partly spot-shaped infiltrates suggestive of granulomatous-lymphocytic lung disease

pulmonary manifestations as outlined above [11, 69]. No typical pulmonary manifestation has been reported, but patients have an increased risk for EBV-induced illness [69]. One patient developed EBV-induced pulmonary lymphomatoid granulomatosis [70], and anti-EBV-directed therapy was successful in this case. Patients should be monitored closely for symptoms of HLH and EBV infection. However, HSCT is the curative option.

5.7 Hermansky-Pudlak Syndrome (Type 2, Type 9, Type 10)

Clinical manifestations in Hermansky-Pudlak syndrome (HPS) include bleeding abnormalities, neutropenia, oculocutaneous albinism, and, in some cases, facial dysmorphisms, hepatosplenomegaly, and susceptibility to bacterial infections. As yet ten different subtypes of HPS have been described.

Pulmonary fibrosis has been reported in patients with HPS types 1, 2, and 4, which carries a high mortality risk in combination with pneumonia [71–75]. Other subtypes of HPS might have a lower risk for pulmonary complications.

HPS type 2 (OMIM#608233) due to mutations in *AP3B1* (OMIM*603401) has a severe immunological phenotype. Affected children are at high risk to develop pulmonary fibrosis – in contrast to patients with HPS type 1. These patients suffer from less infectious complications and only develop the disease as middle-aged adults [71]. The observed pathology in affected individuals could also be demonstrated in animal models (pale ear/pearl mice). Mice showed enlargement of type II pneumocytes, increased levels of surfactant protein-B and protein-C in lung tissue, pulmonary fibrosis, and increased levels of TGF-beta in bronchoalveolar lavage [76–78]. Dysregulated surfactant trafficking and secretion and alveolar epithelial cell type II stress and apoptosis were also reported [79].

One of the two patients so far reported with HPS type 9 showed increased cutaneous infections, but none had a clear pulmonary phenotype [80, 81].

One patient has been reported with a homozygous mutation in *AP3D1* (OMIM*607246) causing HPS type 10 (OMIM#617050). He had a similar phenotype like HPS type 2 but with severe neurological manifestations. This patient also demonstrated chronic interstitial pneumonia [82].

The risk for HLH is not as high as in Griscelli syndrome type 2, so a preemptive HSCT cannot be recommended at this point [83]. Patients with HPS, especially types 1, 2, 4, and 10, should be closely monitored for changes in pulmonary function tests or in radiographic imaging. Early infection control and appropriate treatment might halt or delay the development of pulmonary fibrosis.

5.8 Other Immunodeficiencies Associated with Hypopigmentation (p14 Deficiency, Vici Syndrome)

Vici syndrome (OMIM#242840) is a multisystem disorder of defective autophagy caused by mutations in *EPG5* (OMIM*615068) and presents with hypopigmentation and immunodeficiency as well as severe neurological manifestations [84, 85].

P14-deficient patients (OMIM#610798) have oculocutaneous albinism, hypogammaglobulinemia, neutropenia, and impaired function of cytotoxic T-cells [86]. The underlying cause is mutations in untranslated regions of the adaptor molecule *P14* (OMIM*610389) that leads to false procession of p14 mRNA.

Due to the underlying immunodeficiency in both conditions, patients can present with infections, including severe bronchopulmonary infections, as did the patients with p-14 deficiency reported so far [86]. Especially in the patients who also suffered from hypogammaglobulinemia, immunoglobulin replacement therapy is an option.

5.9 X-Linked Lymphoproliferative Syndromes (SH2D1A Deficiency, XIAP Deficiency, MAGT1 Deficiency)

Three different diseases caused by mutations in X-chromosome-encoded genes have been described so far that present with EBV-triggered lymphoproliferation.

SAP deficiency (OMIM#308240) or X-linked lymphoproliferative syndrome 1 (XLP-1) occurs due to loss-of-function mutations in *SAP/SH2D1A* (OMIM*300490), and the patients have over 50% risk to develop HLH after EBV infection [87]. When patients survive the marked infectious mononucleosis, they sometimes do develop dys- or hypogammaglobulinemias which carry an increased risk for bronchopulmonary infections and their sequelae.

Mutations in *XIAP/BIRC4* (OMIM*300079) cause XIAP deficiency or XLP-2 (OMIM#300635). Up to 80% of affected individuals experience HLH episodes that can reoccur, but other autoimmune phenomena might be present in over 60% of patients as the initial manifestation [88]. Some authors warrant the term "X-linked familiar HLH" to highlight the risk of recurring HLH [89].

Both XLP-1 and XLP-2 therefore carry the risk of pulmonary involvement in HLH as outlined above. For patients with XLP-1, granulomatous-lymphocytic interstitial lung disease has been reported as well [90]. Patients with XLP-1 should receive HSCT, because they are at risk of developing not only HLH but also lymphoma [91]. For XLP-2, HSCT is also a treatment option, but results on outcome have been mixed. Therefore, patients may overcome their risk for recurrent HLH episodes with conservative treatment [88, 92]. In cases presenting with uncontrolled autoimmune conditions, e.g., Crohn's-like disease, HSCT might also be curative [88, 93].

Patients with mutations in the magnesium transporter *MAGT1* (OMIM*300715) causing magnesium defect, EBV infection, and neoplasia (XMEN) (OMIM#300853) show respiratory tract infections, viral pneumonias, chronic diarrhea, and chronic EBV infection leading to EBV-associated lymphoma [94]. Infection control and close monitoring are the therapeutic recommendations until data on more patients become available.

5.10 Autosomal-Recessive Lymphoproliferative Syndromes (ITK Deficiency, CD27 Deficiency, CD70 Deficiency)

Molecular defects in the IL-2-inducable T-cell kinase (*ITK*, OMIM*186973) or mutations in *CD27* (OMIM*186711) can show similar clinical manifestations like the X-linked lymphoproliferative syndromes but are transmitted in an autosomal-recessive fashion (Sect. 5.8).

All patients with ITK deficiency reported so far did present with EBV-induced lymphoproliferation. Many patients suffered from early manifestation of Hodgkin's lymphoma. In the majority of patients reported with ITK deficiency, pulmonary involvement with large interstitial nodules as sign of EBV-induced lymphoproliferation could be identified [95–97].

HSCT is a curative option for patients with ITK deficiency, but the B-cell lymphoproliferative lung involvement can (at least transiently) respond to rituximab as well [97].

CD27 deficiency may present more variably with asymptomatic memory B-cell deficiency, chronic symptomatic EBV viremia, and lymphoma induced by EBV [98–100]. At least three patients with CD27 deficiency did suffer from recurrent pneumonias or episodes of bronchitis in the context of hypogammaglobulinemia [99]. They might benefit from immunoglobulin replacement therapy. Experience on HSCT in CD27 deficiency is limited to two patients who were transplanted successfully.

CD70 deficiency is a clinical phenocopy of CD27 deficiency, and patients may suffer from bronchopulmonary infections related to hypogammaglobulinemia. A typical manifestation is the susceptibility to EBV-related diseases [101].

5.11 Immune Dysregulation, Polyendocrinopathy, Enteropathy, X-Linked (IPEX)

In immune dysregulation, polyendocrinopathy, enteropathy, X-linked (IPEX, OMIM#304790) syndrome due to mutations in *FOXP3* (OMIM*300292) instable *FOXP3* expression leads to dysfunction of regulatory T-cells (Tregs). Immunodysregulative features are the hallmark of the disease, mainly pronounced diarrhea, insulin-dependent diabetes mellitus, and eczema typically in the first few months of life. One recent publication demonstrated pulmonary involvement without specifying its nature, in more detail in 16/96 patients with IPEX syndrome. Under immunosuppressive therapy alone, pulmonary complications increased over time from 15% to 24% in a cohort of 34 IPEX patients. Episodes of acute respiratory distress syndrome and pneumonia accounted for two out of four deaths in this cohort. Patients with pulmonary involvement before HSCT also have a worse outcome than those without pulmonary involvement [102]. Immunosuppressive therapy is only warranted for short-term symptom control and seems to be unable to control pulmonary involvement. HSCT is the only curative option available for patients with IPEX syndrome [102, 103].

Animal data on FOXP3-deficient mice could show that chronic antigen stimulation through the airways leads to a similar picture of lymphoid involvement in the lung suggesting a pivotal role of regulatory T-cells in autoimmune lung disease [104]. Both CD25 (Sect. 5.11) and STAT5b (Sect. 5.12) play a role in the activation of Tregs, and their respective deficiency can cause pulmonary involvement.

5.12 CD25 Deficiency

CD25 deficiency (OMIM#606367) has features of both SCID-like immunodeficiency and immune dysregulation. Mutations in *IL2RA*/CD25 (OMIM*147730) cause defects in the α chain of the high-affinity interleukin-2 (IL-2) receptor. Clinical presentation includes pronounced chronic diarrhea manifesting in the first year of life, insulin-dependent diabetes mellitus, and other autoimmune features. Early-onset CMV pneumonitis, susceptibility to other bronchopulmonary infections, and follicular bronchiolitis with lymphocytic hyperplasia have been reported in CD25-deficient patients [105–108]. A combination of supportive care, immunosuppression, and HSCT was applied to these patients. Pulmonary symptoms improved under a combined immunosuppressive protocol in one patient [108]. Therapy with IL-2 might also be an option (Fig. 5.5).

5.13 STAT5b Deficiency

Growth failure insensitive to therapy with growth hormone, autoimmune features, and immunodeficiency are hallmarks of STAT5b deficiency (OMIN#245590) [109]. Severe, sometimes fatal, pneumonitis or lymphoid interstitial pneumonia has been reported in nine out of ten patients with STAT5b deficiency [110].

The pneumonitis remains difficult to treat and no standard concept could be established so far. All patients with STAT5b deficiency should undergo regular pulmonary function tests and clinical examination for follow-up and to attempt early treatment. Symptomatic therapy is warranted and especially the growth failure

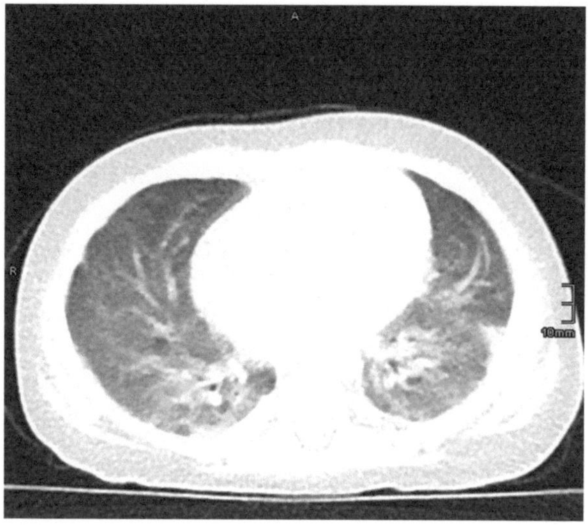

Fig. 5.5 (**a**) Chest CT of a 10-month-old patient with CD25 deficiency. Focal hyperinflation and ground-glass opacities as well as chronic changes to the lung parenchyma. Reactive lymphoproliferation

remains difficult to treat. Future therapy might be able to enhance specific targets in the STAT5b pathway and provide an interesting therapeutic approach [110, 111].

5.14 ITCH Deficiency

ITCH deficiency (OMIM#613385) has been reported in an extended Amish family and is characterized by failure to thrive, developmental delay, relative macrocephaly, hepatosplenomegaly, and chronic lung disease. Three of the ten patients reported so far died following respiratory complications in early childhood (under 3 years of age). The pulmonary phenotype showed an obstructive pattern that resembled asthmatic patients. In one biopsy chronic interstitial bronchitis was described [112]. Immunosuppressive treatment can alleviate some of the autoimmune phenomena, but no data are available on optimal management of the pulmonary complications apart from supportive and possibly inhalative care.

5.15 COPA Deficiency

Individuals with coatomer protein complex subunit alpha (COPA) deficiency (OMIM#616414) experience autoimmune phenomena such as interstitial lung disease and joint or kidney involvement caused by production of autoantibodies due to dysregulation in the COPA protein by mutations in the *COPA* gene (OMIM*601924) [113]. So far, five families with interstitial lung disease have been described; 14/21 of reported patients presented with respiratory symptoms including tachypnea, cough, or hemoptysis on initial presentation; and all patients were found to have interstitial lung disease. Lung biopsies revealed marked interstitial lymphocytic infiltration comparable to lung involvement in other systemic autoimmune diseases [114]. Immunosuppressive treatment is needed to control the autoimmunity.

5.16 Conclusion

In conclusion not enough is known about pulmonary manifestations and complications in genetic disorders of immune regulation. Consequently, it is sensible to order pulmonary function tests including spirometry, body plethysmography, and CO-diffusion even in asymptomatic patients at least once per year to identify pathological changes early in the course of disease. Many syndromes presented in this chapter show an increased rate of malignancies that might be further elevated by the use of ionizing radiation. Chest X-rays are not sensitive enough to capture all abnormalities. Gold standard for the diagnosis of interstitial lung diseases is a chest CT, but its use is only warranted if, e.g., a reduced diffusion capacity could be demonstrated in a patient. Pathological lung function test results should be discussed with a pulmonologist interested in immunology.

References

1. Filipovich AH. Hemophagocytic lymphohistiocytosis (HLH) and related disorders. Hematology Am Soc Hematol Educ Program. 2009:127–31. https://doi.org/10.1182/asheducation-2009.1.127.
2. Stepp SE, Dufourcq-Lagelouse R, Kumar V. Pillars article: Perforin gene defects in familial hemophagocytic lymphohistiocytosis. Science. 1999. 286: 1957–1959. J Immunol. 2015;194(11):5044–6.
3. Stepp SE, Dufourcq-Lagelouse R, Le Deist F, Bhawan S, Certain S, Mathew PA, et al. Perforin gene defects in familial hemophagocytic lymphohistiocytosis. Science. 1999;286(5446):1957–9.
4. Feldmann J, Callebaut I, Raposo G, Certain S, Bacq D, Dumont C, et al. Munc13-4 is essential for cytolytic granules fusion and is mutated in a form of familial hemophagocytic lymphohistiocytosis (FHL3). Cell. 2003;115(4):461–73.
5. zur Stadt U, Schmidt S, Kasper B, Beutel K, Diler AS, Henter JI, et al. Linkage of familial hemophagocytic lymphohistiocytosis (FHL) type-4 to chromosome 6q24 and identification of mutations in syntaxin 11. Hum Mol Genet. 2005;14(6):827–34.
6. Cote M, Menager MM, Burgess A, Mahlaoui N, Picard C, Schaffner C, et al. Munc18-2 deficiency causes familial hemophagocytic lymphohistiocytosis type 5 and impairs cytotoxic granule exocytosis in patient NK cells. J Clin Invest. 2009;119(12):3765–73.
7. zur Stadt U, Rohr J, Seifert W, Koch F, Grieve S, Pagel J, et al. Familial hemophagocytic lymphohistiocytosis type 5 (FHL-5) is caused by mutations in Munc18-2 and impaired binding to syntaxin 11. Am J Hum Genet. 2009;85(4):482–92.
8. Ohadi M, Lalloz MR, Sham P, Zhao J, Dearlove AM, Shiach C, et al. Localization of a gene for familial hemophagocytic lymphohistiocytosis at chromosome 9q21.3-22 by homozygosity mapping. Am J Hum Genet. 1999;64(1):165–71.

9. Bode SF, Lehmberg K, Maul-Pavicic A, Vraetz T, Janka G, Stadt UZ, et al. Recent advances in the diagnosis and treatment of hemophagocytic lymphohistiocytosis. Arthritis Res Ther. 2012;14(3):213.
10. Henter JI, Horne A, Arico M, Egeler RM, Filipovich AH, Imashuku S, et al. HLH-2004: Diagnostic and therapeutic guidelines for hemophagocytic lymphohistiocytosis. Pediatr Blood Cancer. 2007;48(2):124–31.
11. Seguin A, Galicier L, Boutboul D, Lemiale V, Azoulay E. Pulmonary involvement in patients with Hemophagocytic Lymphohistiocytosis. Chest. 2016;149(5):1294–301.
12. Ramachandran B, Balasubramanian S, Abhishek N, Ravikumar KG, Ramanan AV. Profile of hemophagocytic lymphohistiocytosis in children in a tertiary care hospital in India. Indian Pediatr. 2011;48(1):31–5.
13. Fitzgerald NE, MacClain KL. Imaging characteristics of hemophagocytic lymphohistiocytosis. Pediatr Radiol. 2003;33(6):392–401.
14. Jin YK, Xie ZD, Yang S, Lu G, Shen KL. Epstein-Barr virus-associated hemophagocytic lymphohistiocytosis: a retrospective study of 78 pediatric cases in mainland of China. Chin Med J (Engl). 2010;123(11):1426–30.
15. Rohr J, Beutel K, Maul-Pavicic A, Vraetz T, Thiel J, Warnatz K, et al. Atypical familial hemophagocytic lymphohistiocytosis due to mutations in UNC13D and STXBP2 overlaps with primary immunodeficiency diseases. Haematologica. 2010;95(12):2080–7.
16. Ost A, Nilsson-Ardnor S, Henter JI. Autopsy findings in 27 children with haemophagocytic lymphohistiocytosis. Histopathology. 1998;32(4):310–6.
17. Yoshida N, Ishii E, Oshima K, Yanai F, Ogawa A, Kataoka S, et al. Engraftment and dissemination of T lymphocytes from primary haemophagocytic lymphohistiocytosis in scid mice. Br J Haematol. 2003;121(2):349–58.
18. Sato K, Misawa N, Nie C, Satou Y, Iwakiri D, Matsuoka M, et al. A novel animal model of Epstein-Barr virus-associated hemophagocytic lymphohistiocytosis in humanized mice. Blood. 2011;117(21):5663–73.
19. Ouachee-Chardin M, Elie C, de Saint Basile G, Le Deist F, Mahlaoui N, Picard C, et al. Hematopoietic stem cell transplantation in hemophagocytic lymphohistiocytosis: a single-center report of 48 patients. Pediatrics. 2006;117(4):e743–50.
20. Bidere N, Su HC, Lenardo MJ. Genetic disorders of programmed cell death in the immune system. Annu Rev Immunol. 2006;24:321–52.
21. Oliveira JB, Bleesing JJ, Dianzani U, Fleisher TA, Jaffe ES, Lenardo MJ, et al. Revised diagnostic criteria and classification for the autoimmune lymphoproliferative syndrome (ALPS): report from the 2009 NIH international workshop. Blood. 2010;116(14):e35–40.
22. Bleesing JJ, Brown MR, Straus SE, Dale JK, Siegel RM, Johnson M, et al. Immunophenotypic profiles in families with autoimmune lymphoproliferative syndrome. Blood. 2001;98(8):2466–73.
23. Lopatin U, Yao X, Williams RK, Bleesing JJ, Dale JK, Wong D, et al. Increases in circulating and lymphoid tissue interleukin-10 in autoimmune lymphoproliferative syndrome are associated with disease expression. Blood. 2001;97(10):3161–70.
24. Fuss IJ, Strober W, Dale JK, Fritz S, Pearlstein GR, Puck JM, et al. Characteristic T helper 2 T cell cytokine abnormalities in autoimmune lymphoproliferative syndrome, a syndrome marked by defective apoptosis and humoral autoimmunity. J Immunol. 1997;158(4):1912–8.
25. Volkl S, Rensing-Ehl A, Allgauer A, Schreiner E, Lorenz MR, Rohr J, et al. Hyperactive mTOR pathway promotes lymphoproliferation and abnormal differentiation in autoimmune lymphoproliferative syndrome. Blood. 2016;128(2):227–38.
26. Price S, Shaw PA, Seitz A, Joshi G, Davis J, Niemela JE, et al. Natural history of autoimmune lymphoproliferative syndrome associated with FAS gene mutations. Blood. 2014;123(13):1989–99.
27. Lau CY, Mihalek AD, Wang J, Dodd LE, Perkins K, Price S, et al. Pulmonary manifestations of the autoimmune lymphoproliferative syndrome. a retrospective study of a unique patient cohort. Ann Am Thorac Soc. 2016;13(8):1279–88.

28. Teachey DT. New advances in the diagnosis and treatment of autoimmune lymphoproliferative syndrome. Curr Opin Pediatr. 2012;24(1):1–8.
29. Niemela J, Kuehn HS, Kelly C, Zhang M, Davies J, Melendez J, et al. Caspase-8 deficiency presenting as late-onset multi-organ lymphocytic infiltration with granulomas in two adult siblings. J Clin Immunol. 2015;35(4):348–55.
30. Chun HJ, Zheng L, Ahmad M, Wang J, Speirs CK, Siegel RM, et al. Pleiotropic defects in lymphocyte activation caused by caspase-8 mutations lead to human immunodeficiency. Nature. 2002;419(6905):395–9.
31. Bolze A, Byun M, McDonald D, Morgan NV, Abhyankar A, Premkumar L, et al. Whole-exome-sequencing-based discovery of human FADD deficiency. Am J Hum Genet. 2010;87(6):873–81.
32. Niemela JE, Lu L, Fleisher TA, Davis J, Caminha I, Natter M, et al. Somatic KRAS mutations associated with a human nonmalignant syndrome of autoimmunity and abnormal leukocyte homeostasis. Blood. 2011;117(10):2883–6.
33. Oliveira JB, Bidere N, Niemela JE, Zheng L, Sakai K, Nix CP, et al. NRAS mutation causes a human autoimmune lymphoproliferative syndrome. Proc Natl Acad Sci U S A. 2007;104(21):8953–8.
34. Liu L, Okada S, Kong XF, Kreins AY, Cypowyj S, Abhyankar A, et al. Gain-of-function human STAT1 mutations impair IL-17 immunity and underlie chronic mucocutaneous candidiasis. J Exp Med. 2011;208(8):1635–48.
35. Dotta L, Scomodon O, Padoan R, Timpano S, Plebani A, Soresina A, et al. Clinical and immunological data of nine patients with chronic mucocutaneous candidiasis disease. Data Brief. 2016;7:311–5.
36. Toubiana J, Okada S, Hiller J, Oleastro M, Lagos Gomez M, Aldave Becerra JC, et al. Heterozygous STAT1 gain-of-function mutations underlie an unexpectedly broad clinical phenotype. Blood. 2016;127(25):3154–64.
37. Puel A, Cypowyj S, Marodi L, Abel L, Picard C, Casanova JL. Inborn errors of human IL-17 immunity underlie chronic mucocutaneous candidiasis. Curr Opin Allergy Clin Immunol. 2012;12(6):616–22.
38. Leiding JW, Okada S, Hagin D, Abinun M, Shcherbina A, Balashov DN, et al. Hematopoietic stem cell transplantation in patients with gain-of-function signal transducer and activator of transcription 1 mutations. J Allergy Clin Immunol. 2018;141(2):704–717.e5. https://doi.org/10.1016/j.jaci.2017.03.049. Epub 2017 Jun 7.
39. Consonni F, Dotta L, Todaro F, Vairo D, Badolato R. Signal transducer and activator of transcription gain-of-function primary immunodeficiency/immunodysregulation disorders. Curr Opin Pediatr. 2017;29(6):711–7.
40. Weinacht KG, Charbonnier LM, Alroqi F, Plant A, Qiao Q, Wu H, et al. Ruxolitinib reverses dysregulated T helper cell responses and controls autoimmunity caused by a novel signal transducer and activator of transcription 1 (STAT1) gain-of-function mutation. J Allergy Clin Immunol. 2017;139(5):1629–40 e2.
41. Notarangelo LD, Fleisher TA. Targeted strategies directed at the molecular defect: toward precision medicine for select primary immunodeficiency disorders. J Allergy Clin Immunol. 2017;139(3):715–23.
42. Milner JD, Vogel TP, Forbes L, Ma CA, Stray-Pedersen A, Niemela JE, et al. Early-onset lymphoproliferation and autoimmunity caused by germline STAT3 gain-of-function mutations. Blood. 2015;125(4):591–9.
43. Forbes LR, Milner J, Haddad E. Signal transducer and activator of transcription 3: a year in review. Curr Opin Hematol. 2016;23(1):23–7.
44. Siveen KS, Sikka S, Surana R, Dai X, Zhang J, Kumar AP, et al. Targeting the STAT3 signaling pathway in cancer: role of synthetic and natural inhibitors. Biochim Biophys Acta. 2014;1845(2):136–54.
45. Lucas CL, Chandra A, Nejentsev S, Condliffe AM, Okkenhaug K. PI3Kdelta and primary immunodeficiencies. Nat Rev Immunol. 2016;16(11):702–14.

46. Zhang KJ, Husami A, Marsh R, Jordan MB. Identification of a phosphoinositide 3-kinase (PI-3K) p110δ (PIK3CD) deficient individual. J Clin Immunol. 2013;33:673–4.
47. Conley ME, Dobbs AK, Quintana AM, Bosompem A, Wang YD, Coustan-Smith E, et al. Agammaglobulinemia and absent B lineage cells in a patient lacking the p85alpha subunit of PI3K. J Exp Med. 2012;209(3):463–70.
48. Coulter TI, Chandra A, Bacon CM, Babar J, Curtis J, Screaton N, et al. Clinical spectrum and features of activated phosphoinositide 3-kinase delta syndrome: a large patient cohort study. J Allergy Clin Immunol. 2017;139(2):597–606 e4.
49. Angulo I, Vadas O, Garcon F, Banham-Hall E, Plagnol V, Leahy TR, et al. Phosphoinositide 3-kinase delta gene mutation predisposes to respiratory infection and airway damage. Science. 2013;342(6160):866–71.
50. Lucas CL, Kuehn HS, Zhao F, Niemela JE, Deenick EK, Palendira U, et al. Dominant-activating germline mutations in the gene encoding the PI(3)K catalytic subunit p110delta result in T cell senescence and human immunodeficiency. Nat Immunol. 2014;15(1):88–97.
51. Lucas CL, Zhang Y, Venida A, Wang Y, Hughes J, McElwee J, et al. Heterozygous splice mutation in PIK3R1 causes human immunodeficiency with lymphoproliferation due to dominant activation of PI3K. J Exp Med. 2014;211(13):2537–47.
52. Deau MC, Heurtier L, Frange P, Suarez F, Bole-Feysot C, Nitschke P, et al. A human immunodeficiency caused by mutations in the PIK3R1 gene. J Clin Invest. 2015;125(4):1764–5.
53. Elkaim E, Neven B, Bruneau J, Mitsui-Sekinaka K, Stanislas A, Heurtier L, et al. Clinical and immunologic phenotype associated with activated phosphoinositide 3-kinase delta syndrome 2: a cohort study. J Allergy Clin Immunol. 2016;138(1):210–8 e9.
54. Rao VK, Webster S, Dalm V, Sediva A, van Hagen PM, Holland S, et al. Effective "activated PI3K delta syndrome"-targeted therapy with the PI3K delta inhibitor leniolisib. Blood. 2017;130(21):2307–16.
55. Schubert D, Bode C, Kenefeck R, Hou TZ, Wing JB, Kennedy A, et al. Autosomal dominant immune dysregulation syndrome in humans with CTLA4 mutations. Nat Med. 2014;20(12):1410–6.
56. Kuehn HS, Ouyang W, Lo B, Deenick EK, Niemela JE, Avery DT, et al. Immune dysregulation in human subjects with heterozygous germline mutations in CTLA4. Science. 2014;345(6204):1623–7.
57. Verma N, Burns SO, Walker LSK, Sansom DM. Immune deficiency and autoimmunity in patients with CTLA-4 (CD152) mutations. Clin Exp Immunol. 2017;190(1):1–7.
58. Lee S, Moon JS, Lee CR, Kim HE, Baek SM, Hwang S, et al. Abatacept alleviates severe autoimmune symptoms in a patient carrying a de novo variant in CTLA-4. J Allergy Clin Immunol. 2016;137(1):327–30.
59. Shields CL, Say EA, Mashayekhi A, Garg SJ, Dunn JP, Shields JA. Assessment of CTLA-4 deficiency-related autoimmune choroidopathy response to abatacept. JAMA Ophthalmol. 2016;134(7):844–6.
60. Slatter MA, Engelhardt KR, Burroughs LM, Arkwright PD, Nademi Z, Skoda-Smith S, et al. Hematopoietic stem cell transplantation for CTLA4 deficiency. J Allergy Clin Immunol. 2016;138(2):615–9 e1.
61. Lopez-Herrera G, Tampella G, Pan-Hammarstrom Q, Herholz P, Trujillo-Vargas CM, Phadwal K, et al. Deleterious mutations in LRBA are associated with a syndrome of immune deficiency and autoimmunity. Am J Hum Genet. 2012;90(6):986–1001.
62. Gamez-Diaz L, August D, Stepensky P, Revel-Vilk S, Seidel MG, Noriko M, et al. The extended phenotype of LPS-responsive beige-like anchor protein (LRBA) deficiency. J Allergy Clin Immunol. 2016;137(1):223–30.
63. Azizi G, Abolhassani H, Mahdaviani SA, Chavoshzadeh Z, Eshghi P, Yazdani R, et al. Clinical, immunologic, molecular analyses and outcomes of Iranian patients with LRBA deficiency: a longitudinal study. Pediatr Allergy Immunol. 2017;28(5):478–84.

64. Panchabhai TS, Farver C, Highland KB. Lymphocytic interstitial pneumonia. Clin Chest Med. 2016;37(3):463–74.
65. Lo B, Zhang K, Lu W, Zheng L, Zhang Q, Kanellopoulou C, et al. AUTOIMMUNE DISEASE. Patients with LRBA deficiency show CTLA4 loss and immune dysregulation responsive to abatacept therapy. Science. 2015;349(6246):436–40.
66. Kaplan J, De Domenico I, Ward DM. Chediak-Higashi syndrome. Curr Opin Hematol. 2008;15(1):22–9.
67. Eapen M, DeLaat CA, Baker KS, Cairo MS, Cowan MJ, Kurtzberg J, et al. Hematopoietic cell transplantation for Chediak-Higashi syndrome. Bone Marrow Transplant. 2007;39(7):411–5.
68. Tang X, Yamanaka S, Miyagi Y, Nagashima Y, Nakatani Y. Lung pathology of pale ear mouse (model of Hermansky-Pudlak syndrome 1) and beige mouse (model of Chediak-Higashi syndrome): severity of giant lamellar body degeneration of type II pneumocytes correlates with interstitial inflammation. Pathol Int. 2005;55(3):137–43.
69. Pachlopnik Schmid J, Moshous D, Boddaert N, Neven B, Dal Cortivo L, Tardieu M, et al. Hematopoietic stem cell transplantation in Griscelli syndrome type 2: a single-center report on 10 patients. Blood. 2009;114(1):211–8.
70. Szczawinska-Poplonyk A, Kycler Z, Breborowicz A, Klaudel-Dreszler M, Pac M, Zegadlo-Mylik M, et al. Pulmonary lymphomatoid granulomatosis in Griscelli syndrome type 2. Viral Immunol. 2011;24(6):471–3.
71. Gochuico BR, Huizing M, Golas GA, Scher CD, Tsokos M, Denver SD, et al. Interstitial lung disease and pulmonary fibrosis in Hermansky-Pudlak syndrome type 2, an adaptor protein-3 complex disease. Mol Med. 2012;18:56–64.
72. White DA, Smith GJ, Cooper JA Jr, Glickstein M, Rankin JA. Hermansky-pudlak syndrome and interstitial lung disease: report of a case with lavage findings. Am Rev Respir Dis. 1984;130(1):138–41.
73. Brantly M, Avila NA, Shotelersuk V, Lucero C, Huizing M, Gahl WA. Pulmonary function and high-resolution CT findings in patients with an inherited form of pulmonary fibrosis, Hermansky-Pudlak syndrome, due to mutations in HPS-1. Chest. 2000;117(1):129–36.
74. Gahl WA, Brantly M, Kaiser-Kupfer MI, Iwata F, Hazelwood S, Shotelersuk V, et al. Genetic defects and clinical characteristics of patients with a form of oculocutaneous albinism (Hermansky-Pudlak syndrome). N Engl J Med. 1998;338(18):1258–64.
75. Gahl WA, Brantly M, Troendle J, Avila NA, Padua A, Montalvo C, et al. Effect of pirfenidone on the pulmonary fibrosis of Hermansky-Pudlak syndrome. Mol Genet Metab. 2002;76(3):234–42.
76. Lyerla TA, Rusiniak ME, Borchers M, Jahreis G, Tan J, Ohtake P, et al. Aberrant lung structure, composition, and function in a murine model of Hermansky-Pudlak syndrome. Am J Physiol Lung Cell Mol Physiol. 2003;285(3):L643–53.
77. Wang L, Lyerla T. Histochemical and cellular changes accompanying the appearance of lung fibrosis in an experimental mouse model for Hermansky Pudlak syndrome. Histochem Cell Biol. 2010;134(2):205–13.
78. Guttentag SH, Akhtar A, Tao JQ, Atochina E, Rusiniak ME, Swank RT, et al. Defective surfactant secretion in a mouse model of Hermansky-Pudlak syndrome. Am J Respir Cell Mol Biol. 2005;33(1):14–21.
79. Mahavadi P, Korfei M, Henneke I, Liebisch G, Schmitz G, Gochuico BR, et al. Epithelial stress and apoptosis underlie Hermansky-Pudlak syndrome-associated interstitial pneumonia. Am J Respir Crit Care Med. 2010;182(2):207–19.
80. Badolato R, Prandini A, Caracciolo S, Colombo F, Tabellini G, Giacomelli M, et al. Exome sequencing reveals a pallidin mutation in a Hermansky-Pudlak-like primary immunodeficiency syndrome. Blood. 2012;119(13):3185–7.
81. Cullinane AR, Curry JA, Carmona-Rivera C, Summers CG, Ciccone C, Cardillo ND, et al. A BLOC-1 mutation screen reveals that PLDN is mutated in Hermansky-Pudlak syndrome type 9. Am J Hum Genet. 2011;88(6):778–87.

82. Ammann S, Schulz A, Krageloh-Mann I, Dieckmann NM, Niethammer K, Fuchs S, et al. Mutations in AP3D1 associated with immunodeficiency and seizures define a new type of Hermansky-Pudlak syndrome. Blood. 2016;127(8):997–1006.
83. Jessen B, Bode SF, Ammann S, Chakravorty S, Davies G, Diestelhorst J, et al. The risk of hemophagocytic lymphohistiocytosis in Hermansky-Pudlak syndrome type 2. Blood. 2013;121(15):2943–51.
84. del Campo M, Hall BD, Aeby A, Nassogne MC, Verloes A, Roche C, et al. Albinism and agenesis of the corpus callosum with profound developmental delay: Vici syndrome, evidence for autosomal recessive inheritance. Am J Med Genet. 1999;85(5):479–85.
85. Finocchi A, Angelino G, Cantarutti N, Corbari M, Bevivino E, Cascioli S, et al. Immunodeficiency in Vici syndrome: a heterogeneous phenotype. Am J Med Genet A. 2012;158A(2):434–9.
86. Bohn G, Allroth A, Brandes G, Thiel J, Glocker E, Schaffer AA, et al. A novel human primary immunodeficiency syndrome caused by deficiency of the endosomal adaptor protein p14. Nat Med. 2007;13(1):38–45.
87. Pachlopnik Schmid J, Canioni D, Moshous D, Touzot F, Mahlaoui N, Hauck F, et al. Clinical similarities and differences of patients with X-linked lymphoproliferative syndrome type 1 (XLP-1/SAP deficiency) versus type 2 (XLP-2/XIAP deficiency). Blood. 2011;117(5):1522–9.
88. Speckmann C, Lehmberg K, Albert MH, Damgaard RB, Fritsch M, Gyrd-Hansen M, et al. X-linked inhibitor of apoptosis (XIAP) deficiency: the spectrum of presenting manifestations beyond hemophagocytic lymphohistiocytosis. Clin Immunol. 2013;149(1):133–41.
89. Marsh RA, Madden L, Kitchen BJ, Mody R, McClimon B, Jordan MB, et al. XIAP deficiency: a unique primary immunodeficiency best classified as X-linked familial hemophagocytic lymphohistiocytosis and not as X-linked lymphoproliferative disease. Blood. 2010;116(7):1079–82.
90. Steele CL, Dore M, Ammann S, Loughrey M, Montero A, Burns SO, et al. X-linked inhibitor of apoptosis complicated by granulomatous lymphocytic interstitial lung disease (GLILD) and granulomatous hepatitis. J Clin Immunol. 2016;36(7):733–8.
91. Booth C, Gilmour KC, Veys P, Gennery AR, Slatter MA, Chapel H, et al. X-linked lymphoproliferative disease due to SAP/SH2D1A deficiency: a multicenter study on the manifestations, management and outcome of the disease. Blood. 2011;117(1):53–62.
92. Marsh RA, Rao K, Satwani P, Lehmberg K, Muller I, Li D, et al. Allogeneic hematopoietic cell transplantation for XIAP deficiency: an international survey reveals poor outcomes. Blood. 2013;121(6):877–83.
93. Worthey EA, Mayer AN, Syverson GD, Helbling D, Bonacci BB, Decker B, et al. Making a definitive diagnosis: successful clinical application of whole exome sequencing in a child with intractable inflammatory bowel disease. Genet Med. 2011;13(3):255–62.
94. Li FY, Chaigne-Delalande B, Kanellopoulou C, Davis JC, Matthews HF, Douek DC, et al. Second messenger role for Mg2+ revealed by human T-cell immunodeficiency. Nature. 2011;475(7357):471–6.
95. Stepensky P, Weintraub M, Yanir A, Revel-Vilk S, Krux F, Huck K, et al. IL-2-inducible T-cell kinase deficiency: clinical presentation and therapeutic approach. Haematologica. 2011;96(3):472–6.
96. Huck K, Feyen O, Niehues T, Ruschendorf F, Hubner N, Laws HJ, et al. Girls homozygous for an IL-2-inducible T cell kinase mutation that leads to protein deficiency develop fatal EBV-associated lymphoproliferation. J Clin Invest. 2009;119(5):1350–8.
97. Mansouri D, Mahdaviani SA, Khalilzadeh S, Mohajerani SA, Hasanzad M, Sadr S, et al. IL-2-inducible T-cell kinase deficiency with pulmonary manifestations due to disseminated Epstein-Barr virus infection. Int Arch Allergy Immunol. 2012;158(4):418–22.
98. Salzer E, Daschkey S, Choo S, Gombert M, Santos-Valente E, Ginzel S, et al. Combined immunodeficiency with life-threatening EBV-associated lymphoproliferative disorder in patients lacking functional CD27. Haematologica. 2013;98(3):473–8.

99. Alkhairy OK, Perez-Becker R, Driessen GJ, Abolhassani H, van Montfrans J, Borte S, et al. Novel mutations in TNFRSF7/CD27: clinical, immunologic, and genetic characterization of human CD27 deficiency. J Allergy Clin Immunol. 2015;136(3):703–12 e10.
100. van Montfrans JM, Hoepelman AI, Otto S, van Gijn M, van de Corput L, de Weger RA, et al. CD27 deficiency is associated with combined immunodeficiency and persistent symptomatic EBV viremia. J Allergy Clin Immunol. 2012;129(3):787–93 e6.
101. Abolhassani H, Edwards ES, Ikinciogullari A, Jing H, Borte S, Buggert M, et al. Combined immunodeficiency and Epstein-Barr virus-induced B cell malignancy in humans with inherited CD70 deficiency. J Exp Med. 2017;214(1):91–106.
102. Barzaghi F, Amaya Hernandez LC, Neven B, Ricci S, Kucuk ZY, Bleesing J, et al. Long-term follow up of IPEX syndrome patients after different therapeutic strategies: an international multicenter retrospective study. J Allergy Clin Immunol. 2018;141(3):1036–1049.e5. https://doi.org/10.1016/j.jaci.2017.10.041. Epub 2017 Dec 11.
103. Barzaghi F, Passerini L, Bacchetta R. Immune dysregulation, polyendocrinopathy, enteropathy, x-linked syndrome: a paradigm of immunodeficiency with autoimmunity. Front Immunol. 2012;3:211.
104. Curotto de Lafaille MA, Kutchukhidze N, Shen S, Ding Y, Yee H, Lafaille JJ. Adaptive Foxp3+ regulatory T cell-dependent and -independent control of allergic inflammation. Immunity. 2008;29(1):114–26.
105. Gambineri E, Perroni L, Passerini L, Bianchi L, Doglioni C, Meschi F, et al. Clinical and molecular profile of a new series of patients with immune dysregulation, polyendocrinopathy, enteropathy, X-linked syndrome: inconsistent correlation between forkhead box protein 3 expression and disease severity. J Allergy Clin Immunol. 2008;122(6):1105–12 e1.
106. Goudy K, Aydin D, Barzaghi F, Gambineri E, Vignoli M, Ciullini Mannurita S, et al. Human IL2RA null mutation mediates immunodeficiency with lymphoproliferation and autoimmunity. Clin Immunol. 2013;146(3):248–61.
107. Caudy AA, Reddy ST, Chatila T, Atkinson JP, Verbsky JW. CD25 deficiency causes an immune dysregulation, polyendocrinopathy, enteropathy, X-linked-like syndrome, and defective IL-10 expression from CD4 lymphocytes. J Allergy Clin Immunol. 2007;119(2):482–7.
108. Bezrodnik L, Caldirola MS, Seminario AG, Moreira I, Gaillard MI. Follicular bronchiolitis as phenotype associated with CD25 deficiency. Clin Exp Immunol. 2014;175(2):227–34.
109. Kofoed EM, Hwa V, Little B, Woods KA, Buckway CK, Tsubaki J, et al. Growth hormone insensitivity associated with a STAT5b mutation. N Engl J Med. 2003;349(12):1139–47.
110. Nadeau K, Hwa V, Rosenfeld RG. STAT5b deficiency: an unsuspected cause of growth failure, immunodeficiency, and severe pulmonary disease. J Pediatr. 2011;158(5):701–8.
111. Zeiser R, Leveson-Gower DB, Zambricki EA, Kambham N, Beilhack A, Loh J, et al. Differential impact of mammalian target of rapamycin inhibition on CD4+CD25+Foxp3+ regulatory T cells compared with conventional CD4+ T cells. Blood. 2008;111(1):453–62.
112. Lohr NJ, Molleston JP, Strauss KA, Torres-Martinez W, Sherman EA, Squires RH, et al. Human ITCH E3 ubiquitin ligase deficiency causes syndromic multisystem autoimmune disease. Am J Hum Genet. 2010;86(3):447–53.
113. Watkin LB, Jessen B, Wiszniewski W, Vece TJ, Jan M, Sha Y, et al. COPA mutations impair ER-Golgi transport and cause hereditary autoimmune-mediated lung disease and arthritis. Nat Genet. 2015;47(6):654–60.
114. Strange C, Highland KB. Interstitial lung disease in the patient who has connective tissue disease. Clin Chest Med. 2004;25(3):549–59, vii.

Chapter 6
Pulmonary Manifestations of Defects in Innate Immunity

Persio Roxo-Junior, Isabela Mina, and Catherine Sonaly Ferreira Martins

6.1 Introduction

The immune response consists of mechanisms involved in innate immunity and, when necessary, in adaptive immunity. The innate response is phylogenetically older, of a nonspecific nature, and rapid and is coded within the germline, while the adaptive response is antigen specific, has been first described in vertebrates, is slower and of longer duration, and results from somatic DNA recombination.

Examples of the innate immunity components are epithelial barriers, antimicrobial peptides, soluble factors (chemokines and proteins of the complement system), and cell elements (neutrophils, monocytes, and natural killer cells). The humoral and cellular components of the innate immune system are diverse, and their responses are initiated by pattern recognition receptors (PRR) such as Toll-like receptors (TLRs) and NOD-like receptors (NLR, NOD), which recognize the pathogen-associated molecular patterns (PAMPs).

The innate immune responses play a fundamental role in the control of infections by interfering with the replication and/or viability of the pathogen, in addition to favoring the development of adaptive immunity [1]. The important role of innate immunity in the defense against infections can be clearly seen by the presence of severe infections secondary to the intrinsic defects of this immunity sector.

The way the innate immune system detects and responds to infections has been clarified at the molecular level; and the function of the system in the defense against various types of pathogens, as well as its importance in the physiopathology of PIDs, is currently being revealed [2].

P. Roxo-Junior (✉) · I. Mina · C. S. F. Martins
Division of Immunology and Allergy, Department of Pediatrics, Ribeirão Preto Medical School, University of São Paulo, São Paulo, Brazil
e-mail: persiorj@fmrp.usp.br

S. A. Mahdaviani, N. Rezaei (eds.), *Pulmonary Manifestations of Primary Immunodeficiency Diseases*, https://doi.org/10.1007/978-3-030-00880-2_6

This chapter will deal with the main respiratory manifestations occurring in the presence of each innate immunity defect according to the molecular changes involved.

(For further information, you may see Parvaneh P, Lilic D, Roesler J, Niehues T, Casanova JL, Picard C. Defects in intrinsic and innate immunity: receptors and signaling components. In: Rezaei N, Aghamohammadi A, Notarangelo LD, editors. *Primary immunodeficiency diseases: definition, diagnosis, and management*, 2nd ed. p. 339–392).

6.2 Anhidrotic Ectodermal Dysplasia with Immunodeficiency

Anhidrotic ectodermal dysplasia with immunodeficiency (AED-ID) is a rare syndrome characterized by changes in the differentiation of ectoderm-derived structures such as the teeth, hair, and sweat glands and by impaired immunological function. The main clinical abnormalities are conical teeth and teeth present in reduced numbers, scarcity of body and scalp hair, reduced or absent sweating, and severe repeated infections.

According to genetic inheritance, AED-ID can be classified into recessive X-linked and autosomal dominant (AD) forms.

X-linked AED-ID is caused by hypomorphic mutations of the gene that codes for the kinase κB inhibitor gene (*IKBKG*), also known as NF-κB essential modulator (*NEMO*), a regulatory component of the IκB (IKK) complex necessary for the activation of the κB nuclear transcription factor (NF-κB) [3]. NF-κB is a regulatory protein of the immunoglobulin gene expression in B lymphocytes, immune response, inflammatory reactions, and protection against apoptosis, among other functions [4].

Members of the NF-κB family are present in the cell cytoplasm, linked to NF-κB inhibitors (IκB). During cellular activation, signals are generated that lead to the activation of IKK, which phosphorylates IκB in specific serine residues, promoting their ubiquitination and degradation by the proteasome, permitting translocation of the NF-κB complex to the nucleus for the activation of its target genes [3].

Approximately 43 mutations that impair NF-κB activation have been reported thus far [5].

The main disorder detected in X-linked AED-ID is related to the NEMO-dependent NF-κB activation by TLR and interleukin 1 (TIR: TLR, IL-1R, and IL-18R) and by tumor necrosis factor receptors (TNF-R: TNF-αR and CD40) [3].

The immunological investigation of patients with this disease may reveal various changes such as deficiency of specific anti-polysaccharide antibodies, low serum IgG levels [3], and variable IgA, IgM, and IgE levels, as well as increased IgM in some cases. Abnormal CD40-CD40L signaling is observed in some individuals [6] and reduced natural killer cell activity in others, causing these patients to be more susceptible to mycobacterial infections. Patients usually have normal numbers of naive and memory T-cells [3].

The degree of impairment of the various pathways of NEMO activation depends on the type of mutation. In general, patients fail to produce IL-10 in response to activation with TNF-α, and many of them show an impaired antibody response, especially glycans, including pneumococcal capsules. These characteristics are the result of defective signaling by the signaling pathway of the ectodysplasin receptor (EDA-R). More recently, mutations in the leucine zipper domain of the *NEMO* gene have been diagnosed as the X-linked form of Mendelian susceptibility to mycobacterial diseases (MSMD), demonstrating the important role of NEMO in the IL-12/IFNγ pathway.

The AD form of AED-ID, also known as IκBα gain-of-function (GOF) mutation, is caused by a hypermorphic heterozygous *IKBA* mutation that prevents the phosphorylation and degradation of the NF-κB α inhibitor (IκBα), resulting in partial retention of NF-κB dimers in the cytoplasm. These dimers are involved in various pathways, including those triggered by members of the TNF-R, IL-1R, TLR, T-cell receptor (TCR), and B-cell receptor (BCR) families [5]. The quantity of mutant IκBα inside the cell, its binding affinity for NF-kB, and its resistance to degradation determine the degree of GOF and consequently the levels of NF-kB inhibition in heterozygous cells [7].

IκBα deficiency involves a severe impairment of TCR signaling. The patients exhibit hypogammaglobulinemia with the absence of production of specific antibodies. Some patients also have low proportions of CD4 and CD8 memory T-cells and of memory B-cells, few or no T γ/δ cells, and severe impairment of T-cell proliferation in response to anti-CD3 [5].

Children with both X-linked and AD forms of AED-ID suffer recurrent infections by variable pathogens such as capsulated pyogenic bacteria, mycobacteria, viruses, and fungi [3], with respiratory manifestations being the most frequent consequences.

Pneumococcal infections are the most frequent ones in these patients, probably due to the impaired responses related to TLR and IL-1R [5, 8], followed by *Haemophilus influenzae* and *Staphylococcus aureus* infections causing recurrent pneumonias and bronchiectasia [5].

Patients with AD mutations in *IKBA* suffer from severe pyogenic bacterial infections, especially pneumonias, due to β hemolytic type A streptococcus, *Staphylococcus aureus*, *Pseudomonas aeruginosa*, *Klebsiella pneumoniae*, and *Serratia marcescens*.

Infections with atypical mycobacteria such as *Mycobacterium avium*, *Mycobacterium bovis*, and *Mycobacterium kansasii* are also frequent in patients with *NEMO* mutations with defects of CD40-CD40L signaling and changes in the immunity mediated by the IL-12/IFNγ pathway [3, 8], with consequent recurrent pneumonias, bronchiectasis, and pulmonary fibrosis. These patients also can present viral respiratory infections, especially those induced by cytomegalovirus and adenovirus, as well as respiratory infections caused by opportunistic fungi such as

Pneumocystis jirovecii [8]. About one-third of *NEMO*-deficient patients can die from invasive infections.

6.3 LUBAC Deficiency

The linear ubiquitin chain assembly complex (LUBAC), consisting of SHANK-associated RH domain-interacting protein (SHARPIN), heme-oxidized IRP2 ubiquitin ligase-1 (HOIL-1), and HOIL-1-interacting protein (HOIP), is an important regulator of inflammation and of the innate response signaling [9]. HOIL-1 L and SHARPIN are accessory HOIP proteins.

Ubiquitination was initially described as a mechanism of protein labeling as targets for degradation by proteasome. However, today we know that ubiquitination is involved in several other cell functions such as activation of the canonic NF-κB pathways, which occurs in a relatively rapid manner through stimuli from proinflammatory cytokines and PAMPs, such as lipoproteins and bacterial liposaccharides (LPS).

The stimulation of retinoic acid-inducible gene (RIG)-like receptors, TLRs, and NOD-like receptors induces NF-κB activation of type I IFN production. Recent studies have indicated that LUBAC regulates the responses of the immune system via TLR, NOD, and RIG.

Rats with spontaneous SHARPIN deficiency, denoted as carriers of chronic proliferative dermatitis in mice (CPDM), exhibit, in addition to dermatitis, splenomegaly, defects of secondary lymphoid organs, and significantly low serum IgG, IgA, and IgE levels. On this basis, it was discovered that SHARPIN is a physiological LUBAC component interacting with HOIP and that the lack of SHARPIN in rats with CPDM causes LUBAC destabilization resulting in impaired NF-κB signaling. The severe immunodeficiency detected in rats with CPDM resembles that of patients with X-linked AED-ID caused by mutation of the *NEMO* gene [10].

The immunological investigation of patients with LUBAC deficiency reveals lymphopenia, memory B-cell deficiency, deficient production of specific antibodies, and hypogammaglobulinemia [11].

Thus, patients with LUBAC deficiency mainly suffer recurrent respiratory infections, especially pneumonias caused by pyogenic bacteria and *Streptococcus pneumoniae*, due to deficient production of specific antibodies against pneumococcal glycans [12].

6.4 IRAK-4 and MyD88 Deficiencies

IRAK-4 is a kinase protein that plays a fundamental role in the signaling of the TLR family (except for TLR3). After recognizing the pathogens, TLRs trigger intracellular signaling pathways resulting in the induction of inflammatory cytokines and type I INF. TLRs share with members of the IL-1R family an intracellular domain denoted Toll-interleukin-1 receptor (TIR) domain. MyD88 is a cytosolic adaptor molecule that connects TLRs and IL-1Rs to the IRAK complex. The MyD88- and IRAK-4-dependent TIR pathways lead to the production of proinflammatory cytokines.

IRAK deficiency is an autosomal recessive (AR) immunodeficiency caused by homozygous or heterozygous *IRAK4* gene mutations.

MyD88 deficiency is an AR immunodeficiency caused by homozygous or heterozygous *MyD88* gene mutations.

The immunological investigation of patients with IRAK4 and MyD88 deficiency does not reveal changes in leukocyte development or in the proliferative responses of B and T-cells to specific antigens. However, patients can show impairment of neutrophil migration, markedly reduced marginal zone B ($IgM^{+}IgD^{+}CD27^{+}$) cells, and impairment of specific IgG and IgM antibody responses to pneumococcal infections and isohemagglutinins (in up to half the patients). Some patients also exhibit increased serum IgE and IgG4 concentrations, although no association with allergic asthma occurs in these individuals [5].

The clinical signs and symptoms of affected patients are variable, with greater susceptibility to severe and invasive infections caused by pyogenic bacteria, but with normal resistance to viruses, fungi, parasites, and other bacteria. The main invasive bacterial infections of these patients are caused by *Streptococcus pneumoniae*, *Staphylococcus aureus*, and *Pseudomonas aeruginosa*. In more than 90% of patients, the first bacterial infection occurs at 2 years of age, with high lethality.

These patients also have noninvasive infections by pyogenic bacteria that affect the upper respiratory tract, manifesting as otitis, sinusitis, tonsillar abscess, necrotizing epiglottitis, pharyngitis, palatine infection, and pneumonia. The principal bacteria involved in this type of infection are also *Staphylococcus aureus*, *Pseudomonas aeruginosa*, and *Streptococcus pneumoniae*.

Both immunodeficiencies tend to improve with age, with the patients no longer suffering invasive infections by pyogenic bacteria after adolescence. However, all patients continue to have noninvasive infections such as sinusitis and pneumonia even during adult life [5].

6.5 Herpes Simplex Encephalitis (TLR3, UNC93B1, TRAF3, TRIF, TBK1, IRF3 Deficiencies)

This group of inherited deficiencies involves defects of TLR3 signaling and susceptibility to herpes simplex encephalitis (HSE) caused by herpes simplex virus-1 (HSV-1) during childhood, a rare and potentially fatal manifestation [13].

The affected patients carry mutations in the *TLR3*, *UNC93B1*, *TRAF3*, *TRIF*, *TBK1*, or *IRF3* genes. The signaling pathway controlled by TRIF is mediated by TLR3 and TLR4 and leads to activation of the transcription factors IRF3 and NF-kB. TRIF recruits TRAF6, activates TAK1 for NF-kB activation, and also recruits a signaling complex consisting of TBK1 and IKKε via TRAF3 for IRF3 activation. This signaling pathway results in the production of inflammatory cytokines and type I and III IFN with an important antiviral response [8].

Single-gene inborn errors of TLR3 immunity such as TLR3, UNC93B1, TRAF3, TRIF, TBK1, and IRF3 deficiencies predispose some individuals to HSE [14]. Heterozygous mutations of *TLR3* have been reported to cause HSE in children. The AD form is the most common trait. AR UNC93B deficiency has been identified as the first genetic etiology of isolated HSE. AD TRAF3 deficiency and HSE have been described in a French patient 7 years ago. TRIF deficiency associated with HSE was recently described in two kindreds (the first patient with a homozygous nonsense mutation resulting in complete absence of protein and the other with a heterozygous missense mutation). TBK1 deficiency associated with HSE has been reported in two kindreds that carried different heterozygous mutations, both associated with an AD trait. In a 2015 report, heterozygous mutation of *IRF3* was found to be associated with HSE, leading to impaired signaling trough the TLR3-TRIF pathway [15].

The peripheral blood mononuclear cells of patients with TLR3, UNC93B1, TRAF3, TRIF, TBK1, and IRF3 deficiency do not produce type I or III IFN (especially IFNα, β, and λ) [8, 16] in an appropriate manner or fibroblasts after infection with HSV-1 or vesicular stomatitis virus. Deficient IFN production by fibroblasts and induced pluripotent stem cells (iPSC) derived from the central nervous system (CNS) results in viral replication and increased cell death [13].

Despite their multiple affected TLRs, patients with UNC93B1, TLR3, TRAF3, TRIF, TBK1, and TRF3 deficiency seem to suffer only herpes simplex encephalitis, with no systemic or cutaneous HSV-1 and without any other severe viral infections [8]. Some patients are asymptomatic, while others may have neurological sequelae such as blindness and epilepsy.

6.6 Mendelian Susceptibility to Mycobacterial Diseases (IFNγ Receptor 1/2 Deficiencies, IL-12/23 Receptor β1 Chain Deficiency, IL-12p40 Deficiency, AD STAT1 Deficiency, LZ-NEMO Deficiency, Macrophage-Specific CYBB Deficiency, AD IRF8 Deficiency, ISG15 Deficiency)

Most PIDs exhibit Mendelian inheritance, with mutation in single genes. However, many factors contribute to the phenotypic expression of Mendelian PIDs in addition to gene mutations, such as possible mitochondrial and somatic mutations and the infectious environment.

The MSMD is a rare genetic syndrome that predisposes to infections caused by mycobacteria of low virulence such as strains of the BCG vaccine and nontuberculous environmental mycobacteria (EM). However, compromised individuals are also vulnerable to more virulent species such as *Mycobacterium tuberculosis*. On the other hand, most patients are resistant to infections caused by all other pathogens, except for isolated cases of disease caused by intracellular bacteria such as *Nocardia* and *Listeria*, intracellular fungi such as *Paracoccidioides* and *Histoplasma*, intracellular parasites such as *Leishmania*, and some viruses such as herpes virus [8]. Some of these infections must share pathogenic mechanisms with MSMD because of their similar tropism for macrophages and clinical manifestations [17].

After contact with these intracellular mechanisms, macrophages secrete IL-12, which binds to its receptors (IL-12Rβ1 and IL-12Rβ2) on the surface of T and NK cells, culminating with the secretion of IFNγ by these cells. IFNγ, in turn, binds to its receptors (IFNγR1 and IFNγR2) on macrophages, activating genes such as IL-12 and respiratory burst NADPH oxidase, which permit the macrophages to destroy the pathogen. On this basis, IFNγR1 and IFNγR2, STAT1, IL-12B, and IL-12Rβ1 are involved in the immunity mediated by the IFNγ-dependent pathway of IL-12/23. Mutations in *IFNGR1*, *IFNGR2*, and *STAT1* impair the cellular response to IFNγ, while mutations in *IL12B* and *IL12Rβ1* impair the production of IL-12-/23-dependent IFNγ.

In addition, *IRF8* mutations have been reported to impair IL-12 secretion by monocytes and dendritic cells. Furthermore, *CYBB* mutations are responsible for X-linked MSMD [18].

6.6.1 *IFNγR1 Deficiency*

The high frequency of parental consanguinity and the occurrence of MSMD among siblings born to unaffected parents are more probably inherited as an AR trait, although there are cases of AD IFNγR1 deficiency.

The AR complete IFNγR1 deficiency was the first genetic etiology of MSMD to be identified at the molecular level in patients with lack of receptor expression. The lack or dysfunction of IFNγR1 does not permit the recognition of IFNγ, which is detected at high levels in the cytoplasm of affected patients. Patients with AR complete IFNγR1 deficiency suffer early, severe, and fatal infections with BCG and EM pathogens such as *Mycobacterium fortuitum*, *Mycobacterium chelonae*, *Mycobacterium smegmatis*, and *Mycobacterium peregrinum*, which are the most frequent among these patients. Other infections caused by viruses such as herpes virus 8, cytomegalovirus, respiratory syncytial virus, and *Listeria monocytogenes* have been separately detected in patients.

Patients with AR partial IFNγR1 deficiency, in turn, have residual responses to high IFNγ concentrations and for this reason have less severe clinical manifestations.

Patients with dominant IFNγR1 deficiency commonly suffer from recurrent EM and BCG infections with less severe clinical signs and symptoms than patients with complete deficiency. In addition, mycobacterial infection usually occurs later, and the intervals between infections are longer. Other infections caused by pathogens such as *Histoplasma capsulatum* have been detected as isolated infections in patient with this type of alteration [17].

6.6.2 IFNγR2 Deficiency

Based on the cellular response to IFNγ, IFNγ2R deficiency may be complete (undetectable response to IFNγ) or partial (residual response to IFNγ).

The clinical manifestations are similar to those of patients with AR IFNγR1 deficiency, and the major pathogens detected include *Mycobacterium bovis* of BCG, *Mycobacterium avium*, and *Mycobacterium fortuitum* [17].

6.6.3 IL-12/23 Receptor β1 Chain Deficiency

IL-12 comprises two subunits, p35 and p40, respectively, encoded by the *IL12A* and *IL12B* genes. IL-23 also comprises the p40 subunit. Both IL-12 and IL-23 bind to the IL-12 receptor β-subunit chain (IL-12Rβ1).

IL-12 binding to IL-12Rβ1 in T lymphocytes and NK cells induces the production of IFNγ, while IL-23 binding to IL-12Rβ1 and IL-23R promotes the production of IL-17.

IL-12Rβ1 deficiency is the most frequent known genetic cause of MSMD and can be seen in about 40% of the patients. The mutations are of the loss-of-function type and cause complete recessive deficiency [18, 19]. The activated T and NK lymphocytes of affected patients do not express IL-12Rβ1 on their surface.

BCG diseases and salmonellosis are the infections most frequently affecting these patients. Severe tuberculosis conditions may also appear in affected patients. Granulomas can still be formed in the lungs but are often multibacillary.

Other infections such as leishmaniasis and paracoccidioidomycosis have been detected in isolated cases [17].

6.6.4 IL-12p40 Deficiency

Deficiency of the *IL12B* gene, which codes for the IL-12p40 subunit, causes greater predisposition to BCG, *Mycobacterium tuberculosis*, and EM infections. Fungal *Candida* infections and infections with bacteria such as *Klebsiella* and *Nocardia* appear in isolated cases [17, 19]. The clinical picture is similar to that of IL-12Rβ1 deficiency but is mostly more severe.

6.6.5 AD STAT1 Deficiency

STAT1 is required for cellular responses to both type I (IFNα/β) and type II (IFNγ) interferons. Heterozygous missense mutations in *STAT1* cause partial dominant STAT1 deficiency. These mutations mostly compromise IFNγ. Thus, the patients show predisposition only to mycobacterial infections, without increased susceptibility to severe viral infections.

The disease resembles that induced by partial forms of AR IFNγR1 and IFNγR2 deficiencies, and the patients may exhibit conditions ranging from atypical mycobacterial infections to more severe types of pulmonary tuberculosis [17].

6.6.6 LZ-NEMO Deficiency

Mutations in the leucine zipper domain of the *NEMO* gene (LZ-NEMO) were identified in the 1990 decade in male patients of the same family with *Mycobacterium avium* infections and no other opportunistic infections, defining a recessive X-linked cause of MSMD [17].

Patients selectively exhibit reduction of CD40-dependent IL-12 induction in mononuclear cells [20] resulting in deficient IFNγ production.

Most of the infections detected in these patients are limited to mycobacteria, especially *Mycobacterium avium*. Infection with *Haemophilus influenzae* b has been described in isolated cases [17].

6.6.7 Macrophage-Specific CYBB Deficiency

Chronic granulomatous disease (CGD) is characterized by the failure of phagocyte NADPH oxidase to generate superoxides in order to fight the pathogens and is due to mutations in the *CYBB* gene. Patients with mutations in this gene are more susceptible to infection with various catalase-positive pathogens, mainly in the mucocutaneous and respiratory systems.

One of the mutations in the *CYBB* gene causes an impaired respiratory burst in monocyte-derived macrophages, but not in granulocytes. Patients with this alteration only exhibit mycobacterial infections, without the remaining infections characteristic of patients with CGD. Therefore, this mutation selectively affects the respiratory burst in macrophages, which is a crucial mechanism for protective immunity to tuberculous mycobacteria [21].

6.6.8 AD IRF8 Deficiency

The interferon regulatory factor 8 (IRF8) is a member of the family of IFN regulator factors that is expressed in high levels in mononuclear phagocytes and regulates the differentiation of macrophages and granulocytes and the development of dendritic cells. It can activate or suppress gene transcription under stimulation by IFNγ, lipopolysaccharides (LPS), and other microbial stimuli. Thus, it plays an important role in the defense against intracellular pathogens, activating IL-12 production in response to IFNγ.

Patients with AD IRF8 deficiency suffer recurrent infections related to BCG, as well as pulmonary tuberculosis due to *Mycobacterium tuberculosis*, with a rapid development of granulomas [22].

6.6.9 ISG15 Deficiency

The ISG15 (interferon-stimulated gene 15) is an intracellular protein produced by neutrophils, monocytes, lymphocytes, and granulocytes, which acts on T and NK cells, inducing IFNγ production.

Thus, its deficiency impairs the synthesis of IFNγ, rendering ISG15-deficient patients susceptible to mycobacterial infections [23].

6.7 AR STAT1 and STAT2 Deficiency

Signal transducer and activator of transcription-1 (STAT-1) is a protein involved in the transduction of cell responses to IFNα/β, λ, and γ and IL-27 through the formation of two transcriptor factor complexes: the interferon-stimulated gamma factor 3 (ISGF3) composed of STAT1-STAT2-p48/IRF9 trimers and the gamma-activated factor (GAF) comprised of STAT1 homodimers.

Complete AR mutations of *STAT1* lead to a full loss of the STAT1 proteins, and, as a consequence, there is no STAT-dependent response to IFNα/β, λ, and γ. This favors infections with several viruses [8] such as HSV-1, CMV, and respiratory syncytial virus (RSV) [24] and with intracellular bacteria, mainly low-virulence mycobacteria such as BCG vaccine and *Mycobacterium kansasii* [8, 24]. Some infections are similar to those detected in patients with combined T-cell immunodeficiencies but with normal lymphocyte numbers and function of T-cells [24].

A milder form of partial AR STAT1 deficiency has been described in some patients [8], whose cells produce residual quantities of functional STAT1 corresponding to approximately 10–25% of the normal levels, depending on the mutation. The clinical signs and symptoms of these patients are less severe compared to the complete form, with lighter infections with intracellular bacteria such as *Salmonella*, *Mycobacterium avium*, and BCG and with viruses such as CMV, VSR, and HSV-1 [24].

AR STAT2 deficiency is associated with impaired type I IFN signaling and shows incomplete penetrance for various viral infections with diverse signs and symptoms. Severe pneumonitis caused by the measles vaccine strain has been described.

The impaired response to IFNα and infections with more aggressive viruses in patients with AR STAT2 deficiency is part of the phenotype of patients with complete AR STAT1 deficiency, although with a less severe clinical presentation [25].

6.8 Warts, Hypogammaglobulinemia, Infections, Myelokathexis (WHIM Syndrome)

WHIM syndrome is a rare immunodeficiency characterized by warts, hypogammaglobulinemia, infections, and myelokathexis (retention of mature neutrophils in the bone marrow).

Most patients carry heterozygous gain-of-function mutations in the *CXCR4* gene.

The disease should be suspected in any patient with warts, leukopenia, and severe neutropenia. Examination of the bone marrow shows myeloid hypercellularity and morphologic abnormalities consistent with apoptosis (hypersegmented nuclei with long filaments connecting nuclear lobes). Patients can also have variable hypogammaglobulinemia that may affect all isotypes, marked reduction of CD27+ memory B-cells, reduction of T lymphocyte subsets and a proliferative response to mitogens (in some patients only), and reduction in the number and function of dendritic cells contributing to the high susceptibility to specific viral infections [26].

The clinical manifestations usually start in childhood, and in general bacterial infections (especially those due to encapsulated germs) are more frequent than viral ones [27].

Although it has been proposed that infection by human papilloma virus (HPV) is the only one to which patients with WHIM syndrome are susceptible, lymphoproliferative disorders associated with Epstein-Barr virus (EBV), as well as herpes zoster and recurrent serious oral and genital herpes simplex infections, have been reported, demonstrating that these patients have a greater generalized susceptibility to viruses of the herpes family.

Bacterial infections are recurrent, mainly involving the respiratory, gastrointestinal, and cutaneous systems [26]. The respiratory infections mainly manifest as pneumonias and sinusitis due to pathogens such as *Haemophilus influenzae*, *Streptococcus pneumoniae*, *Klebsiella pneumoniae*, *Staphylococcus aureus*, and *Proteus mirabilis*. In some cases, recurrent pneumonias may lead to severe bronchiectasis with the possible occurrence of chronic *Pseudomonas aeruginosa* or *Burkholderia cepacia* [27] infection.

6.9 Epidermodysplasia Verruciformis (EV)

Epidermodysplasia verruciformis (EV) is a rare disorder of genetic heterogeneity characterized by abnormal susceptibility to skin infections caused by HPV, whose serotypes are not pathogenic for the healthy population. There is a specific susceptibility to HPV 3 and 10 in plane warts and to HPV 5 and 8 in skin carcinomas. UV light is likely to be involved in the progression from benign warts to malignancy. However, cancers develop slowly, but progressive lesions and metastases have been observed in some patients.

The lesions usually arise in childhood or at the beginning of adolescence and are highly resistant to treatment.

The main manifestations of EV are hypo- and hyperpigmented reddish squamous maculae, wart-like papillomatous lesions, seborrheic keratosis lesions, and versicolor pityriasis lesions. Skin lesions tend to disseminate throughout the body, although the mucosal membranes are spared.

The *EVER1* (*TMC6*) and *EVER2* (*TMC8*) genes are involved in resistance against skin infections caused by HPV mostly by regulating the distribution of intracellular zinc and by inducing TNF-α, which is important for the prevention of HPV persistence inside the cells.

Most patients present mutations in the *EVER1* and *EVER2* genes. Both mutations code for proteins that inhibit essential transcription factors and that negatively regulate cell-mediated immunity.

EV-like disease has been described in some T-cell deficiencies such as SCID and mutations in the *RHOH*, *MST1*, *CORO1A*, and *IL-7* genes.

Patients with mutations in *RHOH* suffer bronchopulmonary diseases, patients with mutations in *CORO1A* have a high risk of bronchiectasis, and a patient with mutation in *MST1* has been reported to suffer recurrent chronic pulmonary infections [28].

6.10 Chronic Mucocutaneous Candidiasis (IL-17RA Deficiency, IL-17F Deficiency, ACT1 Deficiency, STAT1 Gain of Function)

Chronic mucocutaneous candidiasis (CMC) is a term that describes a group of clinical phenotype presenting as recurring or persistent infections of the skin, nails, and mucous membranes caused by yeast *Candida*, mostly *albicans*, but alternatively by other strains (*C. glabrata*, *C. krusei*, *C. dubliniensis*).

Resistance and tolerance mechanisms participate to the interplay between host and pathogens. IL-17- mediated response has been shown to be crucial for host resistance to respiratory infections, whereas its role in host tolerance during chronic airway colonization is still unclear.

Evidence suggests that CMC can be present in patients with primary defects affecting both the adaptive and innate immunities that activate Th17 pathway. IL-17-mediated immunity plays a double-edged activity during chronic airway infection: on one side, it contributes to the control of *Pseudomonas aeruginosa* burden, modulating host resistance, while, on the other, it alters host tolerance, propagating exacerbated pulmonary neutrophilia and tissue remodeling [29].

6.10.1 IL-17RA and IL17F Deficiency

Studies of Th17 cells and IL-17A have revealed important roles for IL-17A in the development of allergic and autoimmune diseases as well as in protective mechanisms against bacterial and fungal infections, functions that were previously believed to be mediated by Th1 or Th2 cells [30].

Th17 cytokines protect hosts from pathogens at epithelial and mucosal tissues including the skin, lungs, and intestine. Both IL-17A and IL-17F enhance protective immune responses by inducing the production of CXC chemokines, G-CSF, and antimicrobial peptides in epithelial cells and keratinocytes. Indeed, studies using cytokine- and receptor-deficient mice showed that IL-17A and IL-17F were required for responses to *Klebsiella pneumoniae* in the lungs [31].

6.10.2 ACT1 Deficiency

ACT1 is an adaptor protein acting downstream from IL-17RA, IL-17RC, and IL-17RB in humans [32]. Mouse fibroblasts lacking ACT1 display low levels of KC/CXCL1 and IL-6 expression in response to stimulation with IL-17A and IL-17F [33]. In addition, abolition of the IL-25-/IL-17E-induced expression of IL-4, IL-5, IL-13, eotaxin-1 (CCL11), and pulmonary eosinophilia has also been observed in the lung tissues of ACT1-deficient mice [34].

6.10.3 STAT1 Gain-of-Function (GOF) Mutation

GOF mutation reduces the dephosphorylation of activated STAT1 protein, leading to accumulation of phosphorylated STAT1 in the nucleus. Persistently activated STAT1 may shift the immune response toward STAT1-dependent interleukin-17 inhibitors and away from STAT3-mediated induction of IL-17 T-cell generation [35]. GOF mutations affecting STAT1 lead to defective IL-17 T-cell development, characterized by reduced production of IL- 17 and IL-22; these cytokines are essential for the antifungal defense of the skin and mucosa. Patients with AD GOF *STAT1* mutations present with CMC [35]. Clinical manifestations include chronic oropharyngeal candidiasis, cutaneous dermatophytosis, and autoimmune phenomena, such as hypothyroidism and autoimmune hepatitis [36].

Respiratory viral infections have been reported like respiratory syncytial virus (RSV) bronchiolitis and influenza infections [37, 38]. Bacterial infections, mostly caused by *S. aureus*, have also frequently been reported [37].

6.11 CARD9 Deficiency

Human CARD9 deficiency is an AR PID caused by biallelic mutations in the gene *CARD9*, which encodes a signaling protein that was found downstream of many C-type lectin receptors (CLRs). CLRs encompass a large family of innate recognition receptors, expressed predominantly by myeloid and epithelial cells, which bind fungal carbohydrates and initiate antifungal immune responses. Although other receptor families are involved in innate antifungal recognition, only mutations in the CLR pathway have thus far been associated with the spontaneous development of fungal infections in humans. CARD9 deficiency is associated with the spontaneous development of persistent and severe fungal infections that primarily localize to the skin and subcutaneous tissue, mucosal surface, and/or central nervous system (CNS) [39].

The first manifestation associated with CARD9 deficiency affects the skin and subcutaneous tissues. Patients in this category present with severe persistent fungal infections of the skin, nails, and scalp, with occasional contiguous dissemination to the subcutaneous layers, lymph nodes, and bones [40].

The second predominant manifestation of human CARD9 deficiency is systemic fungal disease, which primarily manifests as fungal meningoencephalitis caused by *Candida* species. Some patients have also developed bone infection of the vertebra [41]. Less often, CARD9-deficient patients develop phaeohyphomycosis caused by *Exophiala* species that targets the CNS and/or other deep tissues including the liver, bones, and lungs [42].

In relation to the role of CARD9 in neutrophil accumulation during fungal disease, it was demonstrated a neutrophil recruitment defect to the *Aspergillus fumigatus*-infected lung in CARD9−/− mice, which was also linked to poor CXC chemokine production in the lungs [43]. However, in that model, CARD9 was only partially required in the later stages of infection for neutrophil accumulation in the infected lung.

Thus, the collective dependence on CARD9 for neutrophil recruitment during pulmonary mold infections appears relatively mild compared to the universal reliance required for neutrophil accumulation and protection against *Candida* infection in the CNS [44]. This dichotomy observed in mice between the CARD9 dependence for protection against molds and yeasts may help justify why human CARD9 deficiency does not appear to associate with pulmonary fungal infections, despite the continuous environmental exposure to fungal spores.

6.12 Autoimmune Polyendocrinopathy with Candidiasis and Ectodermal Dystrophy (APECED)

Autoimmune polyendocrinopathy-candidiasis-ectodermal dystrophy (APECED) is a rare disorder caused by mutations in the autoimmune regulator (*AIRE*) gene.

Patients with APECED progressively develop multiple organ-specific autoimmunity of endocrine and nonendocrine tissues. Loss of function of the AIRE protein results in decreased expression of self-antigens in medullary thymic epithelial cells and in failure to establish central tolerance to a range of different autoantigens [45].

Although the underlying mechanism is not well understood, some APECED patients have significant pulmonary disease. Recently, in several APECED patients with autoimmune pulmonary disease, a potassium channel regulating protein (KCNRG) preferentially expressed in the epithelial cells of terminal bronchioles was identified as the putative target antigen [46].

Lung disease was described in two Sicilian brothers with APECED. They were compound heterozygotes with R203X/R257X. The elder brother had experienced recurrent lower respiratory infections since 5 years of age and over the years developed severe obstructive lung disease resulting in bronchiectasis, *cor pulmonale*, and terminal respiratory failure, which led to death at 18 years of age. Both brothers had circulating autoantibodies against tryptophan hydroxylase, and serotonin-producing cells were absent in the duodenal mucosa [46].

An obliterating bronchiolitis has been described also in a Hispanic child [47], and another severe fatal chest disease was observed in an adult woman [48].

Finally, in two short reports, other respiratory illnesses were described. Asthma and chronic hypersensitivity pneumonitis were described in a young girl [19, 49] and autoimmune bronchiolitis in four French children and adolescents [9, 50]. In this last report, the authors concluded that autoimmune bronchiolitis is a very rare but potentially life-threatening component of APECED, emphasizing the diversity of autoimmune targets in this disorder.

6.13 Monocyte Deficiencies (GATA2 Deficiency, IRF8 Deficiency)

6.13.1 GATA2 Deficiency

GATA2 is a zinc finger transcription factor essential for differentiation of immature hematopoietic cells. Among many other functions, GATA2 regulates the phagocytosis of alveolar macrophages [51].

GATA2 deficiency is a recently described disorder of hematopoiesis, lymphatics, and immunity, caused by heterozygous mutations leading to haplo-insufficiency of the transcription factor GATA2. The deficiency presents with a complex array of diagnoses and symptoms of varying extent including myelodysplastic syndrome; acute myelomonocytic leukemia; chronic myelomonocytic leukemia; severe viral, disseminated mycobacterial and invasive fungal infections; pulmonary arterial hypertension; warts; panniculitis; human papillomavirus (HPV)-positive tumors; Epstein-Barr virus (EBV)-positive tumors; venous thrombosis; lymphedema; sensorineural hearing loss; miscarriage; and hypothyroidism. Lymphopenia, monocytopenia, and primary lymphedema also must be considered as part of the disease [52]. Most patients have unremarkable childhood vaccination and infection histories. In relation to infections, nontuberculous mycobacterial infections and general warts are the most common manifestations.

However, *Pneumocystis jiroveci* is not a part of the spectrum of the pathogens that affect these patients; *Pneumocystis jiroveci* pneumonia (PCP) must be considered in patients with profound CD4 dysfunction or lymphopenia. A woman with GATA2 deficiency, lymphedema, lymphopenia, and monocytopenia was described with recurrent PCP, complicated by severe acute respiratory distress syndrome in the setting of influenza A H1N1 coinfection [53]. Experimental mouse models have found a relationship between GATA2 expression and *Pneumocystis jiroveci* infection. Loss of GATA2 production reduces alveolar macrophage phagocytic activity in response to *Pneumocystis jiroveci* infection in mice [52].

Pulmonary alveolar proteinosis is a characteristic feature of *GATA2* mutation that could be reported in about 18% of all subjects with GATA2 deficiency [52].

6.13.2 IRF8 Deficiency

IRF8 is a member of the interferon regulatory factor family that is expressed in myeloid cells such as macrophages and dendritic cells and that activates or represses gene transcription upon stimulation with IFNγ, lipopolysaccharide, and other microbial stimuli. IRF8 plays an important role in several aspects of myeloid cells, including differentiation and maturation of early progenitor cells, expression of intrinsic antimicrobial defenses, and production of the IL-12 cytokine, which is essential for priming of early T-cell-mediated immune response. IRF8 mutant mice are susceptible to a number of intracellular infections including pulmonary tuberculosis [54].

Two types of IRF8 deficiency have been reported. The AR form (due to homozygous K108E mutations) leads to a complete absence of circulating monocytes and dendritic cells. One patient identified with this genotype presented in early infancy with severe disseminated BCG infection, oral candidiasis, severe respiratory viral infection, and striking myeloproliferation [55].

The milder AD form (due to heterozygous T80A mutation) causes selective depletion of circulating dendritic cells. Two patients with this genotype had disseminated BCG disease in early childhood [55].

6.14 NK Cell Deficiencies (MCM4 Deficiency)

Human NK cells play critical role in human innate immune response, particularly the control of viral infection and antitumor surveillance functions. Differing to B and T lymphocytes, NK cells do not possess antigen-receptor rearrangement and do not require pre-activation in order to recognize and lyse target cells.

Patients with genetic defects of human NK cells present a primary immunodeficiency affecting NK cell development (number), function, or both [56]. An important tool in the understanding of human NK cells and NK cell subsets has been the discovery of PIDs that affect the generation or homeostasis of NK cells or specific NK cell subsets as well as those that affect NK cell function. There are over 300 genetic deficiencies of human immunity, and nearly 50 are known to have at least some impact on NK cells [57].

Human NK cell deficiencies can be divided into two categories. Those in the first category are characterized by effects on the number of NK cells in the peripheral blood, while effects on the function of NK cells characterize those in the second one. NK cell deficiencies in the first category have been labeled "classical NK cell deficiencies," and those in the second category have been labeled "functional NK cell deficiencies" [58, 59].

The first example of a classical NK cell deficiency was reported in 1989 in a girl with severe varicella and other complicated herpes virus infections [60]. She was determined to stably lack both NK cells in peripheral blood and peripheral blood NK cell cytotoxic activity against the prototypical human NK cell target cell, the K562 erythroleukemia cell line. The first example of a functional NK cell deficiency was described in 1982 in three siblings with severe Epstein-Barr virus infection [61]. All three individuals in this family presented deficient K562 target cell killing activity, and the surviving affected individual has had persistently deficient function over a 30-year period.

6.14.1 MCM4 Deficiency

MCM4 is a highly conserved DNA helicase that is recruited to origins of replication to promote the unwinding and polymerization of chromosomal DNA and cell proliferation [62]. Patients with AR MCM4 deficiency presented with a developmental syndrome including NK cell deficiency. The analyzed patients shared the same spliced defect [63].

The NK cell pattern in the patients is especially unusual. There is a development defect in transition of $CD56^{bright}$ (immature cells) to $CD56^{dim}$ (mature) NK cells, as evidenced by the lack of $CD56^{dim}$ NK cells in the peripheral blood and the preservation of the small $CD56^{bright}$ NK cells[63,64]. This observation suggests that MCM4 is required for terminal NK cell maturation.

Clinically, patients usually present growth retardation, adrenal insufficiency, and lymphoma. From an infectious standpoint, patients can experience complications from EBV, unusual susceptibility to herpes viruses, and presumed complications of viral illness symptoms clinically consistent with an NK cell deficiency [63, 64].

6.15 Pulmonary Alveolar Proteinosis

Pulmonary alveolar proteinosis (PAP) is a rare syndrome characterized by the accumulation of surfactant in alveolar macrophages and alveoli resulting in hypoxemic respiratory failure. These disorders are defined in the context of abnormalities of surfactant clearance and are caused by disruption of granulocyte-macrophage colony-stimulating factor (GM-CSF) signaling (primary or idiopathic PAP) or by an underlying disease that impairs alveolar macrophage number or functions including surfactant catabolism (secondary PAP) [65].

The primary and the most common clinical form of PAP, which accounts for 90% of cases, is caused by anti-GM-CSF autoantibodies and is considered a primary immunodeficiency [66]. The other form of PAP is often secondary to hematologic diseases (myelodysplastic syndrome, acute myelogenous leukemia, acute lymphoblastic leukemia, chronic myelocytic leukemia, chronic lymphocytic leukemia, aplastic anemia, multiple myeloma, lymphoma, and Waldenstrom macroglobulinemia), nonhematologic malignancies (lung adenocarcinoma, glioblastoma, melanoma), infectious diseases (CMV, *Mycobacterium tuberculosis*, *Nocardia*, *Pneumocystis jirovecii*), and immunosuppressive drugs or encountered in the setting of defined primary immunodeficiency, such as ADA deficiency, GATA2 deficiency, and lysinuric protein intolerance [65].

Usually the onset of clinical manifestations is insidious, and the most important symptom is progressive dyspnea [67]. Patients are also susceptible to pulmonary and extrapulmonary infections frequently caused by opportunistic pathogens [68].

6.16 Trypanosomiasis

The trypanosomiases consist of a group of important animal and human diseases caused by parasitic protozoa of the genera *Trypanosoma* and *Leishmania*. In South and Central America, Chagas's disease (American trypanosomiasis) remains one of the most prevalent infectious diseases.

Chagas's disease is caused by the protozoan *Trypanosoma cruzi* and is endemic in Latin America. This protozoan is most commonly transmitted through the feces of an infected triatomine but can also be congenital, via contaminated blood transfusion or through direct oral contact. In the acute phase, the disease can cause cardiac derangements like myocarditis, conduction system abnormalities, and/or pericarditis. Untreated patients can advance to the chronic phase. Up to one-half of these patients will develop a cardiomyopathy, which can lead to cardiac failure and/or ventricular arrhythmias, both of which are major causes of mortality.

The parasite's ability to escape and/or modulate both innate and adaptive immune responses is crucial for their survival.

Leishmania can escape complement-mediated lysis by targeting host cells through complement activation. Expression of a modified surface lipophosphoglycan (LPG) [69] was found to enhance the synthesis of surface proteinase gp63 [70] and PSA-2 [71] preventing insertion or deposition of the lytic C5b-C9 complex, thereby enhancing tolerance of complement-mediated lysis (CML). *Trypanosoma cruzi* blood forms can also survive complement activation as they express glycoproteins such as gp160, gp58/68, and T-DAF. These proteins can bind to C3b and C4b, which allow evasion of complement [72, 73].

Leishmania sp. and *T. cruzi* are able to resist the antimicrobial mechanisms induced in phagocytic and even in non-phagocytic cells. During the acute phase of infection, *T. cruzi* replicates extensively and releases immunomodulatory molecules (GPI-mucins, trans-sialidase, glycoinositolphospholipids (GPILs), the cysteine proteinase cruzipain), which play an important role in subverting the host's innate immunity. GPI-mucins are responsible for parasite surface variability, leading to differential tissue adherence and evasion of host innate immune responses. Moreover, they render DCs dysfunctional for protective responses [74]. Persistence of *Leishmania* and infection progression are caused by the inability of phagocytes to elicit both effective innate and adaptative responses [75]. *Leishmania* alters some biological functions (retention of intracellular iron, alteration of the DNA methylation status of many host genes with antimicrobial functions, and disruption of cholesterol dynamics) to promote parasite growth.

Ten patients with congenital Chagas's disease were reported with pneumonitis. Amastigotes were found in the lungs in seven of these cases, and in two of these patients, parasitized cells were seen in the alveolar lumen. Parasites were found both in the lungs and in the amniotic epithelium of the extraplacental membranes and umbilical cord in five patients. Probably the infection of the amniotic epithelium in the lungs was carried by the amniotic fluid [76].

6.17 Isolated Congenital Asplenia (ICA)

The spleen represents the largest accumulation of lymphoid tissue in the human body. It also filters the blood; splenic red pulp is primarily dedicated to picking up foreign particles, in addition to worn-out, damaged, or otherwise altered erythrocytes. Meanwhile, the white pulp activates the immune response when antigens and their antibodies are present in the blood [77].

Splenic phagocytes play a crucial role in removal of complement-opsonized pneumococci from the blood, a process that is enhanced by the presence of specific antibody against the polysaccharide capsule of the organism. These immunological observations are supported by clinical experience in which deficiency of specific antibody or hyposplenism led to an increase in the risk of pneumococcal disease [78, 79].

Congenital asplenia often occurs in the context of a recognized malformation syndrome and is associated with complex visceral defects as part of heterotaxy syndromes with bilateral right sidedness [80, 81].

In contrast, isolated congenital asplenia (ICA) is characterized by the absence of heterotaxy or cardiac defects and was first thought to be very rare and sporadic [82]. Studies of case reports suggested probably autosomal dominant inheritance pattern.

Clinical presentation of ICA can be varied based on the age of presentation with increased severity in infants and decreasing severity with age likely due to maturation of cell-mediated immunity beyond 2 years of age [83]. The most frequent pathogens are encapsulated bacteria, especially *Streptococcus pneumonia*.

Infants and young children with ICA presenting with overwhelming sepsis have a high mortality, and the diagnosis is made after autopsy [84]. The Howell-Jolly bodies are intraerythrocytic remnants of an immature erythrocyte, which is normally removed in the spleen. Their presence is considered to signify a high likelihood of splenic dysfunction [85]. The presence of Howell-Jolly bodies in the peripheral blood smear may provide a clue for early diagnosis in patient presenting with sepsis or recurrent febrile illness and trigger an evaluation of splenic function [86].

References

1. Hambleton S, Goodbourn S, Young DF, Dickinson P, Mohamad SM, Valappil M, et al. STAT2 deficiency and susceptibility to viral illness in humans. Proc Natl Acad Sci. 2013;110(8):3053–8.
2. Turvey SE, Broide DH. Innate immunity. J Allergy Clin Immunol. 2010;125(2):S24–32.
3. Courtois G, Smahi A, Reichenbach J, Döffinger R, Cancrini C, Bonnet M, et al. A hypermorphic IκBα mutation is associated with autosomal dominant anhidrotic ectodermal dysplasia and T cell immunodeficiency. J Clin Invest. 2003;112(7):1108–15.
4. Ghosh S, May MJ, Kopp EB. NF-kappa B and Rel proteins: evolutionarily conserved mediators of immune responses. Annu Rev Immunol. 1998;16:225–60.
5. Picard C, Casanova J-L, Puel A. Infectious diseases in patients with IRAK-4, MyD88, NEMO, or IκBα deficiency. Clin Microbiol Rev. 2011;24(3):490–7.
6. Abinun M, Flood T, Cant A, Spickett G, Appleton A. Anhidrotic ectodermal dysplasia associated with specific antibody deficiency. Eur J Pediatr. 1996;155(2):146–7.
7. Boisson B, Puel A, Picard C, Casanova J-L. Human IκBα gain of function: a severe and syndromic immunodeficiency. J Clin Immunol. 2017;37(5):397–412.
8. Sancho-Shimizu V, de Diego RP, Jouanguy E, Zhang S-Y, Casanova J-L. Inborn errors of antiviral interferon immunity in humans. Curr Opin Virol. 2011;1(6):487–96.
9. Zinngrebe J, Rieser E, Taraborrelli L, Peltzer N, Hartwig T, Ren H, et al. LUBAC deficiency perturbs TLR3 signaling to cause immunodeficiency and autoinflammation. J Exp Med. 2016;213(12):2671–89.
10. Tokunaga F. Linear ubiquitination-mediated NF-κB regulation and its related disorders. J Biochem. 2013;154(4):313–23.
11. Aksentijevich I, Zhou Q. NF-κB Pathway in autoinflammatory diseases: dysregulation of protein modifications by ubiquitin defines a new category of autoinflammatory diseases. Front Immunol. 2017;8:399.
12. Boisson B, Laplantine E, Prando C, Giliani S, Israelsson E, Xu Z, et al. Immunodeficiency, autoinflammation and amylopectinosis in humans with inherited HOIL-1 and LUBAC deficiency. Nat Immunol. 2012;13(12):1178.
13. Sancho-Shimizu V, de Diego RP, Lorenzo L, Halwani R, Alangari A, Israelsson E, et al. Herpes simplex encephalitis in children with autosomal recessive and dominant TRIF deficiency. J Clin Invest. 2011;121(12):4889–902.
14. Herman M, Ciancanelli M, Ou Y-H, Lorenzo L, Klaudel-Dreszler M, Pauwels E, et al. Heterozygous TBK1 mutations impair TLR3 immunity and underlie herpes simplex encephalitis of childhood. J Exp Med. 2012;209(9):1567–82.
15. Andersen LL, Mørk N, Reinert LS, Kofod-Olsen E, Narita R, Jørgensen SE, et al. Functional IRF3 deficiency in a patient with herpes simplex encephalitis. J Exp Med. 2015;212(9):1371–9.
16. Casrouge A, Zhang S-Y, Eidenschenk C, Jouanguy E, Puel A, Yang K, et al. Herpes simplex virus encephalitis in human UNC-93B deficiency. Science. 2006;314(5797):308–12.
17. Al-Muhsen S, Casanova J-L. The genetic heterogeneity of mendelian susceptibility to mycobacterial diseases. J Allergy Clin Immunol. 2008;122(6):1043–51.

18. Galal N, Boutros J, Marsafy A, Kong XF, Feinberg J, Casanova JL, et al. Mendelian susceptibility to mycobacterial disease in Egyptian children. Mediterr J Hematol Infect Dis. 2012;4(1):e2012033.
19. Fieschi C, Bosticardo M, De Beaucoudrey L, Boisson-Dupuis S, Feinberg J, Santos OF, et al. A novel form of complete IL-12/IL-23 receptor β1 deficiency with cell surface-expressed nonfunctional receptors. Blood. 2004;104(7):2095–101.
20. Bustamante J, Picard C, Boisson-Dupuis S, Abel L, Casanova JL. Genetic lessons learned from X-linked Mendelian susceptibility to mycobacterial diseases. Ann N Y Acad Sci. 2011;1246(1):92–101.
21. Lee W-I, Huang J-L, Yeh K-W, Jaing T-H, Lin T-Y, Huang Y-C, et al. Immune defects in active mycobacterial diseases in patients with primary immunodeficiency diseases (PIDs). J Formos Med Assoc. 2011;110(12):750–8.
22. Rocca S, Schiavoni G, Sali M, Anfossi AG, Abalsamo L, Palucci I, et al. Interferon regulatory factor 8-deficiency determines massive neutrophil recruitment but T cell defect in fast growing granulomas during tuberculosis. PLoS One. 2013;8(5):e62751.
23. Bogunovic D, Byun M, Durfee LA, Abhyankar A, Sanal O, Mansouri D, et al. Mycobacterial disease and impaired IFN-γ immunity in humans with inherited ISG15 deficiency. Science. 2012;337(6102):1684–8.
24. Boisson-Dupuis S, Kong X-F, Okada S, Cypowyj S, Puel A, Abel L, et al. Inborn errors of human STAT1: allelic heterogeneity governs the diversity of immunological and infectious phenotypes. Curr Opin Immunol. 2012;24(4):364–78.
25. Moens L, Van Eyck L, Jochmans D, Mitera T, Frans G, Bossuyt X, et al. A novel kindred with inherited STAT2 deficiency and severe viral illness. J Allergy Clin Immunol. 2017;139(6):1995–7.e9.
26. Rezaei N, Hedayat M, Aghamohammadi A, Nichols KE. Primary immunodeficiency diseases associated with increased susceptibility to viral infections and malignancies. J Allergy Clin Immunol. 2011;127(6):1329–41.e2.
27. Kawai T, Malech HL. WHIM syndrome: congenital immune deficiency disease. Curr Opin Hematol. 2009;16(1):20.
28. Przybyszewska J, Zlotogorski A, Ramot Y. Re-evaluation of epidermodysplasia verruciformis: reconciling more than 90 years of debate. J Am Acad Dermatol. 2017;76(6):1161–75.
29. Lorè NI, Cigana C, Riva C, De Fino I, Nonis A, Spagnuolo L, et al. IL-17A impairs host tolerance during airway chronic infection by Pseudomonas aeruginosa. Sci Rep. 2016;6:25937.
30. Iwakura Y, Ishigame H, Saijo S, Nakae S. Functional specialization of interleukin-17 family members. Immunity. 2011;34(2):149–62.
31. Aujla SJ, Chan YR, Zheng M, Fei M, Askew DJ, Pociask DA, et al. IL-22 mediates mucosal host defense against Gram-negative bacterial pneumonia. Nat Med. 2008;14(3):275.
32. Boisson B, Wang C, Pedergnana V, Wu L, Cypowyj S, Rybojad M, et al. An ACT1 mutation selectively abolishes interleukin-17 responses in humans with chronic mucocutaneous candidiasis. Immunity. 2013;39(4):676–86.
33. Swaidani S, Bulek K, Kang Z, Liu C, Lu Y, Yin W, et al. The critical role of epithelial-derived Act1 in IL-17-and IL-25-mediated pulmonary inflammation. J Immunol. 2009;182(3):1631–40.
34. Claudio E, Sønder SU, Saret S, Carvalho G, Ramalingam TR, Wynn TA, et al. The adaptor protein CIKS/Act1 is essential for IL-25-mediated allergic airway inflammation. J Immunol. 2009;182(3):1617–30.
35. Liu L, Okada S, Kong X-F, Kreins AY, Cypowyj S, Abhyankar A, et al. Gain-of-function human STAT1 mutations impair IL-17 immunity and underlie chronic mucocutaneous candidiasis. J Exp Med. 2011;208(8):1635–48.
36. Engelhardt KR, Grimbacher B. Mendelian traits causing susceptibility to mucocutaneous fungal infections in human subjects. J Allergy Clin Immunol. 2012;129(2):294–305.
37. Uzel G, Sampaio EP, Lawrence MG, Hsu AP, Hackett M, Dorsey MJ, et al. Dominant gain-of-function STAT1 mutations in FOXP3 wild-type immune dysregulation–polyendocrinopathy–enteropathy–X-linked–like syndrome. J Allergy Clin Immunol. 2013;131(6):1611–23.e3.

38. Lee PP, Mao H, Yang W, Chan K-W, Ho MH, Lee T-L, et al. Penicillium marneffei infection and impaired IFN-γ immunity in humans with autosomal-dominant gain-of-phosphorylation STAT1 mutations. J Allergy Clin Immunol. 2014;133(3):894–6.e5.
39. Drummond RA, Lionakis MS. Mechanistic insights into the role of C-type lectin receptor/CARD9 signaling in human antifungal immunity. Front Cell Infect Microbiol. 2016;6:39.
40. Lanternier F, Pathan S, Vincent QB, Liu L, Cypowyj S, Prando C, et al. Deep dermatophytosis and inherited CARD9 deficiency. N Engl J Med. 2013;369(18):1704–14.
41. Gavino C, Cotter A, Lichtenstein D, Lejtenyi D, Fortin C, Legault C, et al. CARD9 deficiency and spontaneous central nervous system candidiasis: complete clinical remission with GM-CSF therapy. Clin Infect Dis. 2014;59(1):81–4.
42. Lanternier F, Barbati E, Meinzer U, Liu L, Pedergnana V, Migaud M, et al. Inherited CARD9 deficiency in 2 unrelated patients with invasive Exophiala infection. J Infect Dis. 2014;211(8):1241–50.
43. Jhingran A, Kasahara S, Shepardson KM, Junecko BAF, Heung LJ, Kumasaka DK, et al. Compartment-specific and sequential role of MyD88 and CARD9 in chemokine induction and innate defense during respiratory fungal infection. PLoS Pathog. 2015;11(1):e1004589.
44. Whibley N, Jaycox JR, Reid D, Garg AV, Taylor JA, Clancy CJ, et al. Delinking CARD9 and IL-17: CARD9 protects against Candida tropicalis infection through a TNF-α–dependent, IL-17–independent mechanism. J Immunol. 2015; https://doi.org/10.4049/jimmunol.1500870.
45. Anderson MS, Venanzi ES, Klein L, Chen Z, Berzins SP, Turley SJ, et al. Projection of an immunological self shadow within the thymus by the aire protein. Science. 2002;298(5597):1395–401.
46. Popler J, Alimohammadi M, Kämpe O, Dalin F, Dishop MK, Barker JM, et al. Autoimmune polyendocrine syndrome type 1: utility of KCNRG autoantibodies as a marker of active pulmonary disease and successful treatment with rituximab. Pediatr Pulmonol. 2012;47(1):84–7.
47. Martinez Lopez MM, Gonzales Casado I, Alvarez Doforno R, et al. AIRE gene mutation in polyglandular syndrome type 1. An Pediatr (Barc). 2006;64(6):583–7.
48. Korniszewski L, Kurzyna M, Stolarski B, Torbicki A, Smerdel A, Ploski R. Fatal primary pulmonary hypertension in a 30-yr-old female with APECED syndrome. Eur Respir J. 2003;22(4):709–11.
49. Milenkovic T, Zdravkovic D, Djordjevic M, Podkrajsek K, Minic P, Battelino T. A novel AIRE gene mutation in an APS1 patient with adrenal failure, hypoparathyroidism, ovarian failure, growth hormone deficiency, asthma and chronic otitis with effusion (abstract). Horm Res. 2007;68(1):61.
50. Dubois N, Tardivel I, Kajosaari M, Vialettes B, Carel J. Autoimmune bronchiolitis is a life threatening component of autoimmune polyendocrine syndrome type 1 (APS-1). Horm Res. 2007;68(1):61.
51. Tang X, Lasbury ME, Davidson DD, Bartlett MS, Smith JW, Lee C-H. Down-regulation of GATA-2 transcription during Pneumocystis carinii infection. Infect Immun. 2000;68(8):4720–4.
52. Lasbury ME, Tang X, Durant PJ, Lee C-H. Effect of transcription factor GATA-2 on phagocytic activity of alveolar macrophages from Pneumocystis carinii-infected hosts. Infect Immun. 2003;71(9):4943–52.
53. González-Lara MF, Wisniowski-Yáñez A, Pérez-Patrigeon S, Hsu AP, Holland SM, Cuellar-Rodríguez JM. Pneumocystis jiroveci pneumonia and GATA2 deficiency: expanding the spectrum of the disease. J Infect. 2017;74(4):425–7.
54. Marquis J-F, Kapoustina O, Langlais D, Ruddy R, Dufour CR, Kim B-H, et al. Interferon regulatory factor 8 regulates pathways for antigen presentation in myeloid cells and during tuberculosis. PLoS Genet. 2011;7(6):e1002097.
55. Hambleton S, Salem S, Bustamante J, Bigley V, Boisson-Dupuis S, Azevedo J, et al. IRF8 mutations and human dendritic-cell immunodeficiency. N Engl J Med. 2011;365(2):127–38.
56. Jouanguy E, Gineau L, Cottineau J, Béziat V, Vivier E, Casanova J-L. Inborn errors of the development of human natural killer cells. Curr Opin Allergy Clin Immunol. 2013;13(6):589.

57. Mace EM, Orange JS. Genetic causes of human NK cell deficiency and their effect on NK cell subsets. Front Immunol. 2016;7:545.
58. Orange JS. Human natural killer cell deficiencies and susceptibility to infection. Microbes Infect. 2002;4(15):1545–58.
59. Orange JS. Human natural killer cell deficiencies. Curr Opin Allergy Clin Immunol. 2006;6(6):399–409.
60. Biron CA, Byron KS, Sullivan JL. Severe herpesvirus infections in an adolescent without natural killer cells. N Engl J Med. 1989;320(26):1731–5.
61. Fleisher G, Starr S, Koven N, Kamiya H, Douglas SD, Henle W. A non-X-linked syndrome with susceptibility to severe Epstein-Barr virus infections. J Pediatr. 1982;100(5):727–30.
62. Bochman ML, Schwacha A. The Mcm complex: unwinding the mechanism of a replicative helicase. Microbiol Mol Biol Rev. 2009;73(4):652–83.
63. Gineau L, Cognet C, Kara N, Lach FP, Dunne J, Veturi U, et al. Partial MCM4 deficiency in patients with growth retardation, adrenal insufficiency, and natural killer cell deficiency. J Clin Invest. 2012;122(3):821–32.
64. Orange JS. Unraveling human natural killer cell deficiency. J Clin Invest. 2012;122(3):798–801.
65. Borie R, Danel C, Debray M, Taille C, Dombret M, Aubier M, et al. Pulmonary alveolar proteinosis. Eur Respir Rev. 2011;20(120):98–107.
66. Browne SK, Holland SM. Immunodeficiency secondary to anti-cytokine autoantibodies. Curr Opin Allergy Clin Immunol. 2010;10(6):534.
67. Suzuki T, Sakagami T, Young LR, Carey BC, Wood RE, Luisetti M, et al. Hereditary pulmonary alveolar proteinosis: pathogenesis, presentation, diagnosis, and therapy. Am J Respir Crit Care Med. 2010;182(10):1292–304.
68. Seymour JF, Presneill JJ. Pulmonary alveolar proteinosis: progress in the first 44 years. Am J Respir Crit Care Med. 2002;166(2):215–35.
69. McConville M, Ralton J. Developmentally regulated changes in the cell surface architecture of Leishmania parasites. Behring Inst Mitt. 1997;99:34–43.
70. Brittingham A, Morrison CJ, McMaster WR, McGwire BS, Chang K-P, Mosser DM. Role of the Leishmania surface protease gp63 in complement fixation, cell adhesion, and resistance to complement-mediated lysis. J Immunol. 1995;155(6):3102–11.
71. Lincoln LM, Ozaki M, Donelson JE, Beetham JK. Genetic complementation of Leishmania deficient in PSA (GP46) restores their resistance to lysis by complement. Mol Biochem Parasitol. 2004;1(137):185–9.
72. Zambrano-Villa S, Rosales-Borjas D, Carrero JC, Ortiz-Ortiz L. How protozoan parasites evade the immune response. Trends Parasitol. 2002;18(6):272–8.
73. Cestari I, Evans-Osses I, Schlapbach LJ, de Messias-Reason I, Ramirez MI. Mechanisms of complement lectin pathway activation and resistance by trypanosomatid parasites. Mol Immunol. 2013;53(4):328–34.
74. Chaussabel D, Pajak B, Vercruysse V, Bisseyé C, Garzé V, Habib M, et al. Alteration of migration and maturation of dendritic cells and T-cell depletion in the course of experimental Trypanosoma cruzi infection. Lab Investig. 2003;83(9):1373.
75. Freitas-Teixeira P, Silveira-Lemos D, Giunchetti R, Baratta-Masini A, Mayrink W, Peruhype-Magalhães V, et al. Distinct pattern of immunophenotypic features of innate and adaptive immunity as a putative signature of clinical and laboratorial status of patients with localized cutaneous leishmaniasis. Scand J Immunol. 2012;76(4):421–32.
76. Bittencourt AL, de Freitas LAR, de Araujo MOG, Jácomo K. Pneumonitis in congenital Chagas' disease. Am J Trop Med Hyg. 1981;30(1):38–42.
77. Cesta MF. Normal structure, function, and histology of the spleen. Toxicol Pathol. 2006;34(5):455–65.
78. Bisno AL, Freeman JC. The syndrome of asplenia, pneumococcal sepsis, and disseminated intravascular coagulation. Ann Intern Med. 1970;72(3):389–93.
79. Ellis EF, Smith RT. The role of the spleen in immunity: with special reference to the post-splenectomy problem in infants. Pediatrics. 1966;37(1):111–9.

80. Freedom RM. The asplenia syndrome: a review of significant extracardiac structural abnormalities in 29 necropsied patients. J Pediatr. 1972;81(6):1130–3.
81. Ivemark B. Implications of agenesis of the spleen on the pathogenesis of conotruncus anomalies in childhood. Acta Paediatr. 1955;44(6):590–2.
82. Myerson RM, Koelle WA. Congenital absence of the spleen in an adult: report of a case associated with recurrent Waterhouse-Friderichsen syndrome. N Engl J Med. 1956;254(24):1131–2.
83. Maddux AB, Douglas IS. Is the developmentally immature immune response in paediatric sepsis a recapitulation of immune tolerance? Immunology. 2015;145(1):1–10.
84. Mahlaoui N, Minard-Colin V, Picard C, Bolze A, Ku C-L, Tournilhac O, et al. Isolated congenital asplenia: a French nationwide retrospective survey of 20 cases. J Pediatr. 2011;158(1):142–8.e1.
85. William BM, Corazza GR. Hyposplenism: a comprehensive review. Part I: basic concepts and causes. Hematology. 2007;12(1):1–13.
86. Mathew H, Dittus C, Malek A, Negroiu A. Howell-Jolly bodies on peripheral smear leading to the diagnosis of congenital hyposplenism in a patient with septic shock. Clin Case Rep. 2015;3(8):714–7.

Chapter 7
Pulmonary Manifestations of Autoinflammatory Disorders

Ahmadreza Jamshidi, Saeed Aslani, and Mahdi Mahmoudi

7.1 Rheumatoid Arthritis

Rheumatoid arthritis (RA) is an autoimmune and systemic inflammatory disorder, which occurs in about 0.5–1% of the general population worldwide. This AID is characterized by immune-mediated inflammatory complications of the synovium [1–3]. Among the common symptoms of the RA are swelling and pain in joints due to inflammation in the synovium, small joints involvement, fatigue, anemia, cardiovascular complications, and osteoporosis. Adalimumab, which is a humanized monoclonal antibody against tumor necrosis factor (TNF), has been reported to be effective at ameliorating the development of structural damage of joints and soothing the disease symptoms [4].

In RA patients, most common radiologic findings about the pulmonary complications are first, reticular unclear patterns with distortion of lung's lobules and traction bronchiolectasis with honeycombing that associate with fibrotic interstitial lung disease (ILD); second, airway-related complications like fuzzy centrilobular nodules of ground-glass attenuation or wall thickening of bronchus with heterogeneous lung abnormalities; third, patchy and peripheral consolidation, which may be accompanied with organizing pneumonia (OP); fourth, random parenchymal nodules; and fifth, pleural effusions [5–7]. Honeycomb cysts, which may be seen frequently, imply to developed phase of disease and represent usual interstitial pneumonia (UIP) pattern on pathological biopsies. Implying to UIP histopathology, fibrosis is seen with heterogeneous appearance [5, 8, 9].

The most usual form of pulmonary involvement in RA patients is pleural effusions with pleuritis. Such histologic manifestations in lung biopsies in patients with ILD suggest the diagnosis of a rheumatic disorder. A wide range of histopathologic

A. Jamshidi · S. Aslani · M. Mahmoudi (✉)
Rheumatology Research Center, Tehran University of Medical Sciences (TUMS), Tehran, Iran
e-mail: jamshida@tums.ac.ir; s-aslani@razi.tums.ac.ir; mahmoudim@tums.ac.ir

S. A. Mahdaviani, N. Rezaei (eds.), *Pulmonary Manifestations of Primary Immunodeficiency Diseases*, https://doi.org/10.1007/978-3-030-00880-2_7

patterns is seen in RA patients with lung complications [8, 10–14]. The most specific presentation of lung involvement by RA is rheumatoid nodules that are more usually seen in the skin. Oftentimes, these nodules are found in the subpleural area and may be restricted by giant cells and palisading histiocytes. Approximately a diffuse, fibrosing lung disease with equal portions of UIP is observed in two-thirds of RA lung biopsies [8, 15].

UIP is defined by remodeling of fibrotic lung that associates with honeycomb modifications with healthy lung, mostly with fibroblastic points at the location of fibrosis. In contrast, the alveolar septal fibrosis in nonspecific interstitial pneumonia (NSIP) occurs with maintained underlying lung structure [16]. Inconclusive diagnosis is observed in a small group of RA patients who develop lung disease prior to their systemic disease is diagnosed, since both patterns of fibrosis can idiopathically be manifested.

Follicular bronchiolitis occurs in approximately 20% of RA cases [15], commonly presented underlying the UIP or NSIP. There is a chance of small airway disease in RA cases that is commonly presented as constrictive bronchiolitis. This presentation is mainly diagnosed before biopsy evaluation due to certain results of pulmonary function examinations and manifestations of bronchiolar disease, demonstrable by the presence of a mosaic pattern on high-resolution tomography by computational approaches [17]. In patients with sudden respiratory failure, acute lung injury patterns can be presented as OP or diffuse alveolar damage (DAD) [11]. In rare conditions, vasculitis and pulmonary hemorrhage are observed in RA patients that are regarded as an acute pulmonary manifestation [18]. Most of the pathologic presentations of RA assumed to be nonspecific [10]; however, some primary specifications are seen in most of the cases of RA-associated ILD. Often, there is a lymphoid accumulation and follicles with germinal centers within the lung tissues. These accumulations of immune cells are seen in follicular bronchiolitis, as well as in the areas of fibrosis in pleura. Moreover, most of the lung biopsies from RA patients demonstrate concurrent histologic changes in acute, subacute, and chronic phases. Concurrence of acute, subacute, and chronic inflammatory reactions such as involvement of the pleura could strongly be considered as lung disease in subjects with RA [19].

7.2 Systemic Sclerosis

Systemic sclerosis (SSc), or scleroderma, is a systemic autoimmune disorder that has been a challenging disease to be treated. While recent advancements have been promising in the treatment of specific complications, such as pulmonary arterial hypertension (PAH) with prostanoids, there are still no disease-modifying drugs controlling the overall disease activity completely [20].

The most common radiologic presentations in SSc-associated ILD include bibasilar ground-glass attenuation, reticulation, superimposed on mild architectural distortion, and different traction bronchiolectasis presented with a homogeneous appearance relating to NSIP. With respect to lung manifestations in SSc, the immediate subpleural lung is commonly spared, but honeycombing is rarely seen [21, 22]. The area of ground-glass attenuation in ILD underlying SSc is usually greater than that in cases with idiopathic pulmonary fibrosis. Moreover, in SSc-associated ILD, the reticular complications are less coarse [23]. On the other hand, the area of radiographic modifications in SSc subjects seems to be associated with the level of pulmonary hypertension. However, this association is not seen in cases with idiopathic pulmonary fibrosis [24, 25]. As a minor presentation, pleural thickening and pleural effusion may also occur. However, esophageal dilatation is seen oftentimes [26]. Multifocal consolidation or ground-glass attenuation in the posterior upper or lower lobes of lungs may represent aspiration pneumonia due to esophageal dysmotility. In contrast to the NSIP, there is segmental distribution pattern in radiologic manifestations of SSc-associated ILD cases.

In SSc patients, the common pattern of ILD is nonspecific interstitial pneumonia [27]. Its morphologic presentation is certain, which is manifested through a bland and paucicellular fibrosis that involves the interstitium, with overall maintenance of lung structure. Common interstitial pneumonia is rarely seen in SSc, and its diagnosis may depend on focal microscopic honeycombing [27, 28]. Occasionally, the centrilobular fibrosis is the main manifestation, possibly associated with recurrent aspiration because of esophageal dysmotility image of the disorder [29–31]. In SSc patients, pulmonary hypertension is frequently seen that may occur without ILD [32, 33]. As a result, biopsies are not necessarily required for careful evaluation of the pulmonary vasculature. The vascular modifications in SSc cases are recognized with intimal thickening of the pulmonary arteries, in which there is a connective tissue presentation with mucopolysaccharide-rich fibromyxoid [33]. Furthermore, OP and DAD are among the characteristics of SSc patients; nonetheless, they are not clearly distinguishable from OP and DAD seen in other disorders [34, 35]. Alternately, alveolar hemorrhage with capillaritis can be seen rarely [36].

7.3 Systemic Lupus Erythematosus

Systemic lupus erythematosus (SLE) is also a systemic autoimmune disorder and characterized particularly by the production of a wide array of autoantibodies [37].

Pleural thickening and pericardial effusions are the most usual radiologic presentation related to pulmonary complications in SLE [38–42]. Acute lupus pneumonitis usually is manifested by bilateral, diffuse, and ground-glass attenuation. These presentations are frequently observed in the lower lobes of lungs, which may be accompanied by minimal or no associated architectural modifications while may be manifested by pleural effusions in about 20% of the cases [43]. Rarely, acute lupus pneumonitis may be accompanied with normal findings based on chest radiography [44]. In specific cases of pulmonary hemorrhage or vasculitis, centrilobular nodules of ground-glass attenuation may also be presented [45]. In SLE patients, high-resolution computed tomography disorders may be frequently seen [46].

In SLE patients, involvement of the lung is manifested by two main models of injury, namely, acute lupus pneumonitis and cellular NSIP variation. Acute lupus pneumonitis is presented by a damage with diffuse alveolar pattern, which may occur with or without hemorrhage, different levels of interstitial inflammation, as well as edema. In some cases, capillaritis may also occur, particularly during alveolar hemorrhage and hemosiderin-laden macrophages [47, 48]. In some cases, diffuse alveolar hemorrhage may frequently be seen with capillaritis. Furthermore, acute fibrinous pleuritis may be observed in diffuse alveolar hemorrhage, implying to the diagnosis of SLE or, rarely, RA. On the other side, SLE is seen with pulmonary hypertension [49–51]. A number of pathogenetic approaches have been suggested for underlying pulmonary hypertension in various subsets of SLE patients. After chronic thromboembolic disease, some SLE patients are affected with pulmonary hypertension, which is presented by pulmonary arteries intimal thickening as well as complex intraluminal architecture [52, 53]. Some other SLE cases may develop a vasculopathy, which is characterized by vascular remodeling without inflammation that finally results in plexiform lesions [54]. However, in some cases, SLE may be presented by an immune-mediated vasculopathy, which is accompanied by pulmonary vasculitis [55]. Another lung complication pattern seen in SLE patients is NSIP, manifested by an increased infiltration of lymphocytes and plasma cells as well as cellular interstitial pneumonia with interstitial fibrosis [56].

Pulmonary hemorrhage negatively impresses the prognosis of SLE patients [57, 58]. Sometimes, OP is seen and can be the first presentation of the disease [59–61]. Among the other pulmonary complications in SLE patients which are rarely seen include lymphoid interstitial pneumonia, acute fibrinous and OP, and pulmonary fibrosis [57, 58, 62–65].

7.4 Polymyositis-Dermatomyositis

Polymyositis (PM) and dermatomyositis (DM) are considered as systemic inflammatory disorders that are characterized by symmetric muscle weakness. Based on diagnostic criteria, the prevalence of ILD in PM-DM has been established to be ranged from 5% to 30% [66, 67].

Radiologic specifications in PM-DM are presented by an increased incidence of airspace consolidation and a decreased incidence of honeycombing [67]. Typically, modifications involve the lung bases as well as the peripheral regions [68]. Ground-glass and linear opacities in 92%, airspace consolidation in 52%, irregular interfaces in 88%, honeycombing in 16%, and parenchymal micronodules in 28% of patients have been reported [67]. Among the radiographic changes occurred in PM-DM are consolidation and peribronchovascular thickening, which seems to be improvable by medications [69]. The most significant radiologic presentation in PM-DM is the development of airspace consolidation, which associates with acute clinical manifestations and acute lung injury in biopsies [70].

In idiopathic inflammatory myopathies, lung involvement is the most usual extramuscular presentation. Based on their clinical characteristics, patients with idiopathic inflammatory myopathies are traditionally subclassified as PM and DM. In these patients, NSIP is the most frequent form of lung abnormality [71, 72] with a prevalence in biopsies fourfold higher than that of UIP in PM and a somewhat lower predominance in DM [72–74]. It is hard to discriminate the NSIP from the idiopathic subtypes of NSIP. However, in case of further clinical specifications, such as follicular bronchiolitis, diagnosis chance of rheumatic disorder is increased. On the other hand, if there is extensive fibrosis, it can often be distinguishable from idiopathic UIP, which occurs without centrilobular sparing. Approximately 50% of the cases of fibrosing ILD exhibit superimposed OP, which sometimes is primary manifestation [75–77]. Classification of PM-DM patients into distinct clinical subsets has been facilitated through identification of myositis-specific antibodies. Studies show that detection of antibodies against aminoacyl-transfer RNA synthetases, namely, anti-synthetase antibodies such as PL-7, PL-12, Jo-1, EJ, KS, and OJ, has been associated with ILD [78]. It has been stablished that the most prevalent autoantibody, namely, anti-synthetase antibody of Jo-1, is detected in about 20% of myositis patients, suggesting a greater prevalence of UIP than NSIP [79]. A bulk of these patients seems to manifest a rapidly progressive hypoxemia and display superimposed and acute lung injury models [80–82]. In PM-DM individuals, pulmonary hypertension and pulmonary capillaritis have been seen rarely [83, 84]. However, bronchiolitis, pleuritis, and vascular changes are rarely presented in PM/DM [85–87].

7.5 Sjogren's Syndrome

Sjogren's syndrome (SjS) is the second most common multisystem autoimmune disorder after rheumatoid arthritis and is characterized by dryness of the eye and mouth and lymphocytic infiltration of the salivary glands [88].

In SjS patients, the radiographic presentations are mostly nonspecific. However, oftentimes it demonstrates lower lobe-predominant, homogeneous, and ground-glass attenuation with minimum structure modification that displays no honeycombing with subpleural sparing, suggesting the NSIP model [89–92]. In a study evaluating 60 patients with primary SjS, centrilobular nodule was found in 78% of patients, ground-glass opacity in 92% of patients, nonseptal linear opacity in 75% of patients, bronchiectasis in 38% of patients, interlobular septal thickening in 55% of patients, and cyst in 30% of patients [91]. Honeycombing has been less reported in primary SjS (7%), while in secondary SjS is more common (29%) [93]. To diagnose LIP, some manifestations such as thin-walled cysts and small nodules, particularly when concurred with ground-glass attenuation, are contributing [94]. In case of pleural effusions or hilar and mediastinal lymphadenopathy, the risk of lymphoma in SjS patients increases [95].

Diffuse, cellular interstitial pneumonia is the most common ILD in SjS that can be categorized as NSIP or LIP based upon the severity of inflammatory mediatory infiltration [96]. Parambil et al. evaluated 15 SjS patients and identified NSIP in 5 cases, OP in 4 cases, UIP in 3 cases, LIP in 3 cases, primary pulmonary lymphoma in 2 cases, and finally diffuse interstitial amyloidosis in only 1 patient [97]. On the other side, some evaluations have reported the lack of LIP in patients with SjS [96]. Chronic bronchiolitis is another typical morphologic presentation in SjS patients that is represented with follicular lymphoid hyperplasia, which is then called follicular bronchiolitis. With respect to LIP pattern, small, nonnecrotizing, interstitial granulomas are seen that indicate the hypersensitivity pneumonitis and frequently are seen during lymphoid infiltration. Moreover, cysts may be prevalent in LIP-associated SjS. These patients also have an increased chance of developing lymphoproliferative disorders [98–101].

7.6 Ankylosing Spondylitis

Ankylosing spondylitis (AS) is known as a chronic multisystem inflammatory disease, which is presented with articular and extra-articular characteristics. AS primarily affects the joints of the axial skeleton [102, 103]. Inflammation and arthritis of the joints lead to pain and developing stiffening of the spine, pelvis, and chest [104]. In addition to the joint-related complications, pulmonary, ocular, cardiovascular, renal, and neurologic manifestations have been the presentation of AS patients. AS can involve the tracheobronchial airways as well as the pulmonary parenchyma and is manifested by several certain pulmonary manifestations, like chest wall limitations as well as upper lobe fibrocystic disease.

Chest radiographic findings of AS patients may present the severity of clinical involvement. However, upper lobe fibrosis, apical nodular or linear infiltrates, and pleural thickening may be manifested in patients lacking pulmonary implications [103, 105]. Despite some modifications resulted from radiography, examinations may be unilateral or asymmetric during the initial phases, and most of the patients develop bilateral disease in the end [103]. In case of unilateral manifestations, the right apex may more frequently be involved in comparison to the left upper lobe of the lung [104]. Rarely, infiltration of the lower half of the lung lobes is seen [103].

In AS patients, pulmonary parenchymal abnormalities are usually progressive. Oftentimes, nodules coalesce into larger opacities [106] and cavitation, cyst formation, and fibrosis are presented in developed phases [103]. Intense fibrosis can eventuate in bronchiectasis of upper lobe and upward retraction of the hila [105, 107]. In an examination of the chest radiographs of 42 AS cases, the presence of upper lobe fibrosis in 6 patients (14%) and focal parenchymal changes in 13 patients (31%) were reported [108]. In another study, pulmonary modifications via radiography were detected in 5 of 39 AS patients that were 3 cases of apical fibrosis and 2 cases of cavitary lesions [109].

7.7 Behçet's Disease

Behçet's disease (BD) is an autoimmune multisystem vasculitis in which pulmonary involvement has been associated with complex clinical manifestations. Two major types of pulmonary vascular involvement in BD patients are pulmonary artery aneurysms (PAA) and pulmonary artery thrombus (PAT). Nonetheless, other complications related to parenchyma lesions, such as ground-glass opacity, nodules, consolidations, and cavitations, have also been reported [110]. Misinterpretation of these radiographic parenchyma lesions is possible, and there are limited bodies of studies evaluating these radiographic parenchymal modifications in patients.

Evaluation of 106 patients with BD demonstrated 15 patients (14%) with pulmonary involvement. Pulmonary artery aneurysms (PAA) were seen in six patients (5.6%), which also manifested thrombi, attenuation, or occlusion of Pas. Moreover, five (4.7%) of them demonstrated radiographic parenchymal modifications. Three patients (2.8%) had only pulmonary artery thrombus (PAT) without PAA. Patients with PAA or PAT were presented with more frequency of hemoptysis and extrapulmonary vascular lesions in comparison to isolated parenchymal involvement. Radiographic parenchyma modifications were nonspecific, presented with ill-defined ground-glass opacity, which were the most prevailing pulmonary radiographic parenchymal modulation. It was also observed that patients with isolated parenchymal changes had better prognosis in comparison to those with PAA or PAT. It seems that BD with pulmonary involvement displays a wide range of aberrant clinical and radiographic manifestations, and several pulmonary lesions may be present in the same patient.

7.8 Autoimmune Pancreatitis

Autoimmune pancreatitis is a benign autoimmune disorder characterized by swelling of the pancreas, abnormal narrowing of the pancreatic duct, increased immune cell infiltration, and fibrosis [111]. Autoimmune pancreatitis has not been limited to the involvement of pancreas and is considered as a systemic autoimmune disorder [112].

In a study, 30 patients with autoimmune pancreatitis were evaluated, among which, pulmonary involvement was observed in 4 patients. Of these four patients, two of them displayed respiratory failure. However, they indicated good response to treatment with steroid, but a higher dose of prednisolone was required to maintain remission in comparison to required dose in biliary involvement. Pulmonary involvement of these patients was determined through increased Krebs von den Lungen-6 and immunoglobulin G4 (IgG4) levels [113].

7.9 Wegener Granulomatosis

Wegener granulomatosis is a systemic autoimmune disorder, which prevalently affects males. The disease is characterized by granulomatous vasculitis complications seen in upper and lower respiratory tracts, small-vessel vasculitis, and glomerulonephritis. Histopathologically, the hallmark of Wegener granulomatosis is a necrotizing vasculitis of veins and small arteries accompanied with granuloma formation [114].

Studies have demonstrated that most of the patients with Wegener granulomatosis develop pulmonary disease. The most typical radiographic presentation of Wegener granulomatosis is multiple nodules or abnormal marginated masses with no predominance of zonal manifestations [115, 116]. Multiple nodules or masses are commonly seen but can be seen in single spots in approximately 25% of patients [116]. Moreover, the nodule cavitation, with irregular and thick walls, has been reported in about 50% of subjects. The nodules commonly show a pattern of irregular margins and typically possess a peribronchovascular distribution, as observed in CT scans [117, 118]. Stiffness of airspace in localized or diffuse patterns might be seen. These areas commonly exhibit pulmonary hemorrhage [116]. Involvement of the bronchial or tracheal walls commonly manifests with granulomatous thickness of mucosa or submucosa. Tracheal or bronchial wall thickness may be smooth or nodular. The thickening may become intense, which may eventuate in narrowing of the tracheal or bronchial lumen and, sometimes, calcification.

7.10 Churg-Strauss Syndrome

Churg-Strauss syndrome is a granulomatous necrotizing vasculitis and an allergic angiitis that is exclusively seen in patients with asthma, aged 30–50 years, without gender predominance. Patients commonly demonstrate asthmatic manifestations, eosinophilia, allergic rhinitis, and fever [119]. Chest radiography outcomes are usually irregular containing patchy and non-segmental consolidation areas lacking zonal predominance [120].

Consolidation areas may demonstrate an edged distribution pattern and are usually temporary. While the cavitation is rarely seen, nodules may occur more frequently. Moreover, the pleural effusions are seen in about 30% of cases with Churg-Strauss syndrome [120]. The marked findings in evaluation of 17 patients were consolidation or ground-glass attenuation in 10 (59%) subjects. Other pulmonary manifestations of these cases were less prevalent, including interlobular septal thickening, pulmonary nodules, and thickness in bronchial wall [121].

7.11 Adult-Onset Still's Disease

Adult-onset Still's disease (AOSD), which is similar to the juvenile idiopathic arthritis (JIA), has a systemic inflammatory presentation. Among the clinical manifestations of this disease are arthritis, spiking fevers, transient rash, increased liver enzymes, hepatosplenomegaly, lymphadenopathy, and serositis. Despite difficulties in precise prognosis of AOSD during the onset of the disease with initial presentations, clinical presentations of the disease may imply to a more complicated disease. Pulmonary microangiopathy has been observed in AOSD patients and may result in thrombotic thrombocytopenic purpura and renal involvement [122–124].

Inflammatory mechanisms are involved in autoimmune disease-associated PAH, in spite of different mechanisms in AOSD, in which players of innate immunity have a main role. Autoantibodies against nuclear antigens, rheumatoid factor (RF), IgG, and deposition of complement proteins in the walls of pulmonary vessels have been reported in autoimmune disease-associated PAH [125]. Furthermore, microthrombi formation, which is called veno-occlusive disease, and pulmonary fibrosis have frequently been seen in AOSD patients. Among the key histological manifestations of AOSD are plexiform lesion formation, intimal thickening, and hypertrophy of the pulmonary arteries. Nonetheless, autoimmune diseases-associated as well as sporadic forms of PAH are presented with endothelial proliferation in AOSD cases [126].

Cardiopulmonary complications have been reported in 30–40% of cases with AOSD. Pulmonary manifestations of AOSD are ILD, aseptic pneumonitis, serositis alongside with pleural effusion, and in seldom cases acute respiratory distress syndrome (ARDS). AOSD patients may suffer from pleuritic chest pain, cough, and dyspnea [127]. The association of PAH with AOSD was first described in a 29-year-old Japanese woman who manifested precapillary, progressive severe hypertension almost 2.5 years before the diagnosis of AOSD [128]. Afterward, in a case series evaluating 19 patients, other 2 cases of PAH were reported in AOSD patients from northern Taiwan, in which co-occurrence of PAH and several connective tissue diseases was reported [129]. In a 29-year-old woman from the USA, a 9-year history of AOSD was reported. The patient had developed PAH and died 2.5 months after PAH diagnosis [126]. Moreover, an 18-year-old female case was reported from India in 2009, who was newly diagnosed with AOSD and immediately developed severe PAH manifestations [128]. A 27-year-old female case with a 7-year history of AOSD was reported to have PAH, which was responsive to therapy with anakinra [130].

7.12 Familial Mediterranean Fever

Familial Mediterranean fever (FMF) is genetically an autosomal recessive disorder. The disease is specifically seen in Mediterranean populations but is seldom in the rest of the world, particularly Asia. FMF is characterized by arthritis, recurrent attacks of pyrexia, erysipelas-like skin lesions, and secondary amyloidosis. In a case report study, a FMF patient demonstrated nephropathic and pulmonary amyloidosis of the secondary amyloidosis of AA type [131]. FMF coexistence has been implied with disorders, such as ulcerative colitis, spondyloarthritis, and various types of systemic vasculitis [132]. A few reports have implied the lung involvement in FMF patients, like amyloidosis, transient pleuritis during attacks, and mesothelioma of the pleura [133]. A case report described a FMF patient with pulmonary necrotizing granuloma with the *MEFV* mutation of S503C in exon5 [134].

7.13 Inflammatory Bowel Disease

Inflammatory bowel disease (IBD) describes two distinct diseases, namely, ulcerative colitis (UC) and Crohn's disease (CD) [135]. Although the etiology and pathogenesis of IBD have not been fully characterized, there is consensus, nowadays, that the disease arises from an abnormal immune response against the normal flora present in the gut in a genetically susceptible individual [136].

IBD has been reported with several respiratory complications, such as bronchitis, tracheobronchitis [137–142], bronchiectasis [137, 143, 144], and bronchiolitis [145, 146]. None of these manifestations are specifically seen neither in UC nor CD. Nonetheless, most of the cases display complications in distal or proximal conducting airways in UC patients. Respiratory manifestations may occur alongside with exacerbation in IBD complications [138, 147].

According to bronchoscopy, bronchoalveolar lavage, and biopsy finding reports, hyperemia and mucosal edema are frequently seen [138, 140, 141]. Moreover, suppurative bronchitis is prevalently reported and chronic purulent expectoration is the major manifestation [141, 147]. Restriction of airways in the trachea or bronchus has been reported that may result from inflammatory nodules [141], widespread submucosal fibrosis [141, 148], or mucosal infiltration [149]. Bronchial biopsy demonstrated several symptoms, including thickening of basal membrane and angioectasia [139], mucosal hyperplasia [141], cellular infiltrations of T and B lymphocytes and granulocytes [140, 141], or other chronic inflammatory infiltrates [139]. Despite lymphocytosis dominance in the bronchoalveolar lavage (BAL) fluid of IBD patients, BAL fluid may frequently be infiltrated by neutrophils during tracheobronchial involvement [141].

Interstitial disease may occur before the initial symptoms of IBD and mostly is revealed in patients with chronic form of the disease [150]. Moreover, interstitial manifestations of disease are not associated with IBD activity and may also occur in cases with inactive IBD [151–154]. General manifestations during interstitial disease are prevalently described, including fever or subfebrile state, malaise, arthralgia, and weight loss [151, 155, 156]. Alternately, the respiratory symptoms may manifest as breathlessness on exertion or at rest, dry cough, and chest tightness.

Radiological findings of interstitial lung involvement in IBD patients have diversity. Opacities like pneumonia are very prevalent [157, 158], particularly in cases with OP [155, 159]. Pulmonary nodules with different count, size, and location may be seen. Moreover, small cavitations demonstrating central necrosis may also be reported [160]. However, tumors with central necrosis reflecting granulomatosis with polyangiitis (GPA) may need complete differentiation alongside with the disease progression, particularly in UC patients who are positive for anti-neutrophil cytoplasmic antibodies (ANCA) in the serum samples [161–166]. Interstitial pneumonitis may be considered as another radiological finding. The high-resolution computed tomography (HRCT) scans in these cases present alveolar filling, ground-glass opacities, or a reticular pattern [167–170]. Lung opacities may spontaneously migrate [171]. HRCT findings have also depicted that all the cases may share patterns like bronchiectasis, air-trapping, and "tree-in-bud" [167]. These observations as well as several case reports have shown the coexistence of different forms of lung involvement in IBD cases. Nonetheless, most of the patients with abnormal HRCT findings do not present respiratory symptoms [165, 172].

7.14 Cherubism

Cherubism is characterized by bilateral overgrowth of mandible and maxilla because of substitution of bone fibers with fibrotic stromal cells and osteoclast-like cells. The disease phenotype spans from lack of clinical symptoms to severe mandibular and maxillary enlargement alongside with ocular, auditory, respiratory, and swallowing complications [173]. In Cherubism, the respiratory complications can result in obstructive sleep apnea and upper airway obstruction due to backward displacement of the tongue [174].

7.15 Chronic Atypical Neutrophilic Dermatosis with Lipodystrophy and Elevated Temperature (CANDLE) Syndrome

A retrospective case series evaluation of patients with CANDLE syndrome and C1q-deficient SLE identified respiratory problems. Of the evaluated cases, two of them had unusual characteristics, including uveitis and pulmonary involvement. Moreover, chest CT scan indicated diffuse pulmonary nodules [175].

7.16 Conclusion

Pulmonary complications in patients with AID may stem from various sources, including either inherent presentations of the disease itself or infection in the treated patient as well as adverse reactions to toxic medications. In order to obtain a contribution, the surgical pathologist is better to be familiar with the pre-specified patterns of pulmonary complications and distribution of the disorder concurred with AID involving the pleura and the lungs. Being armed with this knowledge can be helpful in estimation of occult AID as a possible cause and guide for serologic and clinical evaluations.

References

1. Müller-Ladner U, Pap T, Gay RE, Neidhart M, Gay S. Mechanisms of disease: the molecular and cellular basis of joint destruction in rheumatoid arthritis. Nat Rev Rheumatol. 2005;1(2):102.
2. McInnes IB, O'dell JR. State-of-the-art: rheumatoid arthritis. Ann Rheum Dis. 2010;69(11):1898–906.
3. de Kleer IM, Wedderburn LR, Taams LS, Patel A, Varsani H, Klein M, et al. CD4+ CD25bright regulatory T cells actively regulate inflammation in the joints of patients with the remitting form of juvenile idiopathic arthritis. J Immunol. 2004;172(10):6435–43.
4. Keystone EC, Kavanaugh AF, Sharp JT, Tannenbaum H, Hua Y, Teoh LS, et al. Radiographic, clinical, and functional outcomes of treatment with adalimumab (a human anti–tumor necrosis factor monoclonal antibody) in patients with active rheumatoid arthritis receiving concomitant methotrexate therapy: a randomized, placebo-controlled, 52-week trial. Arthritis Rheumatol. 2004;50(5):1400–11.
5. Akira M, Sakatani M, Hara H. Thin-section CT findings in rheumatoid arthritis-associated lung disease: CT patterns and their courses. J Comput Assist Tomogr. 1999;23(6):941–8.
6. Tanaka N, Kim JS, Newell JD, Brown KK, Cool CD, Meehan R, et al. Rheumatoid arthritis–related lung diseases: CT findings. Radiology. 2004;232(1):81–91.
7. White ES, Tazelaar HD, Lynch Iii JP, editors. Bronchiolar complications of connective tissue diseases. Semin Respir Crit Care Med; 2003. Copyright© 2003 by Thieme Medical Publishers, Inc., 333 Seventh Avenue, New York, NY 10001, USA. Tel.:+ 1 (212) 584-4662.
8. Lee H-K, Kim DS, Yoo B, Seo JB, Rho J-Y, Colby TV, et al. Histopathologic pattern and clinical features of rheumatoid arthritis-associated interstitial lung disease. Chest J. 2005;127(6):2019–27.
9. Remy-Jardin M, Remy J, Cortet B, Mauri F, Delcambre B. Lung changes in rheumatoid arthritis: CT findings. Radiology. 1994;193(2):375–82.
10. Colby TV. Pulmonary pathology in patients with systemic autoimmune diseases. Clin Chest Med. 1998;19(4):587–612.
11. Yousem SA, Colby TV, Carrington CB. Lung biopsy in rheumatoid arthritis 1, 2. Am Rev Respir Dis. 1985;131(5):770–7.
12. Lamblin C, Bergoin C, Saelens T, Wallaert B. Interstitial lung diseases in collagen vascular diseases. Eur Respir J. 2001;18(32 suppl):69s–80s.
13. Yoshinouchi T, Ohtsuki Y, Fujita J, Yamadori I, Bandoh S, Ishida T, et al. Nonspecific interstitial pneumonia pattern as pulmonary involvement of rheumatoid arthritis. Rheumatol Int. 2005;26(2):121–5.
14. Hakala M, Pääkkö P, Huhti E, Tarkka M, Sutinen S. Open lung biopsy of patients with rheumatoid arthritis. Clin Rheumatol. 1990;9(4):452–60.
15. Tansey D, Wells A, Colby TV, Ip S, Nikolakoupolou A, Du Bois R, et al. Variations in histological patterns of interstitial pneumonia between connective tissue disorders and their relationship to prognosis. Histopathology. 2004;44(6):585–96.
16. Katzenstein AL, Fiorelli RF. Nonspecific interstitial pneumonia/fibrosis. Histologic features and clinical significance. Am J Surg Pathol. 1994;18(2):136–47.
17. Devouassoux G, Cottin V, Lioté H, Marchand E, Frachon I, Schuller A, et al. Characterisation of severe obliterative bronchiolitis in rheumatoid arthritis. Eur Respir J. 2009;33(5):1053–61.
18. Schwarz MI, Zamora MR, Hodges TN, Chan ED, Bowler RP, Tuder RM. Isolated pulmonary capillaritis and diffuse alveolar hemorrhage in rheumatoid arthritis and mixed connective tissue disease. Chest. 1998;113(6):1609–15.
19. Rice AJ, Wells AU, Bouros D, du Bois RM, Hansell DM, Polychronopoulos V, et al. Terminal diffuse alveolar damage in relation to interstitial pneumonias: an autopsy study. Am J Clin Pathol. 2003;119(5):709–14.

20. Hoogen F, Khanna D, Fransen J, Johnson SR, Baron M, Tyndall A, et al. 2013 classification criteria for systemic sclerosis: an American College of Rheumatology/European League against Rheumatism collaborative initiative. Arthritis Rheumatol. 2013;65(11):2737–47.
21. Kim EA, Johkoh T, Lee KS, Ichikado K, Koh E-M, Kim TS, et al. Interstitial pneumonia in progressive systemic sclerosis: serial high-resolution CT findings with functional correlation. J Comput Assist Tomogr. 2001;25(5):757–63.
22. Cozzi F, Corona MC, Rizzi M, Dus C, Durigon N, Mancin S, et al. Lung fibrosis quantified by HRCT in scleroderma patients with different disease forms and ANA specificities. Reumatismo. 2001;53(1):55–62.
23. Desai SR, Veeraraghavan S, Hansell DM, Nikolakopolou A, Goh NS, Nicholson AG, et al. CT features of lung disease in patients with systemic sclerosis: comparison with idiopathic pulmonary fibrosis and nonspecific interstitial pneumonia. Radiology. 2004;232(2):560–7.
24. Zisman DA, Karlamangla AS, Ross DJ, Keane MP, Belperio JA, Saggar R, et al. High-resolution chest CT findings do not predict the presence of pulmonary hypertension in advanced idiopathic pulmonary fibrosis. Chest J. 2007;132(3):773–9.
25. Pandey AK, Wilcox P, Mayo JR, Sin D, Moss R, Ellis J, et al. Predictors of pulmonary hypertension on high-resolution computed tomography of the chest in systemic sclerosis: a retrospective analysis. Can Assoc Radiol J. 2010;61(5):291–6.
26. Bhalla M, Silver R, Shepard J, McLoud T. Chest CT in patients with scleroderma: prevalence of asymptomatic esophageal dilatation and mediastinal lymphadenopathy. AJR Am J Roentgenol. 1993;161(2):269–72.
27. Kim DS, Yoo B, Lee JS, Kim EK, Lim CM, Lee SD, et al. The major histopathologic pattern of pulmonary fibrosis in scleroderma is nonspecific interstitial pneumonia. Sarcoidosis Vasc Diffuse Lung Dis. 2002;19(2):121–7.
28. Fujita J, Tokuda M, Bandoh S, Yang Y, Fukunaga Y, Hojo S, et al. Primary lung cancer associated with polymyositis/dermatomyositis, with a review of the literature. Rheumatol Int. 2001;20(2):81–4.
29. De Souza RB, Borges CT, Capelozzi VL, Parra ER, Jatene FB, Kavakama J, et al. Centrilobular fibrosis: an underrecognized pattern in systemic sclerosis. Respiration. 2009;77(4):389–97.
30. Johnson DA, Drane WE, Curran J, Cattau EL, Ciarleglio C, Khan A, et al. Pulmonary disease in progressive systemic sclerosis: a complication of gastroesophageal reflux and occult aspiration? Arch Intern Med. 1989;149(3):589–93.
31. Montesi A, Pesaresi A, Cavalli ML, Ripa G, Candela M, Gabrielli A. Oropharyngeal and esophageal function in scleroderma. Dysphagia. 1991;6(4):219–23.
32. Yousem SA. The pulmonary pathologic manifestations of the CREST syndrome. Hum Pathol. 1990;21(5):467–74.
33. Launay D, Mouthon L, Hachulla E, Pagnoux C, de Groote P, Remy-Jardin M, et al. Prevalence and characteristics of moderate to severe pulmonary hypertension in systemic sclerosis with and without interstitial lung disease. J Rheumatol. 2007;34(5):1005–11.
34. Bridges AJ, Hsu K, Dias-Arias AA, Chechani V. Bronchiolitis obliterans organizing pneumonia and scleroderma. J Rheumatol. 1992;19(7):1136–40.
35. Muir TE, Tazelaar HD, Colby TV, Myers JL, editors. Organizing diffuse alveolar damage associated with progressive systemic sclerosis. Mayo Clin Proc. 1997;72:639–42. Elsevier.
36. Griffin M, Robb J, Martin J. Diffuse alveolar haemorrhage associated with progressive systemic sclerosis. Thorax. 1990;45(11):903–4.
37. Tan EM, Cohen AS, Fries JF, Masi AT, Mcshane DJ, Rothfield NF, et al. The 1982 revised criteria for the classification of systemic lupus erythematosus. Arthritis Rheumatol. 1982;25(11):1271–7.
38. Bankier AA, Kiener HP, Wiesmayr MN, Fleischmann D, Kontrus M, Herold CJ, et al. Discrete lung involvement in systemic lupus erythematosus: CT assessment. Radiology. 1995;196(3):835–40.
39. Fenlon H, Doran M, Sant S, Breatnach E. High-resolution chest CT in systemic lupus erythematosus. AJR Am J Roentgenol. 1996;166(2):301–7.

40. Sant S, Doran M, Fenelon H, Breatnach E. Pleuropulmonary abnormalities in patients with systemic lupus erythematosus: assessment with high resolution computed tomography, chest radiography and pulmonary function tests. Clin Exp Rheumatol. 1996;15(5):507–13.
41. Ooi G, Ngan H, Peh W, Mok M, Ip M. Systemic lupus erythematosus patients with respiratory symptoms: the value of HRCT. Clin Radiol. 1997;52(10):775–81.
42. Cheema GS, Quismorio FP Jr. Interstitial lung disease in systemic lupus erythematosus. Curr Opin Pulm Med. 2000;6(5):424–9.
43. Matthay RA, Schwarz MI, Petty TL, Stanford RE, Gupta RC, Sahn SA, et al. Pulmonary manifestations of systemic lupus erythematosus: review of twelve cases of acute lupus pneumonitis. Medicine. 1975;54(5):397–410.
44. Susanto I, Peters JI. Acute lupus pneumonitis with normal chest radiograph. Chest. 1997;111(6):1781–3.
45. Gruden JF, Webb WR, Warnock M. Centrilobular opacities in the lung on high-resolution CT: diagnostic considerations and pathologic correlation. AJR Am J Roentgenol. 1994;162(3):569–74.
46. Oki H, Aoki T, Saito K, Yamashita Y, Hanamiya M, Hayashida Y, et al. Thin-section chest CT findings in systemic lupus erythematosus with antiphospholipid syndrome: a comparison with systemic lupus erythematosus without antiphospholipid syndrome. Eur J Radiol. 2012;81(6):1335–9.
47. Haupt HM, Moore GW, Hutchins GM. The lung in systemic lupus erythematosus: analysis of the pathologic changes in 120 patients. Am J Med. 1981;71(5):791–8.
48. Myers JL, Katzenstein A-LA. Microangiitis in lupus-induced pulmonary hemorrhage. Am J Clin Pathol. 1986;85(5):552–6.
49. Pope J. An update in pulmonary hypertension in systemic lupus erythematosus–do we need to know about it? Lupus. 2008;17(4):274–7.
50. Johnson S, Granton J. Pulmonary hypertension in systemic sclerosis and systemic lupus erythematosus. Eur Respir Rev. 2011;20(122):277–86.
51. Wakaki K, Koizumi F, Fukase M. Vascular lesions in systemic lupus erythematosus (SLE) with pulmonary hypertension. Pathol Int. 1984;34(3):593–604.
52. Asherson R, Hackett D, Gharavi A, Harris E, Kennedy H, Hughes G. Pulmonary hypertension in systemic lupus erythematosus: a report of three cases. J Rheumatol. 1986;13(2):416–20.
53. Yokoi T, Tomita Y, Fukaya M, Ichihara S. Pulmonary hypertension associated with systemic lupus erythematosus: predominantly thrombotic arteriopathy accompanied by plexiform lesions. Arch Pathol Lab Med. 1998;122(5):467.
54. Roncoroni AJ, Alvarez C, Molinas F. Plexogenic arteriopathy associated with pulmonary vasculitis in systemic lupus erythematosus. Respiration. 1992;59(1):52–6.
55. Simonson J, Schiller N, Petri M, Hellmann D. Pulmonary hypertension in systemic lupus erythematosus. J Rheumatol. 1989;16(7):918–25.
56. Fayemi A. The lung in systemic lupus erythematosus: a clinico-pathologic study of 20 cases. Mt Sinai J Med New York. 1974;42(2):110–8.
57. Yood R, Steigman D, Gill L. Lymphocytic interstitial pneumonitis in a patient with systemic lupus erythematosus. Lupus. 1995;4(2):161–3.
58. Marenco J, Sanchez-Burson J, Campos JR, Jimenez M, Garcia-Bragado F. Pulmonary amyloidosis and unusual lung involvement in SLE. Clin Rheumatol. 1994;13(3):525–7.
59. Min J, Hong Y, Park S, Park J, Lee S, Lee Y, et al. Bronchiolitis obliterans organizing pneumonia as an initial manifestation in patients with systemic lupus erythematosus. J Rheumatol. 1997;24(11):2254–7.
60. Gammon RB, Bridges TA, Al-Nezir H, Alexander CB, Kennedy JI. Bronchiolitis obliterans organizing pneumonia associated with systemic lupus erythematosus. Chest. 1992;102(4):1171–4.
61. Filipek MS, Thompson ME, Wang P-L, Gosselin MV, Primack SL. Lymphocytic interstitial pneumonitis in a patient with systemic lupus erythematosus: radiographic and high-resolution CT findings. J Thorac Imaging. 2004;19(3):200–3.

62. Harvey Eisenberg M, Sherwin RP. Diffuse interstitial lung disease in systemic lupus erythematosus. Ann Intern Med. 1973;79:37–45.
63. Koh W, Boey M. Open lung biopsy in systemic lupus erythematosus patients with pulmonary disease. Ann Acad Med Singap. 1993;22(3):323–5.
64. Benisch B, Peison B. The association of lymphocytic interstitial pneumonia and systemic lupus erythematosus. Mt Sinai J Med New York. 1978;46(4):398–41.
65. Hariri LP, Unizony S, Stone J, Mino-Kenudson M, Sharma A, Matsubara O, et al. Acute fibrinous and organizing pneumonia in systemic lupus erythematosus: a case report and review of the literature. Pathol Int. 2010;60(11):755–9.
66. Schwarz MI. Pulmonary and cardiac manifestations of polymyositis-dermatomyositis. J Thorac Imaging. 1992;7(2):46–54.
67. Ikezoe J, Johkoh T, Kohno N, Takeuchi N, Ichikado K, Nakamura H. High-resolution CT findings of lung disease in patients with polymyositis and dermatomyositis. J Thorac Imaging. 1996;11(4):250–9.
68. Arakawa H, Yamada H, Kurihara Y, Nakajima Y, Takeda A, Fukushima Y, et al. Nonspecific interstitial pneumonia associated with polymyositis and dermatomyositis: serial high-resolution CT findings and functional correlation. Chest J. 2003;123(4):1096–103.
69. Mino M, Noma S, Taguchi Y, Tomii K, Kohri Y, Oida K. Pulmonary involvement in polymyositis and dermatomyositis: sequential evaluation with CT. AJR Am J Roentgenol. 1997;169(1):83–7.
70. Tazelaar HD, Viggiano RW, Pickersgill J, Colby TV. Interstitial lung disease in polymyositis and dermatomyositis. Am Rev Respir Dis. 1990;141(3):727–31.
71. Selva-O'Callaghan A, Labrador-Horrillo M, Munoz-Gall X, Martinez-Gomez X, Majo-Masferrer J, Solans-Laque R, et al. Polymyositis/dermatomyositis-associated lung disease: analysis of a series of 81 patients. Lupus. 2005;14(7):534–42.
72. Fujisawa T, Suda T, Nakamura Y, Enomoto N, Ide K, Toyoshima M, et al. Differences in clinical features and prognosis of interstitial lung diseases between polymyositis and dermatomyositis. J Rheumatol. 2005;32(1):58–64.
73. Cottin V, Thivolet-Bejui F, Reynaud-Gaubert M, Cadranel J, Delaval P, Ternamian P, et al. Interstitial lung disease in amyopathic dermatomyositis, dermatomyositis and polymyositis. Eur Respir J. 2003;22(2):245–50.
74. Marie I, Hachulla E, Cherin P, Dominique S, Hatron PY, Hellot MF, et al. Interstitial lung disease in polymyositis and dermatomyositis. Arthritis Care Res. 2002;47(6):614–22.
75. Ito M, Kaise S, Suzuki S, Kazuta Y, Sato Y, Miyata M, et al. Clinico-laboratory characteristics of patients with dermatomyositis accompanied by rapidly progressive interstitial lung disease. Clin Rheumatol. 1999;18(6):462–7.
76. Fata F, Rathore R, Schiff C, Herzlich BC. Bronchiolitis obliterans organizing pneumonia as the first manifestation of polymyositis. South Med J. 1997;90(2):227–30.
77. Hsue Y, Paulus H, Coulson W. Bronchiolitis obliterans organizing pneumonia in polymyositis. A case report with longterm survival. J Rheumatol. 1993;20(5):877–9.
78. Labirua A, Lundberg IE. Interstitial lung disease and idiopathic inflammatory myopathies: progress and pitfalls. Curr Opin Rheumatol. 2010;22(6):633–8.
79. Yousem SA, Gibson K, Kaminski N, Oddis CV, Ascherman DP. The pulmonary histopathologic manifestations of the anti-Jo-1 tRNA synthetase syndrome. Modern Pathol. 2010;23(6):874.
80. Lee C-S, Chen T-L, Tzen C-Y, Lin F-J, Peng M-J, Wu C-L, et al. Idiopathic inflammatory myopathy with diffuse alveolar damage. Clin Rheumatol. 2002;21(5):391–6.
81. Mukae H, Ishimoto H, Sakamoto N, Hara S, Kakugawa T, Nakayama S, et al. Clinical differences between interstitial lung disease associated with clinically amyopathic dermatomyositis and classic dermatomyositis. Chest J. 2009;136(5):1341–7.
82. Bonnefoy O, Ferretti G, Calaque O, Coulomb M, Begueret H, Beylot-Barry M, et al. Serial chest CT findings in interstitial lung disease associated with polymyositis–dermatomyositis. Eur J Radiol. 2004;49(3):235–44.

83. Schwarz MI, Sutarik JM, Nick JA, Leff JA, Emlen JW, Tuder RM. Pulmonary capillaritis and diffuse alveolar hemorrhage. A primary manifestation of polymyositis. Am J Respir Crit Care Med. 1995;151(6):2037–40.
84. Bunch TW, Tancredi RG, Lie J. Pulmonary hypertension in polymyositis. Chest. 1981;79(1):105–7.
85. Aisa Y, Yokomori H, Kashiwagi K, Nagata S, Yanagisawa R, Takahashi M, et al. Polymyositis, pulmonary fibrosis and malignant lymphoma associated with hepatitis C virus infection. Intern Med. 2001;40(11):1109–12.
86. Marie I, Lahaxe L, Benveniste O, Delavigne K, Adoue D, Mouthon L, et al. Long-term outcome of patients with polymyositis/dermatomyositis and anti-PM-Scl antibody. Br J Dermatol. 2010;162(2):337–44.
87. Castañeda-Pomeda M, Prieto-González S, Grau JM. Antisynthetase syndrome and malignancy: our experience. JCR J Clin Rheumatol. 2011;17(8):458.
88. Shiboski S, Shiboski C, Criswell L, Baer A, Challacombe S, Lanfranchi H, et al. American College of Rheumatology classification criteria for Sjögren's syndrome: a data-driven, expert consensus approach in the Sjögren's International Collaborative Clinical Alliance Cohort. Arthritis Care Res. 2012;64(4):475–87.
89. Meyer CA, Pina JS, Taillon D, Godwin JD. Inspiratory and expiratory high-resolution CT findings in a patient with Sjögren's syndrome and cystic lung disease. AJR Am J Roentgenol. 1997;168(1):101–3.
90. Franquet T, Gimenez A, Monill JM, Diaz C, Geli C. Primary Sjögren's syndrome and associated lung disease: CT findings in 50 patients. AJR Am J Roentgenol. 1997;169(3):655–8.
91. Koyama M, Johkoh T, Honda O, Mihara N, Kozuka T, Tomiyama N, et al. Pulmonary involvement in primary Sjögren's syndrome: spectrum of pulmonary abnormalities and computed tomography findings in 60 patients. J Thorac Imaging. 2001;16(4):290–6.
92. Uffmann M, Kiener HP, Bankier AA, Baldt MM, Zontsich T, Herold CJ. Lung manifestation in asymptomatic patients with primary Sjögren syndrome: assessment with high resolution CT and pulmonary function tests. J Thorac Imaging. 2001;16(4):282–9.
93. Watanabe M, Naniwa T, Hara M, Arakawa T, Maeda T. Pulmonary manifestations in Sjögren's syndrome: correlation analysis between chest computed tomographic findings and clinical subsets with poor prognosis in 80 patients. J Rheumatol. 2010;37(2):365–73.
94. Lohrmann C, Uhl M, Warnatz K, Ghanem N, Kotter E, Schaefer O, et al. High-resolution CT imaging of the lung for patients with primary Sjögren's syndrome. Eur J Radiol. 2004;52(2):137–43.
95. Hansen LA, Prakash UB, Colby TV, editors. Pulmonary lymphoma in Sjögren's syndrome. Mayo Clin Proc. 1989;64:920–31. Elsevier.
96. Ito I, Nagai S, Kitaichi M, Nicholson AG, Johkoh T, Noma S, et al. Pulmonary manifestations of primary Sjogren's syndrome: a clinical, radiologic, and pathologic study. Am J Respir Crit Care Med. 2005;171(6):632–8.
97. Parambil JG, Myers JL, Lindell RM, Matteson EL, Ryu JH. Interstitial lung disease in primary Sjogren syndrome. Chest J. 2006;130(5):1489–95.
98. Kassan SS, Thomas TL, Moutsopoulos HM, Hoover R, Kimberly RP, Budman DR, et al. Increased risk of lymphoma in sicca syndrome. Ann Intern Med. 1978;89(6):888–92.
99. Jeong YJ, Lee KS, Chung MP, Han J, Chung MJ, Kim K-I, et al. Amyloidosis and lymphoproliferative disease in Sjögren syndrome: thin-section computed tomography findings and histopathologic comparisons. J Comput Assist Tomogr. 2004;28(6):776–81.
100. Lee I-J, Kim SH, Koo SH, Kim HB, Hwang DH, Lee KS, et al. Bronchus-associated lymphoid tissue (BALT) lymphoma of the lung showing mosaic pattern of inhomogeneous attenuation on thin-section CT: a case report. Korean J Radiol. 2000;1(3):159–61.
101. Nakamura N, Yamada G, Itoh T, Suzuki A, Morita-Ichimura S, Teramoto S, et al. Pulmonary MALT lymphoma with amyloid production in a patient with primary Sjögren's syndrome. Intern Med. 2002;41(4):309–11.
102. Byrd SL, Case BA, Boulware DW. Pulmonary manifestations of rheumatic disease. Postgrad Med. 1993;93(1):149–66.

103. Rumancik WM, Firooznia H, Davis MS, Leitman BS, Golimbu C, Rafii M, et al. Fibrobullous disease of the upper lobes: an extraskeletal manifestation of ankylosing spondylitis. J Comput Tomogr. 1984;8(3):225–9.
104. Gupta S, Johnston W. Apical pulmonary disease in ankylosing spondylitis. N Z Med J. 1978;88(619):186–8.
105. Hunninghake GW, Fauci AS. Pulmonary involvement in the collagen vascular diseases 1, 2. Am Rev Respir Dis. 1979;119(3):471–503.
106. Wolson AH, Rohwedder JJ. Upper lobe fibrosis in ankylosing spondylitis. Am J Roentgenol. 1975;124(3):466–71.
107. Tanoue LT. Pulmonary involvement in collagen vascular disease: a review of the pulmonary manifestations of the Marfan syndrome, ankylosing spondylitis, Sjogren's syndrome, and relapsing polychondritis. J Thorac Imaging. 1992;7(2):62.
108. Chakera T, Howarth F, Kendall M, Lawrence D, Whitfield A. The chest radiograph in ankylosing spondylitis. Clin Radiol. 1975;26:455–9.
109. Appelrouth D, Gottlieb N. Pulmonary manifestations of ankylosing spondylitis. J Rheumatol. 1975;2(4):446–53.
110. Uzun O, Akpolat T, Erkan L. Pulmonary vasculitis in behcet disease: a cumulative analysis. Chest J. 2005;127(6):2243–53.
111. Okazaki K, Chiba T. Autoimmune related pancreatitis. Gut. 2002;51(1):1–4.
112. Kamisawa T, Egawa N, Nakajima H. Autoimmune pancreatitis is a systemic autoimmune disease. Am J Gastroenterol. 2003;98(12):2811.
113. Hirano K, Kawabe T, Komatsu Y, Matsubara S, Togawa O, Arizumi T, et al. High-rate pulmonary involvement in autoimmune pancreatitis. Intern Med J. 2006;36(1):58–61.
114. Hoffman GS, Kerr GS, Leavitt RY, Hallahan CW, Lebovics RS, Travis WD, et al. Wegener granulomatosis: an analysis of 158 patients. Ann Intern Med. 1992;116(6):488–98.
115. Aberle D, Gamsu G, Lynch D. Thoracic manifestations of Wegener granulomatosis: diagnosis and course. Radiology. 1990;174(3):703–9.
116. Cordier J-F, Valeyre D, Guillevin L, Loire R, Brechot J-M. Pulmonary Wegener's granulomatosis: a clinical and imaging study of 77 cases. Chest. 1990;97(4):906–12.
117. Kuhlman JE, Hruban RH, Fishman EK. Wegener granulomatosis: CT features of parenchymal lung disease. J Comput Assist Tomogr. 1991;15(6):948–52.
118. Maskell G, Lockwood C, Flower C. Computed tomography of the lung in Wegener's granulomatosis. Clin Radiol. 1993;48(6):377–80.
119. Stübiger N, Zierhut M. Churg-Strauss syndrome. In: Intraocular inflammation. Berlin: Springer; 2016. p. 761–5.
120. Lanham JG, Elkon KB, Pusey CD, Hughes GR. Systemic vasculitis with asthma and eosinophilia: a clinical approach to the Churg-Strauss syndrome. Medicine. 1984;63(2):65–81.
121. Worthy SA, Müller N, Hansell DM, Flower C. Churg-Strauss syndrome: the spectrum of pulmonary CT findings in 17 patients. AJR Am J Roentgenol. 1998;170(2):297–300.
122. Jaqua NT, Finger D, Hawley JS. Adult-onset Still's disease masquerading as sepsis in an asplenic active duty soldier. Case Rep Med. 2012;2012:349521.
123. Duburcq T, Delannoy P, Sivova N, Leroy O, editors. Adult onset Still's disease revealed by a myocarditis. Ann Fr Anesth Reanim. 2013;32:50–2.
124. Fautrel B. Adult-onset Still disease. Best Pract Res Clin Rheumatol. 2008;22(5):773–92.
125. Sirnes PA, Tendera M, Vardas P, Widimsky P. Guidelines for the diagnosis and treatment of pulmonary hypertension. Eur Heart J. 2009;30:2493–537.
126. Efthimiou P, Kadavath S, Mehta B. Life-threatening complications of adult-onset Still's disease. Clin Rheumatol. 2014;33(3):305–14.
127. Yamaguchi M, Ohta A, Tsunematsu T, Kasukawa R, Mizushima Y, Kashiwagi H, et al. Preliminary criteria for classification of adult Still's disease. J Rheumatol. 1992;19(3):424–30.
128. Zen A, Yamashita N, Ueda M, Asakawa Y, Yoshikawa Y, Funai T, et al. A case of adult Still's disease with pulmonary hypertension. Ryumachi[Rheumatism]. 1990;30(1):45–52.

129. Chen C, Chen H, Wang H, Liao H, Chou C, Huang D. Pulmonary arterial hypertension in autoimmune diseases: an analysis of 19 cases from a medical center in northern Taiwan. J Microbiol Immunol Infect. 2006;39(2):162.
130. Campos M, Schiopu E. Pulmonary arterial hypertension in adult-onset Still's disease: rapid response to anakinra. Case Rep Rheumatol. 2012;2012:537613.
131. Şahan C, Cengiz K. Pulmonary amyloidosis in familial Mediterranean fever. Acta Clin Belg. 2006;61(3):147–51.
132. Ozen S. Mutations/polymorphisms in a monogenetic autoinflammatory disease may be susceptibility markers for certain rheumatic diseases: lessons from the bedside for the benchside. Clin Exp Rheumatol. 2009;27(2 Suppl 53):S29–31.
133. Lidar M, Pras M, Langevitz P, Livneh A. Thoracic and lung involvement in familial Mediterranean fever (FMF). Clin Chest Med. 2002;23(2):505–11.
134. Kushima H, Ishii H, Ishii K, Kadota J-i. Pulmonary necrotizing granulomas in a patient with familial Mediterranean fever. Mod Rheumatol. 2015;25(5):806–9.
135. Ponder A, Long MD. A clinical review of recent findings in the epidemiology of inflammatory bowel disease. Clin Epidemiol. 2013;5:237.
136. Rodriguez-Bores L, Barahona-Garrido J, Yamamoto-Furusho JK. Basic and clinical aspects of osteoporosis in inflammatory bowel disease. World J Gastroenterol WJG. 2007;13(46):6156.
137. Kraft SC, Earle RH, Roesler M, Esterly JR. Unexplained bronchopulmonary disease with inflammatory bowel disease. Arch Intern Med. 1976;136(4):454–9.
138. Spira A, Grossman R, Balter M. Large airway disease associated with inflammatory bowel disease. Chest. 1998;113(6):1723–6.
139. Valletta E, Bertini M, Sette L, Braggion C, Pradal U, Zannoni M. Early bronchopulmonary involvement in Crohn disease: a case report. BMC Gastroenterol. 2001;1(1):13.
140. Iwama T, Higuchi T, Imajo M, Akagawa S, Matsubara O, Mishima Y. Tracheo-bronchitis as a complication of Crohn's disease—a case report—. Surg Today. 1991;21(4):454–7.
141. Kuzniar T, Sleiman C, Brugiere O, Groussard O, Mal H, Mellot F, et al. Severe tracheobronchial stenosis in a patient with Crohn' disease. Eur Respir J. 2000;15(1):209–12.
142. Hamada S, Ito Y, Imai S, Oguma T, Niimi A, Mishima M. Effect of inhaled corticosteroid therapy on CT scan-estimated airway dimensions in a patient with chronic bronchitis related to ulcerative colitis. Chest J. 2011;139(4):930–2.
143. Peradzyńska J, Krenke K, Lange J, Banaszkiewicz A, Łazowska-Przeorek I, Radzikowski A, et al. Low prevalence of pulmonary involvement in children with inflammatory bowel disease. Respir Med. 2012;106(7):1048–54.
144. Desai D, Patil S, Udwadia Z, Maheshwari S, Abraham P, Joshi A. Pulmonary manifestations in inflammatory bowel disease: a prospective study. Indian J Gastroenterol. 2011;30(5):225.
145. Desai SJ, Gephardt GN, Stoller JK. Diffuse panbronchiolitis preceding ulcerative colitis. Chest. 1989;95(6):1342–4.
146. Vandenplas O, Casel S, Delos M, Trigaux J-P, Melange M, Marchand E. Granulomatous bronchiolitis associated with Crohn's disease. Am J Respir Crit Care Med. 1998;158(5):1676–9.
147. Butland R, Cole P, Citron K, Turner-Warwick M. Chronic bronchial suppuration and inflammatory bowel disease. QJM An Int J Med. 1981;50(1):63–75.
148. Wilcox P, Miller R, Miller G, Heath J, Nelems B, Muller N, et al. Airway involvement in ulcerative colitis. Chest. 1987;92(1):18–22.
149. Nakamura M, Inoue T, Ishida A, Miyazu YM, Kurimoto N, Miyazawa T. Endobronchial ultrasonography and magnetic resonance imaging in tracheobronchial stenosis from ulcerative colitis. J Bronchol Intervent Pulmonol. 2011;18(1):84–7.
150. Shulimzon T, Rozenman J, Perelman M, Bardan E, Ben-Dov I. Necrotizing granulomata in the lung preceding colonic involvement in 2 patients with Crohn's disease. Respiration. 2007;74(6):698–702.
151. Piotrowski WJ, Zieliñski KW, Kozłowska A, Górski P. Atypical lung changes in a 19-year-old woman with Crohn's disease. Lung. 2007;185(3):189–90.
152. Golpe R, Mateos A, Pérez-Valcárcel J, Lapeña JA, García-Figueiras R, Blanco J. Multiple pulmonary nodules in a patient with Crohn's disease. Respiration. 2003;70(3):306–9.
153. Lucero PF, Frey WC, Shaffer RT, Morris MJ. Granulomatous lung masses in an elderly patient with inactive Crohn's disease. Inflamm Bowel Dis. 2001;7(3):256–9.

154. Jang EC, Choi SJ, Cho JH, Ryu J-S, Kwak SM, Lee HL, et al. Organizing pneumonia presenting after ulcerative colitis remission. J Thorac Dis. 2013;5(2):E71.
155. Carratù P, Dragonieri S, Nocerino MC, Trabucco SMR, Lacedonia D, Parisi G, et al. A case of cryptogenic organizing pneumonia occurring in Crohn's disease. Can Respir J. 2005;12(8):437–9.
156. Adachi Y, Hinoda Y, Takahashi H, Nakagawa N, Sakamoto H, Itoh F, et al. Rheumatoid arthritis associated with ulcerative colitis. J Gastroenterol. 1996;31(4):590–5.
157. Lu D-G, Ji X-Q, Zhao Q, Zhang C-Q, Li Z-F. Tracheobronchial nodules and pulmonary infiltrates in a patient with Crohn's disease. World J Gastroenterol WJG. 2012;18(39):5653.
158. Calder C, Lacy D, Raafat F, Weller P, Booth I. Crohn9s disease with pulmonary involvement in a 3 year old boy. Gut. 1993;34(11):1636–8.
159. Krishnan S, Banquet A, Newman L, Katta U, Patil A, Dozor AJ. Lung lesions in children with Crohn's disease presenting as nonresolving pneumonias and response to infliximab therapy. Pediatrics. 2006;117(4):1440–3.
160. Freeman HJ, Davis JE, Prest ME, Lawson EJ. Granulomatous 'bronchiolitis with necrobiotic pulmonary nodules in Chrohn's disease. Can J Gastroenterol Hepatol. 2004;18(11):687–90.
161. Kedziora JA, Wolff M, Chang J. Limited form of Wegener's granulomatosis in ulcerative colitis. Am J Roentgenol. 1975;125(1):127–33.
162. Saxon A, Shanahan F, Landers C, Ganz T, Targan S. A distinct subset of antineutrophil cytoplasmic antibodies is associated with inflammatory bowel disease. J Allergy Clin Immunol. 1990;86(2):202–10.
163. Kasuga A, Mandai Y, Katsuno T, Sato T, Yamaguchi T, Yokosuka O. Pulmonary complications resembling Wegener's granulomatosis in ulcerative colitis with elevated proteinase-3 anti-neutrophil cytoplasmic antibody. Intern Med. 2008;47(13):1211–4.
164. Elzouki AN, Eriksson S, Löfberg R, Nässberger L, Wieslander J, Lindgren S. The prevalence and clinical significance of α1-antitrypsin deficiency (PiZ) and anca specificities (proteinase 3, BPI) in patients with ulcerative colitis. Inflamm Bowel Dis. 1999;5(4):246–52.
165. Majewski S, Piotrowski W. Pulmonary manifestations of inflammatory bowel disease. Arch Med Sci AMS. 2015;11(6):1179.
166. Talwar A, Kunst H, Ngatchu T, Trotter S. A case presentation of a pulmonary complication of ulcerative colitis. BMJ Case Rep. 2013;2013:bcr0220125806.
167. Mahadeva R, Walsh G, Flower C, Shneerson J. Clinical and radiological characteristics of lung disease in inflammatory bowel disease. Eur Respir J. 2000;15(1):41–8.
168. Black H, Mendoza M, Murin S. Thoracic manifestations of inflammatory bowel disease. Chest J. 2007;131(2):524–32.
169. Chikano S, Sawada K, Ohnishi K, Fukunaga K, Tanaka J, Shimoyama T. Interstitial pneumonia accompanying ulcerative colitis. Intern Med. 2001;40(9):883–6.
170. Ikehara N, Fujimoto K, Sadohara J, Iwamoto R, Tajiri M, Okamoto M, et al. Interstitial pneumonia associated with ulcerative colitis: high-resolution computed tomography and pathologic findings. J Thorac Imaging. 2013;28(1):W21–W3.
171. Faller M, Gasser B, Massard G, Pauli G, Quoix E. Pulmonary migratory infiltrates and pachypleuritis in a patient with Crohn's disease. Respiration. 2000;67(4):459–63.
172. Songür N, Songür Y, Tüzün M, Dogan I, Tüzün D, Ensari A, et al. Pulmonary function tests and high-resolution CT in the detection of pulmonary involvement in inflammatory bowel disease. J Clin Gastroenterol. 2003;37(4):292–8.
173. Roginsky V, Ivanov A, Ovtchinnikov I, Khonsari R. Familial cherubism: the experience of the Moscow Central Institute for Stomatology and Maxillo-Facial Surgery. Int J Oral Maxillofac Surg. 2009;38(3):218–23.
174. Battaglia A, Merati A, Magit A. Cherubism and upper airway obstruction. Otolaryngol Head Neck Surg. 2000;122(4):573–4.
175. Al-Mayouf SM, AlSaleem A, AlMutairi N, AlSonbul A, Alzaid T, Alazami AM, et al. Monogenic interferonopathies: Phenotypic and genotypic findings of CANDLE syndrome and its overlap with C1q deficient SLE. Int J Rheum Dis. 2018;21:208–13.

Chapter 8
Pulmonary Manifestations of Complement Deficiencies

Anete Sevciovic Grumach and Kathleen E. Sullivan

8.1 Introduction

The complement system has an important role in host defense against infectious agents, in the removal of apoptotic cells and immune complexes, and in the modulation of the adaptive immune system [1]. It has also been described as a "double-edged sword" since it defends the host against infection but can also cause harm when activated in an uncontrolled manner, as in sepsis [2]. Besides numerous experimental studies evaluating knockout mice, complement-deficient patients reveal the role of this system in several functions related to immunity. Clinical data suggest the importance of complement for preventing infections with pyogenic bacteria [3]; and experiments using animal models of disease have confirmed the essential role of complement for innate immunity to *S. pneumoniae* and other gram-positive pathogens such as group B streptococcus [4–6].

There are three activation pathways of the complement system. The classical pathway is activated when the first component, C1q, binds to the Fc region of antibody complexed with antigen. Other serum components such as natural IgM or C-reactive protein can activate classical pathway as well [4, 7]. Component C1q can directly stimulate the phagocyte oxidative burst, chemotaxis, and phagocytosis independently of the whole complement system activation [7]. All protein interactions lead to a conformational change in C1q that allows autoactivation of C1r. Two molecules of active C1r cleave the two molecules of C1s. Once cleaved, the active C1s cleaves C4 into C4a and C4b. C4b is a highly reactive molecule that binds to the pathogen surface near the antibody-C1 complex. The C4b-C1s_2 complex with

A. S. Grumach (✉)
Center of Reference for Rare Diseases, Clinical Immunology, Faculdade de Medicina ABC, Santo Andre, SP, Brazil

K. E. Sullivan
ARC 1216 Children's Hospital of Philadelphia, Philadelphia, PA, USA
e-mail: sullivank@email.chop.edu

S. A. Mahdaviani, N. Rezaei (eds.), *Pulmonary Manifestations of Primary Immunodeficiency Diseases*, https://doi.org/10.1007/978-3-030-00880-2_8

the enzymatically active C1s can cleave C2 into C2a and C2b. The smaller C2b is released, and the C2a becomes incorporated into the complex. The C3-converting enzyme C4bC2a (C3 convertase) is formed, and C3 is cleaved into C3a, which diffuses away, and C3b, which attaches to the pathogen, acting as an opsonin and initiating the activation of the terminal components. C3b deposited on the pathogen surface, which is recognized by specific receptors on neutrophils, can enhance phagocytosis. Cleavage products that result from this activation pathway incite inflammation with erythema (vasodilatation) and edema (vascular leak) [1].

In humans, different pattern recognition molecules (PRMs) activate the lectin pathway: mannose-binding lectin (MBL), ficolin-1 (also called M-ficolin or ficolin/P35-related protein), ficolin-2 (also called L-ficolin, hucolin, EBP-37, or ficolin/P35), ficolin-3 (also called H-ficolin, Hakata antigen, thermolabile β-2 macroglycoprotein, or thermolabile substance), and heteromers of collectin 10 (COLEC10, collectin liver 1, or CL-L1) and collectin 11 (COLEC11, collectin kidney 1, or CL-K1). Besides recognizing and binding different bacterial PAMPs (pathogen-associated molecular patterns) [8], PRMs of the lectin pathway were reported to opsonize bacteria and elicit cytokine release from phagocytes [8]. The ficolins also bind surface structures of various classes of microorganisms and of various acetylated compounds. Moreover, they are involved in sequestration and removal of dying host cells [9]. These pattern recognition molecules – MBL and the three ficolins – circulate in complexes with the MBL-associated serine proteases MASP-1, MASP-2, and MASP-3, with two additional proteins, MAp19 and MAp44 (also termed sMAP and MAP-1, respectively). The MBL or lectin pathway is activated by binding of these molecules to specific patterns of mannose or other sugar residues on the pathogen's surface. Although found sufficient to autoactivate and initiate the lectin pathway of complement, MASP-2 is usually activated by MASP1 at physiological conditions, afterward cleaving the complement components C4 and C2, thus generating the C3 convertase C4bC2b. The anaphylatoxin C4a is released. Once C3 convertase is bound to the pathogen surface, the remaining protein-protein interactions are identical to those in the classical pathway [10]. MASP-1 is required for efficient activation of the lectin pathway. Compared to C1s, the serine protease of the classical pathway, MASP-2, is up to 1000 times more catalytic active and up to 50-fold more rapidly inhibited by C1-inhibitor [10]. Nevertheless PRM-mediated phagocytosis may potentially be inhibited by MASP-3 [11]. Thus, the relative concentration and functional integrity of MASPs may regulate the lectin pathway-mediated antibacterial response balancing complement activation/formation of the membrane attack complex and opsonization/phagocytosis [12].

The alternative pathway is activated by spontaneous hydrolysis of C3 leading to covalent binding of C3b in association with factor B to the hydroxyl groups on cell-surface carbohydrates and proteins. This pathway does not require the existence of preformed antibody. Pathogen specificity is provided by regulatory proteins, such as factor H, which prevents alternative pathway activity against host cells [13]. Only when factor B is complexed with hydrolyzed C3, it can be cleaved by the serum protein factor D. The cleaved factor B is termed Bb; the small fragment liberated in this enzymatic cleavage, known as Ba, is not thought to be biologically active.

C3bBb is the alternative pathway C3-converting enzyme, which is stabilized by properdin and cleaves additional C3 into C3b and C3a.

The central component of the complement system is C3. The activation of each of the three pathways (CP, LP, and AP) results in cleavage of inactive complete C3 protein into the functional fragments C3a and C3b. C3a is an inflammatory mediator and C3b is an opsonin, which can bind covalently and tag any surface in the immediate proximity to the site of its generation [1].

Direct lysis of targets requires the terminal components. Once C3 is cleaved by any of the activation pathways, it becomes a part of the next enzymatic complex, the C5 convertase. This C5 convertase will be either C4b2a3b (in the classical and lectin activation pathways) or $C3b_2Bb$ (in the alternative pathway). The cleavage of C5 follows the typical pattern, with the larger fragment becoming attached to a surface and the smaller fragment diffusing into the fluid phase. C5a has relevance as anaphylatoxin. The C5b fragment bound to the active convertase initiates the terminal pathway, which results in directed, nonenzymatic assembly of the terminal pathway components C5, C6, C7, C8, and C9, leading to formation of the terminal complement complex (TCC) or membrane attack complex (MAC). C5b has a low affinity for lipids, but when bound to C6, C7, and C8, it can firmly insert into a lipid membrane. C5b, which remains more external than the other components, binds directly to C8, which compromises the physical integrity of the membrane, so that leakage of cytoplasmic proteins and ions begins to occur. The addition of C9 leads to formation of a true pore. Multiple C9 molecules can be associated with the C5-C6-C7-C8 complex [1, 14].

In view of the enormous capacity for damage, it is no surprise that a large number of regulatory proteins are involved in controlling complement system. Several fluid-phase and membrane-bound proteins are involved in this regulation.

The main fluid-phase inhibitors of the classical pathway of complement are C1-inhibitor and C4b-binding protein (C4bp); factors H and I inhibit the alternative pathway, while S-protein (vitronectin) and clusterin (SP-40,40/apolipoprotein) regulate the terminal pathway. C1-inhibitor inhibits contact system proteases (factor XII and plasma kallikrein), an intrinsic coagulation protease (factor XI), and the fibrinolytic proteases (plasmin and tissue plasminogen activator) in addition to complement system proteases C1r, C1s, and MASP-2. C4-binding protein displaces C2a and dissociates the classical pathway convertase, and it is a cofactor for factor I cleavage of C4b [1]. Factor I inactivates C3b by cleaving it to iC3b, and its activity is enhanced in the presence of factor H. Both factors act to control spontaneous activation of alternative pathway when an activator surface is not present. Although factor H has always been considered a fluid-phase inhibitor of the alternative pathway, it also plays a key role in regulating complement on tissue surfaces [14].

Membrane-bound regulatory proteins are decay-accelerating factor (DAF/CD55), membrane cofactor protein (MCP/CD46), CD59 (HRF20), C8-binding protein, and complement receptor 1 (CR1/immune adherence receptor, CD35). Other complement receptors, CR2, 3, and 4, have no complement regulatory activity [15]. Membrane-bound regulators control the three major complement activation pathways and inactivate both C3 and C4 (CR1 and CD46).

(For further information, you may see Mahmoudi M, Nilsson PH, Mollnes TE, Roos D, Sullivan KE. Complement deficiencies. In: Rezaei N, Aghamohammadi A, Notarangelo LD. *Primary immunodeficiency diseases: definition, diagnosis, and management*. 2nd ed. p. 437–460).

8.2 Deficiencies of Classical Pathway Components

Homozygous hereditary deficiency of each classical pathway early proteins involved in complement activation is very strongly associated with the development of systemic lupus erythematous (SLE) [14, 16]. The association shows a hierarchy of association with SLE and disease severity according to the position of the protein in the activation pathway. The most prevalent and severe disease is associated with deficiency of the proteins involved in the C1 complex and with total C4 deficiency, where 93% and 75% of C1 and C4 deficient patients have SLE, respectively. C2 deficiency is associated with a much lower prevalence of disease, estimated at approximately 10% [16, 17], and the SLE is typically mild.

The patients with complete deficiencies of classical pathway components (C1q/r/s, C4, and C2) have been reported to be infected mostly with encapsulated bacteria such as *S. pneumoniae*, *Haemophilus influenzae*, and *Neisseria meningitidis*. A similar spectrum of infections is seen in patients with antibody deficiencies, because classical pathway components form the "effector arm" of antibodies against these bacteria [18].

Complement component **C4** is encoded by duplicated genes C4A and C4B within the major histocompatibility complex (MHC) III region in chromosome 6. As reported in the literature, complete C4 deficiency was associated with recurrent respiratory infections, pneumonias, and meningitis [19]. On the other hand, complete deficiency of either C4A or C4B is relatively common and occurs in about 6% of the population [20–22].

The role of C4 isoform (C4A and C4B) deficiency in determining predisposition to infections has been extensively studied. Because the capsules of most bacteria that cause meningitis, such as *N. meningitidis*, *S. pneumoniae*, and *H. influenzae*, all possess OOH groups, but not ONH2 groups, it was hypothesized that deficiency of C4B (which preferentially forms ester linkages) would result in reduced complement activation on these bacterial pathogens and an increased incidence of invasive infections would be the outcome. C4A deficiency was associated with recurrent acute otitis media, sinusitis, and pneumonia in children and adolescents [14, 23].

Homozygous C4B-deficient children with bacterial meningitis and bacteremia caused by *N. meningitidis*, *S. pneumoniae*, and *H. influenzae* have been reported [24, 25]. Nevertheless, bacteremia was only found in Caucasian children [24]. However, another study did not show an association between C4B deficiency and the development of either bacteremia or meningitis [26]. Similarly, there was no increase in the frequency of C4B deficiency in patients with meningococcemia and terminal complement deficiency [27]. Furthermore, no association between homozygous C4 isoform deficiency and patients with pneumococcal bacteremia or recurrent pneumonia was noted either [28]. Regarding fungal infections, Brazilian patients had increased susceptibility to paracoccidioidomycosis with either C4A or C4B deficiencies. In summary, C4 gene deficiency should be evaluated in subjects with recurrent respiratory infections as an additional predisposing factor [29].

Homozygous C2 deficiency is common (1 in 10,000 individuals of Caucasian origin), while heterozygous C2 deficiency occurs in 1% of the population. Individuals with C2 deficiency may remain healthy and not presenting infectious complications. About 10–30% of C2-deficient individuals develop autoimmune disorders, including SLE, cutaneous lupus, and discoid lupus erythematosus [30]. Among the homozygous C2-deficient patients described previously, *N. meningitidis*, *S. pneumoniae* bacteremia, *H. influenzae* meningitis, and recurrent respiratory infections were common [31]. Immunoglobulin (IgA, IgG4) and MBL deficiencies have also been contributed with susceptibility to infections in C2-deficient patients [14, 32].

Observation of 40 individuals with homozygous C2 deficiency from 33 Swedish families over a 25-year period showed the occurrence of severe infections as septicemia or meningitis caused by *S. pneumoniae* and, in addition, recurrent infections as pneumonia [3]. Those authors also identified other bacteria related to invasive infections as *S. aureus*, *H. influenzae type b* (Hib), *Streptococcus agalactiae*, *N. meningitidis*, and others. These infections occurred mostly during infancy and childhood. As mentioned before, SLE, undifferentiated connective tissue disease, or vasculitis developed during the follow-up in some patients [3], and therefore, immune suppression for these conditions may further increase the infectious susceptibility.

8.3 Deficiencies of Lectin Pathway Components

8.3.1 Mannose-Binding Lectin (MBL)

Mannose-binding lectin (MBL) is a soluble pattern recognition protein that contributes to killing of a broad range of pathogenic microorganisms via the lectin complement pathway and through opsonophagocytosis [12, 33].

The serum levels of MBL are genetically determined as a consequence of single-nucleotide polymorphisms (SNPs) embedded into the promoter and the exon 1 of the human MBL2 gene [34, 35]. Homo- and heterozygous combinations of those SNPs give rise to different genotypes responsible for high (A/A, XA/A), intermediate (O/A, XA/XA), or low (O/O, XA/O) serum MBL levels [36]. MBL levels vary widely among individuals, with serum levels ranging from 5 ng/ml to over 10 ug/ml [34, 37].

The frequency of MBL deficiency in the general Caucasian population has been estimated between 5% and 10% [38] and may, therefore, be considered the most common congenital immunodeficiency. Studies that address the correlation of MBL levels with infections must be interpreted with caution [39]. First, the cutoff value that defines MBL deficiency varies from study to study, and values ranging from 50 ng/ml to 1 μg/ml have been used. Second, the finding that MBL levels were genetically determined led to several investigators to use genotyping to correlate MBL levels with disease. It must be noted that MBL levels in individuals with the identical genotype for all MBL variants may significantly differ [14, 34, 40]. Even considering those facts, several studies correlate MBL levels with respiratory infections and suggest its relevance to the defense of the lung. MBL can contribute to respiratory mucosal and bloodstream defenses as it can be shown to bind to numerous important respiratory pathogens, promoting C4 deposition [12, 33]. It may be that in individuals with additional risk factors, MBL deficiency plays a more significant role in predisposition to infection.

MBL is a serum protein produced in the liver, but it is also found at the sites of inflammation, although at levels substantially less than in the blood [33]. No appreciable MBL transcription was found by real-time PCR on lung tissue [41], so MBL present in respiratory secretions most likely represents "leakage" from the serum.

Before the description of MBL, Soothill and Harvey [42] described recurrent infections caused by several etiological agents affecting the skin and respiratory tract and also associated with diarrhea and cutaneous rash. These patients did not opsonize *Saccharomyces cerevisiae* (baker's yeast) adequately, and no antibody deficiency or hemolytic activity was identified either. Subsequently, Super et al. [43] confirmed that about 5–7% of the general population failed to opsonize *S. cerevisiae*, and the addition of purified MBL in a dose-dependent fashion was corrected to the defect. Sumiya et al. indicated association of *mbl2* gene polymorphism, low MBL levels, and infections in children. These studies preceded innumerous investigations looking for the role of MBL deficiency and infections [44], supporting the biological role of MBL and the infectious consequences of low levels.

It has been reported that low concentrations of serum MBL are associated with recurrent infections not only in children but also in adults [14, 45]. Eisen et al. observed higher risk of death due to *S. pneumoniae* sepsis in patients with low MBL levels (less than 0.5 μg/ml) associated to different *mbl2* genotypes [33]. Regarding invasive pneumococcal disease, a higher frequency of MBL genotypes corresponding to low MBL levels was observed [46]. MBL deficiency may not be a risk factor for developing pneumococcal infection, but the prognosis is worst for patients with homozygous variant MBL alleles.

Several studies have linked MBL deficiency, which arises through common mutations in exon-1 of the *mbl2* gene, with susceptibility to invasive pneumococcal disease and severity of community-acquired pneumonia, although these have not been universal findings [39, 47–49].

Aittoniemi et al. [50] first suggested the concomitance of humoral immunodeficiencies and MBL deficiency. IgG subclass deficiency was found in association with MBL deficiency, and this finding was attributed as a risk factor for infection. In contrast, 1 year later, the same group did not find the relationship of MBL and IgG subclass deficiency in patients with IgA deficiency leading to recurrent infections [51]. Cedzynski et al. [52] indicated that children with associated humoral deficiencies and MBL insufficiency are more susceptible to respiratory infections.

Litzman et al. [53] evaluated 94 patients with common variable immunodeficiency, and they observed that low MBL-producing genotypes predisposed CVID patients to pulmonary complications such as bronchiectasis, fibrosis, and respiratory insufficiency. No other clinical manifestations in CVID patients were influenced by MBL genotype. In contrast, Mullighan et al. [54] identified the relationship of early-onset symptoms and autoimmunity in CVID.

Watkins et al. [55] reported a patient with severe X-linked chronic granulomatous disease and very low MBL levels. Although only reported once, the authors suggested that the concomitance of MBL deficiency could worsen the course of the disease.

There appears to be evidence that a critical "intermediate" level of MBL may be protective against intracellular pathogens such as *Mycobacterium tuberculosis*. One possible explanation is that high levels of MBL binding would lead to C3b/iC3b deposition and promote entry of bacteria into phagocytes through complement receptors such as CR1 and CR3. MBL binds to lipoarabinomannan (LAM) on the mycobacterial surface, which is also a mycobacterial ligand for mannose receptors on monocytes and macrophages [56]. Not all mycobacteria bind MBL equally well, e.g., *Mycobacterium africanum* binds recombinant human MBL more efficiently than *M. tuberculosis* [57]. Low levels of MBL would result in limited complement activation but sufficient to bind to LAM and block engagement of mannose receptors. On the other hand, MBL itself can bind to CR1 and could enhance bacterial uptake. In addition, MBL bound to bacteria could improve ligation of macrophage receptors, which can modulate release of cytokines such as IL-12 that play a critical role in host responses to infection [58]. MBL deficiency was shown to increase the susceptibility to Mycobacteria in Northwestern Brazil [59].

Lambourne et al. [60] found lower mean MBL levels in persons with invasive aspergillosis than in a control population. Another study found low MBL levels and chronic necrotizing pulmonary aspergillosis (CNPA) (also known as "semi-invasive aspergillosis"). This form of aspergillosis is usually seen in patients with preexisting damage to the lung parenchyma and/or mild immunocompromised, as may occur with alcoholism, diabetes, malnutrition, or low-dose steroid use [61]. Allergic bronchopulmonary aspergillosis (ABPA) was associated with higher MBL levels, higher levels of circulating eosinophils and IgE, and disease severity [62].

8.3.2 Cystic Fibrosis

Cystic fibrosis (CF) is a hereditary disorder caused by a mutation in the cystic fibrosis transmembrane conductance regulator (*CFTR*) gene and affects the exocrine glands of the lungs, liver, pancreas, and intestines. Pulmonary infections are a major cause of morbidity in CF. Younger children become infected with bacteria such as *H. influenzae* and *S. aureus*, but *P. aeruginosa* and *Burkholderia cepacia* predominate in older children. Several studies have been developed to evaluate the influence of MBL variants in CF. Lung function is significantly impaired in carriers of MBL variant alleles according to some reports [63–65]. MBL genotype does not influence colonization by *P. aeruginosa*; however, children colonized with this bacterium who are carriers of variant MBL alleles have significantly impaired lung function. According to the authors, variant MBL alleles also shorten survival [14, 65]. Other reports did not find an association between MBL levels and disease severity in CF [66, 67].

8.3.3 MASP2 Deficiency

MASP2 deficiency is estimated to affect 0.4–1 individuals in 1000 Europeans and North Africans [68]. Stengaard-Pedersen et al. [69] reported the first patient with *MASP2* deficiency and recurrent infections in adulthood. Pneumococcal pneumonia was the main clinical manifestation associated with this defect in the lectin pathway. Cedzynski et al. [70] found that both MBL deficiency and *MASP2* insufficiency represent risk factors for recurrence of infections independently of allergic disease. In this study, one *MASP2*-deficient patient was identified.

MASP2 deficiency caused by homozygosity for the p.120G amino acid substitution was also recently reported in two patients with pulmonary tuberculosis [71]. Another study including Spaniard volunteers detected two individuals with MASP2 deficiency, homozygous for D105G mutation. No relevant clinical symptoms were present in both, raising the possibility of low penetrance in *MASP2* deficiency [72].

8.3.4 Ficolin Deficiency

The ficolin family of proteins, ficolin-1 (FCN1 or M-ficolin), ficolin-2 (FCN2 or L-ficolin), and ficolin-3 (FCN3 or H-ficolin), comprise the other members of the recognition proteins of the lectin pathway. Human L-ficolin is mainly synthesized in the liver and secreted into blood circulation. H-ficolin is expressed in the lung and liver and can also be found in serum. M-ficolin is a secretory protein from neutrophils and monocytes in peripheral blood and from type II alveolar epithelial cells in the lung [73].

Ficolins act as pattern recognition molecules that specifically bind to many clinically important microorganisms. They also function as opsonins when binding to certain types of oligosaccharides on the surfaces of pathogens via their lectin activity [9, 74]. The role of H-ficolin in *A. fumigatus* defense was demonstrated in vitro. It occurs through the activation of the lectin complement pathway, enhanced fungus-host interactions, and modulated immune responses [73].

L-ficolin (ficolin-2) is a serum lectin with multiple binding sites, able to recognize and bind to various microorganisms [70]. Although inherited deficiencies of ficolins are rare, polymorphisms that influence the concentration and function of ficolin-2 (L-ficolin) have been described [70]. Like MBL, the structure of L-ficolin is based on multimerization of a basic collagen-like helical triplet (mainly 12-mers), and exhibits considerable genetic polymorphism affecting both the promoter region and exon 8, which encodes the fibrinogen (lectin) domain.

It has been reported that both L-ficolin and H-ficolin are able to inhibit influenza A virus infection both in vitro and in vivo [74–76]. While H-ficolin has a role in the airway, reducing viremia of influenza A virus [76], L-ficolin interacts with surface glycoproteins of influenza A virus, hemagglutinin and neuraminidase [75].

Both L-ficolin and M-ficolin have been demonstrated to be associated with gram-positive bacterial infectious diseases such as streptococci (GBS) and *Staphylococcus aureus*. L-ficolin was shown to activate the lectin pathway through binding to carbohydrate on the bacterial surface, and it enhanced the opsonic activity of polymorphonuclear neutrophils [77]. L-ficolin insufficiency was associated with susceptibility to infection of *S. pneumonia.* There was a tendency to fatal or adverse outcome, but these differences were not statistically significant [78]. L-ficolin insufficiency enhances susceptibility to childhood respiratory infections only in patients with allergic asthma or rhinitis [70]. H-ficolin binds to the gram-positive bacterium *Aerococcus viridans* [74].

Low L-ficolin was associated with bronchiectasis, and it was hypothesized that impaired innate immunity might influence susceptibility to this disease process. In this study, no genotyping was performed. It was previously reported that L-ficolin is present in high levels during pneumonia as acute phase reactant. In addition, L-ficolin has variable levels according to the age in contrast with MBL, which has stable concentrations during the life [79].

Munthe-Fog et al. reported a 32-year-old man, homozygous for ficolin-3 mutation, who developed several respiratory infections during childhood, followed by cerebral abscesses at 20 years old. The pulmonary condition progressed to bronchiectasis and pulmonary fibrosis. The authors identified an additional 23 patients, heterozygous for the same mutation, out of 1,282 individuals, expecting 1 person in 10,000 to be homozygous [80]. Further investigation has to be done considering that no other patient was identified with FCN3 mutation [80].

L-ficolin can bind to gram-negative bacteria, such as the rough type of *Salmonella typhimurium* TV119 and *Pseudomonas aeruginosa* [79]. It has an opsonic effect facilitating phagocytosis by polymorphonuclear leukocytes and monocytes. H- and M-ficolins also bind carbohydrate structures of gram-negative bacteria [81].

Tuberculosis (TB) is a disease caused by *Mycobacterium tuberculosis* and remains a major global health problem. It was previously found that L-ficolin (ficolin-2) serum levels were lower in patients with pulmonary TB [82]. The capacity of L-ficolin to bind to virulent *M. tuberculosis* was demonstrated in vitro and that the administration of exogenous L-ficolin had a protective effect in mice [82].

8.3.5 *Collectin 11*

Collectin-11 (CL-11, also known as CL-K1 and encoded by COLEC11) is a recently described component of innate defense that is synthesized by several types of non-immune cells, including epithelial cells of the renal tract and mucosal cells in the intestinal and bronchial tracts. The structure of CL-11 consists of a globular head, followed by a neck region and a N-terminal collagenous domain. Each chain associates to form trimeric CL-11 subunits that combine to give CL-11 oligomers (100–200 kDa). This oligomerization contributes to the high avidity of interaction with monosaccharide ligands. The globular head of CL-11 contains a carbohydrate recognition domain (CRD), which is reported to preferentially bind L-fucose among other possible ligands [83, 84]. Like MBL, CL-11 can interact with the surfaces of bacteria, viruses, and fungi, which indicates a significant role for CL-11 in host defense [83].

It has been reported that MBL does not bind to some investigated *Streptococcus pneumonia* strains, while a clear binding of collectin-11 was observed [85]. These findings clearly show that molecules like collectin-11 may compensate for MBL deficiency and explain why MBL may be partly redundant. Collectin-11 may bind to microorganisms with which MBL cannot interact and vice versa as well.

A role in embryogenesis is apparent in individuals with inherited deficiency of CL-11. Together with CL-K1, MASP-3 seems to have an important role in early embryonic development. Defects in the genes encoding either collectin-11 or MASP-3 have been shown to cause the 3MC developmental syndrome [86]. The 3MC syndrome is a unifying term encompassing the overlapping Carnevale, Mingarelli, Malpuech, and Michels syndromes. These rare autosomal recessive disorders exhibit a spectrum of developmental features, including characteristic facial dysmorphism, cleft lip and/or palate, craniosynostosis, learning disability, and genital, limb, and vesicorenal anomalies. However, it is difficult to reconcile that the 3MC syndrome could be caused by a complement defect per se. COLEC11 RNA knockdown studies using embryonal zebra fish indicated that collectin-11 deficiency hampered neural crest cell migration [86]. Thus, collectin-11 may be considered as the fifth recognition molecule of the lectin pathway besides MBL, ficolin-1, ficolin-2, and ficolin-3.

8.4 Deficiencies of Alternative Pathway Components

The role of the AP in host defense has received great impetus from the identification of individuals with deficiencies of AP components, which include fB, factor D (fD), properdin, and C3.

Partial deficiency of fD was reported in twins who suffered from respiratory infections with *H. influenzae* and *Proteus* and *Pseudomonas* spp. The diagnosis was made in adulthood, but there was a history of recurrent infections since childhood (about 7–8 years of age). The first case of complete deficiency of fD (the mode of inheritance is autosomal recessive) was of an adult with a history of *N. meningitidis* meningitis and two episodes of disseminated gonococcal infection (DGI) [87]. It is worth noting that immunization of all factor D-deficient patients in both of these studies resulted in normal antibody responses.

Properdin deficiency has been described in several families and is the only X-linked complement deficiency. It manifests with complete absence of the molecule (type I), partial deficiency (type II), and normal level of a dysfunctional properdin (type III). The properdin-deficient individuals identified in a substantial number are susceptible to meningococcal disease (MD), emphasizing the important role of the AP to control the growth of meningococci. Meningococcal meningitis is frequently complicated by sepsis; it occurs preferentially in adolescence and it is often caused by uncommon serogroups. Other recurrent infections are rare in these case [88]. Schejbel et al. reported a large Pakistani family with properdin deficiency. The index case had a history of recurrent infections. Screening of 24 available relatives revealed four affected males, four female carriers, and a male heterozygous carrier who was subsequently diagnosed with Klinefelter syndrome. There was a strong association between properdin deficiency and recurrent otitis media and recurrent pneumonia. This study was the first to associate properdin deficiency with infections other than meningococcal disease [89].

8.5 Syndromes Associated with Deficiency of Complement Component C3

8.5.1 C3 Deficiency

C3 occupies a central position in the complement cascade, and it is involved in several critical functions, which include solubilization of immune complexes, enhancing bacterial killing either through membrane attack complex formation or opsonophagocytosis, and potentiation of the humoral immune response.

Alper & Propp first described heterozygous C3 deficiency and C3 levels approximately 50% of normal values [90]. Those patients were healthy, although mild impairment in functions mediated by complement was observed. Homozygous-deficient patients have serum concentration less than 0.1% of normal values [91].

C3-deficient individuals develop autoimmune disorders, infections, or both. Infections tend to be recurrent and severe. Invasive infections (meningitis, bacteremia, pneumonia, and otitis media) with *S. pneumoniae*, *N. meningitidis*, and *H. influenzae* have been reported [92, 93]. Because of its role in bridging innate immunity and adaptive immunity, patients with C3 deficiency show impaired responses to immunization. Immunization of a 2-year-old child with total C3 deficiency and a history of recurrent pyogenic infections did not induce a long-term antibody response [94]. Various aspects of the adaptive immune responses are impaired in C3 deficiency.

Secondary C3 deficiency can also result from excessive activation and consumption of complement. Such a situation arises with deficiencies of factor H or factor I or in the presence of C3 nephritic factor (antibodies against C3 factor). C3 levels under conditions of excessive C3 consumption are less than 10% of normal levels. However, the presence of even small amounts of C3 reduces the severity and frequency of infections.

8.5.2 *Factor I Deficiency*

Total deficiency of the regulatory components of the alternative pathway, factors H and I (both inherited in an autosomal recessive manner), leads to uninhibited activation of the alternative pathway. Factors H and I are primarily responsible for the negative regulation of the fluid phase at the C3 convertase of the alternative pathway. In the absence of one of these proteins, the spontaneous formation of C3 convertase continues, leading to the consumption of C3 and its depletion [95].

The most consistent clinical feature of factor I deficiency is increased susceptibility to infection, particularly by encapsulated bacteria such as *Neisseria meningitidis*, *Haemophilus influenzae*, and/or *Streptococcus pneumoniae*. The most frequently observed clinical consequences of factor I deficiency are respiratory infections (sinusitis, otitis, tonsillitis, bronchitis, pneumonia), meningitis, and arthritis [95, 96].

The spectrum of clinical manifestations of factor I deficiency may range from asymptomatic to severe repeat pyogenic infections. There is no clear explanation for this variability. Until recently, the partial deficiency had not been related to clinical manifestations. In our experience, frequent episodes of less severe infections were observed in heterozygotes, although the functional capacity of the complement system (by hemolytic activity) was not diminished, as previously reported [96].

Factor I-deficient patients appear to develop a greater number of recurrences and also display a broader range of infections. Recurrent otitis media, bronchitis, sinusitis, tonsillitis, and cutaneous abscesses have been described. As seen with C3 deficiency, invasive infections with *S. pneumoniae*, *H. influenzae*, and *N. meningitidis* (groups B, C, and W-135) have been reported, and recurrences are common [97]. Because of uninhibited C3 activation and C3b production, constant stimulation of CR1 on macrophages was thought to be responsible for lower CR1 expression and defective CR1-mediated opsonophagocytosis in factor I-deficient patients [98]. Functional defects of CR3 were also described, although the mechanism for this observation remains undefined. Factor I deficiency also leads to autoimmune disorders, including immune complex glomerulonephritis and vasculitis.

In factor I deficiency, a secondary reduction in circulating factor H levels occurs which is thought to be a consequence of factor H-C3b interactions [99]. In contrast, factor I levels remain normal in factor H deficiency [101].

8.5.3 *Factor H Deficiency*

Complete factor H deficiency is a rare disorder, and it is also associated with an increased incidence of infections, including recurrent otitis media (caused by *H. influenza*) and bronchitis [100], and invasive disease with *N. meningitidis* (groups B and X) [101]. About half of the reported patients with factor H deficiency do not have infectious complications.

All the deficient individuals present hypocomplemententemia, and the clinical manifestations are very different [101]. Complete factor H deficiency results in damage and formation of dense deposits in the glomerular basement membrane as in type II membranoproliferative glomerulonephritis (MPGN II). Factor H mutations characterize several clinical changes that may be polymorphisms associated with advanced macular degeneration, atypical hemolytic uremic syndrome (aHUS), and type II membranoproliferative glomerulonephritis (MPGN II) [102]. Furthermore, recurrent infections have been associated with the deficiency, especially the occurrence of *N. meningitidis*-related processes such as meningitis and septicemia [97]. Despite the severity of some cases, there are reports of asymptomatic individuals with total factor H deficiency, detected through the evaluation of other family members.

8.6 Deficiencies of Terminal Pathway Components

As a major effector mechanism of the complement cascade, MAC is responsible for complement-dependent serum bactericidal activity. MAC can also participate in tissue injury in various diseases. Perhaps, for this reason, a small percentage (approximately 5%) of individuals reported with late component complement deficiency (CDCD) have evidence of rheumatic or immune complex disease [103].

The most representative clinical picture of the terminal component deficiencies is a greater susceptibility to *Neisseria* infections, especially meningococcal meningitis, although gonococcal infections also occur. An important distinction between C5 deficiency and deficiency of the other components of the terminal complement pathway is that C5-deficient patients lack the ability to mount an efficient chemotactic response because of the absence of C5a generation. Despite this additional defect, the bacterial etiology of systemic infections does not differ in these individuals (more than 95% *Neisseria* spp.) [31, 104].

The median age of the first neisserial infection is in the second decade of life, a significant difference in the general population and individuals with deficiencies of classical components of the complement. Complement deficiencies are more related to meningococcal meningitis caused by rare serogroups X, Y, Z, W132, and 29E [105]. Although the incidence of meningococcal infection is much higher, the frequency of death and the percentage of fulminant cases appear to be lower in terminal complement-deficient individuals when compared to normal individuals [105]. Failure to generate the MAC with inability to lyse foreign and autologous cells may lead to milder forms of the disease with lower endotoxin concentration and less damage to the host. In addition, few organisms are required for systemic infection [103].

The genes for C6, C7, C8α, C8β, and C9 were isolated and characterized. Protein and DNA polymorphisms have been identified for members of the MAC protein family. The association between C9 deficiency and neisserial infection is not as strong as in C5-C8 deficiency. Individuals with total C9 deficiency exhibit delayed and diminished bactericidal and hemolytic activity in vitro. C9 deficiency is very common in the Japanese population, it is often asymptomatic, and several findings suggest that the deficiency is a susceptibility factor for the development of meningococcal disease [106].

8.7 Deficiencies of the Soluble Regulatory Proteins[1]

Hereditary angioedema is an autosomal dominant inherited disease resulting in heterozygous deficit of C1-inhibitor and bradykinin accumulation leading to increased vascular permeability and edema. C1-INH is a glycoprotein (serum α-globulin) consisting of 478 amino acids and a signal peptide of 22 hydrophobic amino acids from the protease inhibitor serpin family encoded on chromosome 11. The liver is the main organ responsible for its synthesis, but some other cells also participate. The synthesis is stimulated by interferon-γ, mainly by an increase of its gene transcription and, less frequently, by other cytokines. Its physiological function is to inhibit the catalytic subunits of the first component of the classical complement pathway (C1r-C1s), as well as to inhibit the function of kallikrein, plasmin, α1 antitrypsin, and activated clotting factors XI and XII [107].

Deficient production of C1-inhibitor associated with functional deficit represents 85% of the cases (type I), and normal quantitative production of the inhibitor, but with altered function (type II), corresponds to 15% of case [108]. Another type of hereditary angioedema was described with normal C1 esterase inhibitor and, in these cases, a percentage of families have mutations in exon 9 of coagulation factor XII (Hageman factor). Recently, plasminogen and angiopoietin 1 mutations were also identified in small numbers of cases with hereditary angioedema [109].

Patients with HAE usually become symptomatic as early as childhood and present great variability in the frequency of episodes. Most attacks occur without identification of the triggering factor, in three main sites: subcutaneous tissue (face, hands, arms, genital area), abdominal organs (stomach, intestine, bladder), and upper airways (larynx). The occurrence of laryngeal edema and asphyxia was associated with death in 25–40% of untreated individuals [108, 110]. There is no involvement of the bronchial tree in the symptomatology of angioedema, which may be related to the rapid metabolism of the kinins in the pulmonary circulation and activation of angiotensin. Stimuli that activate the fibrinolytic and contact sys-

[1] Deficiencies of factors H and I have been described with C3 deficiency syndromes, and properdin deficiency has been described with alternative pathway deficiencies.

tem, such as stress, trauma, and anxiety, often precede the attack. There is a tendency to worsen during menstrual cycles and pregnancy or with the use of oral contraceptives.

Laboratory diagnosis relies on quantitative and/or functional C1-INH evaluation. C4 concentration can be a screening test for diagnosis; it is reduced in approximately 95% of the cases, particularly during an episode. In the case of HAE with normal C1-INH, both C4 and C1-INH are normal and gene mutations represent the only markers so far.

Long-term prophylaxis can utilize attenuated androgens, such as danazol, stanozolol, and oxandrolone, which act by increasing the transcription of C1 INH. Androgens have several side effects and are therefore less commonly used in childhood and females. Anti-fibrinolytic agents as tranexamic acid and epsilon-aminocaproic acid are plasmin blockers, and their efficacy is restricted although they have few side effects [111].

Short-term prophylaxis is required for surgical or dental procedures. Plasma derived C1-inhibitor has been used for prophylaxis. It is administrated every 3–4 days intravenously, and recently, subcutaneously for this role [112].

In cases of acute attacks, antihistamines, glucocorticoids, and epinephrine have no effect on angioedema due to C1-INH deficiency. The treatment of choice consists of the replacement of C1-INH, application of the inhibitor of bradykinin receptor 2 (icatibant), or anti-kallikrein (ecallantide) drugs. Due to the possibility to develop upper airway obstruction, early intubation should be considered if no specific therapy is available [112].

8.7.1 Deficiency of C4bp

The C4b-binding protein (C4BP) is a potent circulating soluble complement factor and lectin pathway inhibitor. C4bp binds to C4b and accelerates the decay of C4b2a, acting as a cofactor for C4b factor I inactivation. It is synthesized in the liver and also acts on the coagulation system by binding to protein S and inactivating it. Only one patient with C4bp deficiency was reported, and no specific genetic defect was identified. This patient had angioedema, cutaneous vasculitis, and arthritis.

8.8 Deficiencies of the Regulatory Proteins and Complement Receptors

Genetic deficiencies or mutations that result in altered membrane receptor or protein function or complement inhibitors may be associated with diseases such as uremic hemolytic syndrome, age-related macular degeneration, glomerulonephritis, and nocturnal paroxysmal hemoglobinuria.

The decay-accelerating factor (CD55 or DAF) is a classic and alternative pathway control protein anchored to the erythrocyte, lymphocyte, granulocyte, endothelium, and epithelium membranes. Its primary function is to protect cells from complement-mediated cytolysis, but it also has a role in T-cell activation. Deficiency of DAF is not associated with spontaneous hemolysis, although DAF-deficient erythrocytes are moderately susceptible to hemolysis when complement is activated by the classical route. In patients with paroxysmal nocturnal hemoglobinuria, a proportion of erythrocytes is susceptible to complement-mediated lysis due to deficiency of DAF and other phospholipids anchored to membrane proteins [113]. DAF deficiency is associated with a unique type of protein-losing enteropathy.

CD59 (reactive lysis membrane inhibitor) is anchored in erythrocytes, leukocytes, and endothelial cells, where it prevents intravascular attack of the complement. CD59 deficiency has been described and differs from nocturnal paroxysmal hemoglobinuria, which is an acquired deficiency of all cell-surface glycosylphosphatidylinositol proteins (CR1, CD59, CD55) [113].

Decreased expression of CR1 (complement receptor 1) in erythrocytes and other cell types has been described in patients with SLE and has stimulated extensive investigation of CR1 function in relation to pathogenic events in immune complex disease. CR1 reduction was also found in another disease, the reactive arthritis by *Yersinia enterocolitica*. Patients with SLE also have decreased CR2 expression in B lymphocytes. Evidence suggests that these deficiencies are acquired through mechanisms related to the disease.

Complement receptor 3 (CR3, CD11b/CD18) binds complement and is found on macrophages, neutrophils, and large granular lymphocytes. Complement receptor 4 (CR4, CD11c/CD18) also binds complement and is found on neutrophils, monocytes, and macrophages. Both CR3 and CR4 bind bacterial lipopolysaccharide and β-glucans and promote phagocytosis of unopsonized bacteria and yeast. Additionally, they are upregulated at sites of inflammation and enhance the binding of monocytes and neutrophils to endothelial cells, allowing diapedesis [114].

Leukocyte adhesion deficiency (LAD) syndromes are innate defense defects against bacteria, fungi, and other microorganisms, resulting in the adhesion and arrival of leukocytes to the sites of microbial invasion [115]. LAD is a rare disease, affecting one in one million individuals. In this disorder, it is a failure to synthesize CD18, which then is associated with CD11b to form CR3 and with CD11c to form CR4. LFA-1 (CD11a/CD18), important in cellular adhesion and trafficking, is also deficient. These three receptor proteins are known as β2 integrins, part of the Ig superfamily. LAD-1 inheritance is autosomal recessive with some variability in the amounts of CD18 expressed, resulting in two phenotypes (severe deficiency and moderate deficiency). Omphalitis is a classic presenting infection with delayed separation of the umbilical cord. Infections from birth onward are usually seen with prominent bowel, perirectal, respiratory, and cutaneous infections. Recurrent and chronic bacterial infections are also seen. These are usually localized to the skin and mucosal surfaces and often involve *Staphylococcus aureus* and gram-negative bacilli. The characteristic pathologic finding is the lack of neutrophils at sites of infection and lymphoid tissues lacking lymphocytes. As expected, neutrophil counts in peripheral blood are usually elevated [115].

8.9 Summary and Conclusions

Recurrent and severe respiratory infections are a hallmark of primary immunodeficiencies. Nevertheless, complement deficiencies are often not considered as possible etiologies in this setting due to the much higher frequency of antibody deficiencies in the general population. Recognition of complement deficiencies has enormous implications for the patient because therapy is distinct from that of antibody deficiencies and can be lifesaving. Defects in the terminal complement pathway are associated with neisserial infections, which are generally systemic and abrupt in onset, although chronic meningococcemia can be a presentation. Defects in the activation arms are more likely to be associated with respiratory infections caused by encapsulated organisms. There may be a history of recurrent respiratory infections prior to the diagnosis being established or a single severe episode with sepsis. The severity may drive an intense focus on treatment and supportive care and only in retrospect is there consideration of an underlying complement deficiency. One ongoing impediment to the diagnosis of inherited complement deficiencies is the inconsistent availability of CH50 and AH50 tests. The recent development of a plate-based assay which is technically simpler to execute may improve availability and hence the diagnosis of patients.

The crucial first step in the approach to an individual patient is the consideration of potential etiologies. In the setting of respiratory tract infections that are either recurrent or severe in nature, primary immunodeficiency should be a consideration. Complement deficiencies and antibody disorders should be among the prime considerations with T-cell disorders added to the differential diagnosis in young children. Once a complement deficiency is recognized, education on risks and initiation of therapy is critical to prevent ongoing infections and death.

References

1. Sullivan KE, Grumach AS. The complement system. In: Middleton's allergy: principles and practice. 8th ed. Philadelphia: Elsevier Inc; 2017. p. 113–38.
2. Sjoholm AG, Jonsson G, Braconier JH, Sturfelt G, Truedsson L. Complement deficiency and disease: an update. Mol Immunol. 2006;43(1–2):78–85.
3. Jonsson G, Truedsson L, Sturfelt G, Oxelius VA, Braconier JH, Sjoholm AG. Hereditary C2 deficiency in Sweden: frequent occurrence of invasive infection, atherosclerosis, and rheumatic disease. Medicine (Baltimore). 2005;84(1):23–34.

4. Brown JS, Hussell T, Gilliland SM, Holden DW, Paton JC, Ehrenstein MR, et al. The classical pathway is the dominant complement pathway required for innate immunity to Streptococcus pneumoniae infection in mice. Proc Natl Acad Sci U S A. 2002;99(26):16969–74.
5. Gross GN, Rehm SR, Pierce AK. The effect of complement depletion on lung clearance of bacteria. J Clin Invest. 1978;62(2):373–8.
6. Wessels MR, Butko P, Ma M, Warren HB, Lage AL, Carroll MC. Studies of group B streptococcal infection in mice deficient in complement component C3 or C4 demonstrate an essential role for complement in both innate and acquired immunity. Proc Natl Acad Sci. 1995;92(25):11490–4.
7. Yuste J, Ali S, Sriskandan S, Hyams C, Botto M, Brown JS. Roles of the alternative complement pathway and C1q during innate immunity to Streptococcus pyogenes. J Immunol. 2006;176(10):6112–20.
8. Andrade FA, Lidani KCF, Catarino SJ, Messias-Reason IJ. Serine proteases in the lectin pathway of the complement system. In: Chakraborti S, Dhalla N, editors. Proteases in physiology and pathology. Singapore: Springer; 2017.
9. Endo Y, Matsushita M, Fujita T. Role of ficolin in innate immunity and its molecular basis. Immunobiology. 2007;212(4–5):371–9.
10. Beltrame MH, Boldt AB, Catarino SJ, Mendes HC, Boschmann SE, Goeldner I, et al. MBL-associated serine proteases (MASPs) and infectious diseases. Mol Immunol. 2015;67(1):85–100.
11. Duus K, Thielens NM, Lacroix M, Tacnet P, Frachet P, Holmskov U, et al. CD91 interacts with mannan-binding lectin (MBL) through the MBL-associated serine protease-binding site. FEBS J. 2010;277(23):4956–64.
12. Neth O, Jack DL, Dodds AW, Holzel H, Klein NJ, Turner MW. Mannose-binding lectin binds to a range of clinically relevant microorganisms and promotes complement deposition. Infect Immun. 2000;68(2):688–93.
13. Walport MJ. Complement. Second of two parts. N Engl J Med. 2001;344:1140–4.
14. Ram S, Lewis LA, Rice PA. Infections of people with complement deficiencies and patients who have undergone splenectomy. Clin Microbiol Rev. 2010;23(4):740–80.
15. Zipfel PF, Skerka C. Complement regulators and inhibitory proteins. Nat Rev Immunol. 2009;9(10):729.
16. Pickering MC, Walport MJ. Links between complement abnormalities and systemic lupus erythematosus. Rheumatology (Oxford, England). 2000;39(2):133–41.
17. Macedo AC, Isaac L. Systemic lupus erythematosus and deficiencies of early components of the complement classical pathway. Front Immunol. 2016;7:55.
18. Ross SC, Densen P. Complement deficiency states and infection: epidemiology, pathogenesis and consequences of neisserial and other infections in an immune deficiency. Medicine (Baltimore). 1984;63(5):243–73.
19. Mascart-Lemone F, Hauptmann G, Goetz J, Duchateau J, Delespesse G, Vray B, et al. Genetic deficiency of C4 presenting with recurrent infections and a SLE-like disease. Genetic and immunologic studies. Am J Med. 1983;75(2):295–304.
20. Carroll MC, Campbell RD, Bentley DR, Porter RR. A molecular map of the human major histocompatibility complex class III region linking complement genes C4, C2 and factor B. Nature. 1984;307(5948):237–41.
21. Carroll MC, Fathallah DM, Bergamaschini L, Alicot EM, Isenman DE. Substitution of a single amino acid (aspartic acid for histidine) converts the functional activity of human complement C4B to C4A. Proc Natl Acad Sci U S A. 1990;87(17):6868–72.
22. Samano ES, Ribeiro Lde M, Gorescu RG, Rocha KC, Grumach AS. Involvement of C4 allotypes in the pathogenesis of human diseases. Rev Hosp Clin. 2004;59(3):138–44.
23. Kainulainen L, Peltola V, Seppanen M, Viander M, He Q, Lokki ML, et al. C4A deficiency in children and adolescents with recurrent respiratory infections. Hum Immunol. 2012;73(5):498–501.
24. Bishof NA, Welch TR, Beischel LS. C4B deficiency: a risk factor for bacteremia with encapsulated organisms. J Infect Dis. 1990;162(1):248–50.

25. Rowe PC, McLean RH, Wood RA, Leggiadro RJ, Winkelstein JA. Association of homozygous C4B deficiency with bacterial meningitis. J Infect Dis. 1989;160(3):448–51.
26. Cates KL, Densen P, Lockman JC, Levine RP. C4B deficiency is not associated with meningitis or bacteremia with encapsulated bacteria. J Infect Dis. 1992;165(5):942–4.
27. Fasano MB, Densen P, McLean RH, Winkelstein JA. Prevalence of homozygous C4B deficiency in patients with deficiencies of terminal complement components and meningococcemia. J Infect Dis. 1990;162(5):1220–1.
28. Ekdahl K, Truedsson L, Sjoholm AG, Braconier JH. Complement analysis in adult patients with a history of bacteremic pneumococcal infections or recurrent pneumonia. Scand J Infect Dis. 1995;27(2):111–7.
29. Alves Pedroso M, Boldt A, Pereira-Ferrari L, Steffensen R, Strauss E, Jensenius JC, et al. Mannan-binding lectin MBL2 gene polymorphism in chronic hepatitis C: association with the severity of liver fibrosis and response to interferon therapy. Clin Exp Immunol. 2008;152(2):258–64.
30. Truedsson L, Bengtsson AA, Sturfelt G. Complement deficiencies and systemic lupus erythematosus. Autoimmunity. 2007;40(8):560–6.
31. Figueroa JE, Densen P. Infectious diseases associated with complement deficiencies. Clin Microbiol Rev. 1991;4(3):359–95.
32. Alper CA, Xu J, Cosmopoulos K, Dolinski B, Stein R, Uko G, et al. Immunoglobulin deficiencies and susceptibility to infection among homozygotes and heterozygotes for C2 deficiency. J Clin Immunol. 2003;23(4):297–305.
33. Eisen DP. Mannose-binding lectin deficiency and respiratory tract infection. J Innate Immun. 2010;2(2):114–22.
34. Ferraroni NR, Segat L, Guimaraes RL, Brandao LA, Crovella S, Constantino-Silva RN, et al. Mannose-binding lectin and MBL-associated serine protease-2 gene polymorphisms in a Brazilian population from Rio de Janeiro. Int J Immunogenet. 2012;39(1):32–8.
35. Madsen HO, Garred P, Thiel S, Kurtzhals JA, Lamm LU, Ryder LP, et al. Interplay between promoter and structural gene variants control basal serum level of mannan-binding protein. J Immunol (Baltimore, MD: 1950). 1995;155(6):3013–20.
36. Turner M, Hamvas R. Mannose-binding lectin: structure, function, genetics and disease associations. Rev Immunogenet. 2000;2(3):305–22.
37. Garred P. Mannose-binding lectin genetics: from A to Z. Biochem Soc Trans. 2008;36(Pt 6):1461–6.
38. Turner MW. The role of mannose-binding lectin in health and disease. Mol Immunol. 2003;40(7):423–9.
39. Dahl M, Tybjaerg-Hansen A, Schnohr P, Nordestgaard BG. A population-based study of morbidity and mortality in mannose-binding lectin deficiency. J Exp Med. 2004;199(10):1391–9.
40. Jensenius JC, Jensen PH, McGuire K, Larsen JL, Thiel S. Recombinant mannan-binding lectin (MBL) for therapy. Biochem Soc Trans. 2003;31(Pt 4):763–7.
41. Seyfarth J, Garred P, Madsen HO. Extra-hepatic transcription of the human mannose-binding lectin gene (mbl2) and the MBL-associated serine protease 1-3 genes. Mol Immunol. 2006;43(7):962–71.
42. Soothill JF, Harvey BA. Defective opsonization. A common immunity deficiency. Arch Dis Child. 1976;51(2):91–9.
43. Super M, Thiel S, Lu J, Levinsky RJ, Turner MW. Association of low levels of mannan-binding protein with a common defect of opsonisation. Lancet. 1989;334(8674):1236–9.
44. Sumiya M, Tabona P, Arai T, Summerfield J, Super M, Levinsky R, et al. Molecular basis of opsonic defect in immunodeficient children. Lancet. 1991;337(8757):1569–70.
45. Eisen DP, Dean MM, Boermeester MA, Fidler KJ, Gordon AC, Kronborg G, et al. Low serum mannose-binding lectin level increases the risk of death due to pneumococcal infection. Clin Infect Dis. 2008;47(4):510–6.
46. Munoz-Almagro C, Bautista C, Arias MT, Boixeda R, Del Amo E, Borras C, et al. High prevalence of genetically-determined mannose binding lectin deficiency in young children with invasive pneumococcal disease. Clin Microbiol Infect. 2014;20(10):O745–52.

47. Garcia-Laorden MI, Sole-Violan J, Rodriguez de Castro F, Aspa J, Briones ML, Garcia-Saavedra A, et al. Mannose-binding lectin and mannose-binding lectin-associated serine protease 2 in susceptibility, severity, and outcome of pneumonia in adults. J Allergy Clin Immunol. 2008;122(2):368–74, 74.e1–2.
48. Kronborg G, Weis N, Madsen HO, Pedersen SS, Wejse C, Nielsen H, et al. Variant mannose-binding lectin alleles are not associated with susceptibility to or outcome of invasive pneumococcal infection in randomly included patients. J Infect Dis. 2002;185(10):1517–20.
49. Roy S, Knox K, Segal S, Griffiths D, Moore CE, Welsh KI, et al. MBL genotype and risk of invasive pneumococcal disease: a case-control study. Lancet (London, England). 2002;359(9317):1569–73.
50. Aittoniemi J, Baer M, Soppi E, Vesikari T, Miettinen A. Mannan binding lectin deficiency and concomitant immunodefects. Arch Dis Child. 1998;78(3):245–8.
51. Aittoniemi J, Koskinen S, Laippala P, Laine S, Miettinen A. The significance of IgG subclasses and mannan-binding lectin (MBL) for susceptibility to infection in apparently healthy adults with IgA deficiency. Clin Exp Immunol. 1999;116(3):505–8.
52. Cedzynski M, Szemraj J, Swierzko AS, Bak-Romaniszyn L, Banasik M, Zeman K, et al. Mannan-binding lectin insufficiency in children with recurrent infections of the respiratory system. Clin Exp Immunol. 2004;136(2):304–11.
53. Litzman J, Freiberger T, Grimbacher B, Gathmann B, Salzer U, Pavlik T, et al. Mannose-binding lectin gene polymorphic variants predispose to the development of bronchopulmonary complications but have no influence on other clinical and laboratory symptoms or signs of common variable immunodeficiency. Clin Exp Immunol. 2008;153(3):324–30.
54. Mullighan CG, Marshall SE, Welsh KI. Mannose binding lectin polymorphisms are associated with early age of disease onset and autoimmunity in common variable immunodeficiency. Scand J Immunol. 2000;51(2):111–22.
55. Watkins C, Saleh H, Song E, Bala Jaishankar G, Chi S, Misran N, et al. Concomitant gene mutations of MBL and CYBB in chronic granulomatous disease: implications for host defense. Inflamm Allergy Drug Targets (Form Curr Drug Targets Inflamm Allergy). 2012;11(3):222–6.
56. Garred P, Harboe M, Oettinger T, Koch C, Svejgaard A. Dual role of mannan-binding protein in infections: another case of heterosis? Eur J Immunogenet. 1994;21(2):125–31.
57. Thye T, Niemann S, Walter K, Homolka S, Intemann CD, Chinbuah MA, et al. Variant G57E of mannose binding lectin associated with protection against tuberculosis caused by Mycobacterium africanum but not by M. tuberculosis. PloS One. 2011;6(6):e20908.
58. Sutterwala FS, Noel GJ, Clynes R, Mosser DM. Selective suppression of interleukin-12 induction after macrophage receptor ligation. J Exp Med. 1997;185(11):1977–85.
59. da Cruz HL, da Silva RC, Segat L, de Carvalho MS, Brandao LA, Guimaraes RL, et al. MBL2 gene polymorphisms and susceptibility to tuberculosis in a northeastern Brazilian population. Infect Genet Evol: J Mol Epidemiol Evol Genet Infect Dis. 2013;19:323–9.
60. Lambourne J, Agranoff D, Herbrecht R, Troke PF, Buchbinder A, Willis F, et al. Association of mannose-binding lectin deficiency with acute invasive aspergillosis in immunocompromised patients. Clin Infect Dis. 2009;49(10):1486–91.
61. Crosdale DJ, Poulton KV, Ollier WE, Thomson W, Denning DW. Mannose-binding lectin gene polymorphisms as a susceptibility factor for chronic necrotizing pulmonary aspergillosis. J Infect Dis. 2001;184(5):653–6.
62. Madan T, Kaur S, Saxena S, Singh M, Kishore U, Thiel S, et al. Role of collectins in innate immunity against aspergillosis. Med Mycol. 2005;43(Suppl 1):S155–63.
63. Dorfman R, Sandford A, Taylor C, Huang B, Frangolias D, Wang Y, et al. Complex two-gene modulation of lung disease severity in children with cystic fibrosis. J Clin Invest. 2008;118(3):1040–9.
64. Garred P, Pressler T, Madsen HO, Frederiksen B, Svejgaard A, Hoiby N, et al. Association of mannose-binding lectin gene heterogeneity with severity of lung disease and survival in cystic fibrosis. J Clin Invest. 1999;104(4):431–7.

65. Yarden J, Radojkovic D, De Boeck K, Macek M, Zemkova D, Vavrova V, et al. Polymorphisms in the mannose binding lectin gene affect the cystic fibrosis pulmonary phenotype. J Med Genet. 2004;41(8):629–33.
66. Carlsson M, Sjoholm AG, Eriksson L, Thiel S, Jensenius JC, Segelmark M, et al. Deficiency of the mannan-binding lectin pathway of complement and poor outcome in cystic fibrosis: bacterial colonization may be decisive for a relationship. Clin Exp Immunol. 2005;139(2): 306–13.
67. Olesen HV, Jensenius JC, Steffensen R, Thiel S, Schiotz PO. The mannan-binding lectin pathway and lung disease in cystic fibrosis–dysfunction of mannan-binding lectin-associated serine protease 2 (MASP-2) may be a major modifier. Clin Immunol (Orlando, Fla). 2006;121(3): 324–31.
68. Lozano F, Suarez B, Munoz A, Jensenius JC, Mensa J, Vives J, et al. Novel MASP2 variants detected among north African and sub-Saharan individuals. Tissue Antigens. 2005;66(2):131–5.
69. Stengaard-Pedersen K, Thiel S, Gadjeva M, Moller-Kristensen M, Sorensen R, Jensen LT, et al. Inherited deficiency of mannan-binding lectin-associated serine protease 2. N Engl J Med. 2003;349(6):554–60.
70. Cedzynski M, Atkinson AP, St Swierzko A, MacDonald SL, Szala A, Zeman K, et al. L-ficolin (ficolin-2) insufficiency is associated with combined allergic and infectious respiratory disease in children. Mol Immunol. 2009;47(2–3):415–9.
71. Sokolowska A, Szala A, St Swierzko A, Kozinska M, Niemiec T, Blachnio M, et al. Mannan-binding lectin-associated serine protease-2 (MASP-2) deficiency in two patients with pulmonary tuberculosis and one healthy control. Cell Mol Immunol. 2015;12(1):119–21.
72. Garcia-Laorden MI, Garcia-Saavedra A, de Castro FR, Violan JS, Rajas O, Blanquer J, et al. Low clinical penetrance of mannose-binding lectin-associated serine protease 2 deficiency. J Allergy Clin Immunol. 2006;118(6):1383–6.
73. Bidula S, Sexton DW, Yates M, Abdolrasouli A, Shah A, Wallis R, et al. H-ficolin binds aspergillus fumigatus leading to activation of the lectin complement pathway and modulation of lung epithelial immune responses. Immunology. 2015;146(2):281–91.
74. Ren Y, Ding Q, Zhang X. Ficolins and infectious diseases. Virol Sin. 2014;29(1):25–32.
75. Pan Q, Chen H, Wang F, Jeza VT, Hou W, Zhao Y, et al. L-ficolin binds to the glycoproteins hemagglutinin and neuraminidase and inhibits influenza a virus infection both in vitro and in vivo. J Innate Immun. 2012;4(3):312–24.
76. Verma A, White M, Vathipadiekal V, Tripathi S, Mbianda J, Ieong M, et al. Human H-ficolin inhibits replication of seasonal and pandemic influenza a viruses. J Immunol. 2012;189(5):2478–87.
77. Aoyagi Y, Adderson EE, Min JG, Matsushita M, Fujita T, Takahashi S, et al. Role of L-ficolin/mannose-binding lectin-associated serine protease complexes in the opsonophagocytosis of type III group B streptococci. J Immunol (Baltimore, MD: 1950). 2005;174(1):418–25.
78. Chalmers JD, Fleming GB, Rutherford J, Matsushita M, Kilpatrick DC, Hill AT. Serum ficolin-2 in hospitalised patients with community-acquired pneumonia. Inflammation. 2014;37(5):1635–41.
79. Kilpatrick DC, Chalmers JD, MacDonald SL, Murray M, Mohammed A, Hart SP, et al. Stable bronchiectasis is associated with low serum L-ficolin concentrations. Clin Respir J. 2009;3(1):29–33.
80. Munthe-Fog L, Hummelshoj T, Honore C, Madsen HO, Permin H, Garred P. Immunodeficiency associated with FCN3 mutation and ficolin-3 deficiency. N Engl J Med. 2009;360(25):2637–44.
81. Matsushita M. Ficolins: complement-activating lectins involved in innate immunity. J Innate Immun. 2010;2(1):24–32.
82. Luo F, Sun X, Wang Y, Wang Q, Wu Y, Pan Q, et al. Ficolin-2 defends against virulent mycobacteria tuberculosis infection in vivo, and its insufficiency is associated with infection in humans. PLoS One. 2013;8(9):e73859.

83. Ma YJ, Skjoedt MO, Garred P. Collectin-11/MASP complex formation triggers activation of the lectin complement pathway–the fifth lectin pathway initiation complex. J Innate Immun. 2013;5(3):242–50.
84. Selman L, Hansen S. Structure and function of collectin liver 1 (CL-L1) and collectin 11 (CL-11, CL-K1). Immunobiology. 2012;217(9):851–63.
85. Ali YM, Lynch NJ, Haleem KS, Fujita T, Endo Y, Hansen S, et al. The lectin pathway of complement activation is a critical component of the innate immune response to pneumococcal infection. PLoS Pathog. 2012;8(7):e1002793.
86. Rooryck C, Diaz-Font A, Osborn DP, Chabchoub E, Hernandez-Hernandez V, Shamseldin H, et al. Mutations in lectin complement pathway genes COLEC11 and MASP1 cause 3MC syndrome. Nat Genet. 2011;43(3):197–203.
87. Hiemstra PS, Langeler E, Compier B, Keepers Y, Leijh PC, van den Barselaar MT, et al. Complete and partial deficiencies of complement factor D in a Dutch family. J Clin Invest. 1989;84(6):1957–61.
88. Fijen CA, van den Bogaard R, Schipper M, Mannens M, Schlesinger M, Nordin FG, et al. Properdin deficiency: molecular basis and disease association. Mol Immunol. 1999;36(13–14):863–7.
89. Schejbel L, Rosenfeldt V, Marquart H, Valerius NH, Garred P. Properdin deficiency associated with recurrent otitis media and pneumonia, and identification of male carrier with Klinefelter syndrome. Clin Immunol (Orlando, Fla). 2009;131(3):456–62.
90. Alper CA, Propp RP. Genetic polymorphism of the third component of human complement (C′3). J Clin Invest. 1968;47(9):2181–91.
91. Grumach AS, Vilela MM, Gonzalez CH, Starobinas N, Pereira AB, Dias-da-Silva W, et al. Inherited C3 deficiency of the complement system. Brazilian J Med Biol Res = Rev Brasileira de pesquisas medicas e biologicas. 1988;21(2):247–57.
92. Grumach AS, Kirschfink M. Are complement deficiencies really rare? Overview on prevalence, clinical importance and modern diagnostic approach. Mol Immunol. 2014;61(2):110–7.
93. Hazlewood MA, Kumararatne DS, Webster AD, Goodall M, Bird P, Daha M. An association between homozygous C3 deficiency and low levels of anti-pneumococcal capsular polysaccharide antibodies. Clin Exp Immunol. 1992;87(3):404–9.
94. Ghannam A, Pernollet M, Fauquert JL, Monnier N, Ponard D, Villiers MB, et al. Human C3 deficiency associated with impairments in dendritic cell differentiation, memory B cells, and regulatory T cells. J Immunol (Baltimore, MD: 1950). 2008;181(7):5158–66.
95. Grumach AS, Leitao MF, Arruk VG, Kirschfink M, Condino-Neto A. Recurrent infections in partial complement factor I deficiency: evaluation of three generations of a Brazilian family. Clin Exp Immunol. 2006;143(2):297–304.
96. Leitao MF, Vilela MM, Rutz R, Grumach AS, Condino-Neto A, Kirschfink M. Complement factor I deficiency in a family with recurrent infections. Immunopharmacology. 1997;38(1–2):207–13.
97. Reis ES, Falcao D, Isaac L. Clinical aspects and molecular basis of primary deficiencies of complement component C3 and its regulatory proteins factor I and factor H. Scand J Immunol. 2006;63(3):155–68.
98. Porteu F, Fischer A, Descamps-Latscha B, Halbwachs-Mecarelli L. Defective complement receptors (CR1 and CR3) on erythrocytes and leukocytes of factor I (C3b-inactivator) deficient patients. Clin Exp Immunol. 1986;66(2):463–71.
99. Naked GM, Florido MP, Ferreira de Paula P, Vinet AM, Inostroza JS, Isaac L. Deficiency of human complement factor I associated with lowered factor H. Clin Immunol (Orlando, Fla). 2000;96(2):162–7.
100. Thompson R, Winterborn M. Hypocomplementaemia due to a genetic deficiency of beta 1H globulin. Clin Exp Immunol. 1981;46(1):110.
101. Falcao DA, Reis ES, Paixao-Cavalcante D, Amano MT, Delcolli MI, Florido MP, et al. Deficiency of the human complement regulatory protein factor H associated with low levels of component C9. Scand J Immunol. 2008;68(4):445–55.

102. Saunders RE, Goodship TH, Zipfel PF, Perkins SJ. An interactive web database of factor H-associated hemolytic uremic syndrome mutations: insights into the structural consequences of disease-associated mutations. Hum Mutat. 2006;27(1):21–30.
103. Lappegard KT, Christiansen D, Pharo A, Thorgersen EB, Hellerud BC, Lindstad J, et al. Human genetic deficiencies reveal the roles of complement in the inflammatory network: lessons from nature. Proc Natl Acad Sci U S A. 2009;106(37):15861–6.
104. Botto M, Kirschfink M, Macor P, Pickering MC, Wurzner R, Tedesco F. Complement in human diseases: Lessons from complement deficiencies. Mol Immunol. 2009;46(14):2774–83.
105. Platonov AE, Beloborodov VB, Vershinina IV. Meningococcal disease in patients with late complement component deficiency: studies in the U.S.S.R. Medicine (Baltimore). 1993;72(6):374–92.
106. Fukumori Y, Yoshimura K, Ohnoki S, Yamaguchi H, Akagaki Y, Inai S. A high incidence of C9 deficiency among healthy blood donors in Osaka, Japan. Int Immunol. 1989;1(1):85–9.
107. Kaplan AP, Joseph K. Pathogenic mechanisms of bradykinin mediated diseases: dysregulation of an innate inflammatory pathway. Adv Immunol. 2014;121:41–89.
108. Cicardi M, Aberer W, Banerji A, Bas M, Bernstein JA, Bork K, et al. Classification, diagnosis, and approach to treatment for angioedema: consensus report from the hereditary angioedema international working group. Allergy. 2014;69(5):602–16.
109. Veronez CL, Moreno AS, Constantino-Silva RN, Maia LS, Ferriani MP, Castro FF, et al. Hereditary angioedema with normal C1 inhibitor and F12 mutations in 42 Brazilian families. J Allergy Clin Immunol Pract. 2017;6:1209–1216.e8.
110. Bork K, Hardt J, Witzke G. Fatal laryngeal attacks and mortality in hereditary angioedema due to C1-INH deficiency. J Allergy Clin Immunol. 2012;130(3):692–7.
111. Lang DM, Aberer W, Bernstein JA, Chng HH, Grumach AS, Hide M, et al. International consensus on hereditary and acquired angioedema. Ann Allergy Asthma Immunol. 2012;109(6):395–402.
112. Maurer M, Magerl M, Ansotegui I, Aygoren-Pursun E, Betschel S, Bork K, et al. The international WAO/EAACI guideline for the management of hereditary angioedema-the 2017 revision and update. Allergy. 2018;73:1575–96.
113. Pu JJ, Brodsky RA. Paroxysmal nocturnal hemoglobinuria from bench to bedside. Clin Transl Sci. 2011;4(3):219–24.
114. Roos D, Law SK. Hematologically important mutations: leukocyte adhesion deficiency. Blood Cells Mol Dis. 2001;27(6):1000–4.
115. Hanna S, Etzioni A. Leukocyte adhesion deficiencies. Ann N Y Acad Sci. 2012;1250:50–5.

Chapter 9
Pulmonary Manifestations of Other Well-Defined Immunodeficiencies

Man Amanat, Mona Salehi, and Nima Rezaei

9.1 Introduction

"Other well-defined immunodeficiencies" is a category of primary immunodeficiency (PID) and consisted of different rare diseases with systemic manifestations often combined with immune system dysfunction (Fig. 9.1). Combined immunodeficiencies with associated or syndromic features have a less profound immunophenotype than severe combined immunodeficiencies, and this can make their diagnosis more challenging [1]. Increasing our knowledge about characteristic manifestations of these disorders can ease their diagnosis. For instance, the presence of ichthyosis, hair abnormality, and recurrent infections are characteristics for Netherton syndrome [2].

Respiratory manifestations are common in most PIDs. Recurrent respiratory infections and their concurrent complications such as bronchiectasis have been reported in these conditions, including other well-defined immunodeficiencies. They were also reported as the main cause of death in patients with associated diseases. Therefore, by focusing on respiratory features of PIDs, we can increase the life-span

M. Amanat · M. Salehi
NeuroImmunology Research Association (NIRA), Universal Scientific Education and Research Network (USERN), Tehran, Iran

Students' Scientific Research Center (SSRC), Tehran University of Medical Sciences (TUMS), Tehran, Iran

N. Rezaei (✉)
Research Center for Immunodeficiencies, Children's Medical Center, Tehran University of Medical Sciences (TUMS), Tehran, Iran

Department of Immunology, School of Medicine, Tehran University of Medical Sciences (TUMS), Tehran, Iran

Network of Immunity in Infection, Malignancy and Autoimmunity (NIIMA), Universal Scientific Education and Research Network (USERN), Tehran, Iran

S. A. Mahdaviani, N. Rezaei (eds.), *Pulmonary Manifestations of Primary Immunodeficiency Diseases*, https://doi.org/10.1007/978-3-030-00880-2_9

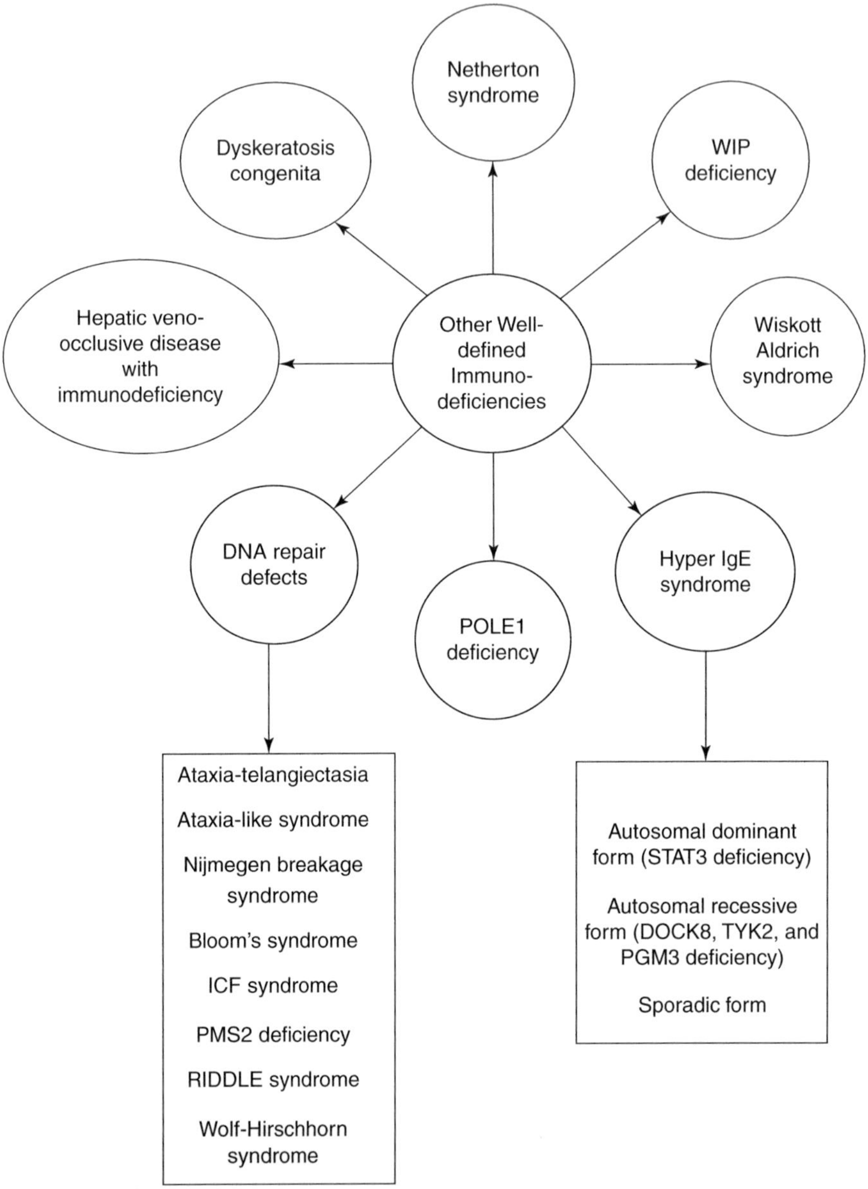

Fig. 9.1 Conditions classified as other well-defined primary immunodeficiencies

and even quality of life of patients. Herein, we describe conditions classified as other well-defined immunodeficiencies and their associated respiratory manifestations.

9.2 Ataxia Telangiectasia

9.2.1 Background

Ataxia telangiectasia (A-T) also known as Louis-Bar syndrome was first described in 1957 as a familial syndrome of progressive cerebellar ataxia, oculocutaneous telangiectasia, and frequent pulmonary infection [3]. It is now well-established that A-T is an autosomal recessive cerebellar ataxia. The worldwide incidence of this rare disease was estimated to be between 1 in 40,000 and 1 in 300,000 people [4]. Different neurological features have been identified in individuals with A-T. Examples include ataxia, impaired coordination of eye movement, dysarthria, loss of tendon reflexes, development of involuntary movements, and extrapyramidal symptoms [5]. Telangiectasia of conjunctiva is another characteristic manifestation of A-T. It can also appear on sun-exposed areas of the skin such as face and ear, in the bladder, and even inside the brain [5, 6]. A-T is also associated with development of many other systemic manifestations. Dysphagia and concurrent insufficient caloric intake, endocrine abnormalities like gonadal dysgenesis, reduced insulin sensitivity, sleep disturbance and cognitive dysfunction are some of the reported manifestations [7–11]. Furthermore, people with A-T were at increased risk of developing malignancies due to chromosomal instability and increased sensitivity to ionizing radiation [12].

Approximately two-third of individuals with A-T suffer from immune system dysfunctions [13]. Defects in both cellular and humeral immunity were recognized. Low total immunoglobulin levels (IgA, IgG, or IgM), defects in making antibody in response to vaccines and infections, and lymphopenia which affects CD4+ cells are the commonest immunological abnormalities in patients with A-T [14]. A-T is correlated with increased risk of developing autoimmune disorders and chronic inflammatory diseases including immune thrombocytopenia, and different types of arthritis,

9.2.2 Respiratory Manifestations

Pulmonary disease is responsible for about half of deaths in A-T patients [3, 17]. Prolonged cough, fever, and abnormal findings on auscultation of chest are the most reported early signs and symptoms of respiratory tract diseases in A-T patients [18]. By ignoring these early findings, severe manifestations including bronchiectasis, recurrent pneumonia, lung fibrosis, and interstitial lung disease (ILD) may occur [18]. Studies on common spirometry indices have demonstrated considerable decrease in forced volume capacity (FVC) which is a feature of restrictive lung disease [19]. Decreased FVC can affect other indices like tidal volume (VT). The progression of A-T leads to more reduction in FVC, and VT/FVC ratio has been shown to be an important marker in an A-T patient's life-span [19]. Obstruction of airway is another respiratory feature of A-T people. However, first second of expiration (FEV1)/FVC ratio is not a suitable index to show this obstruction [20].

Different underlying mechanisms can be postulated for respiratory manifestations in A-T. Immunodeficiency in A-T can increase the risk of infections and leads to different pulmonary conditions. Poor mucociliary clearance and aspiration due to impaired bulbar function and dysphagia are other causal mechanisms for this correlation [5]. Respiratory muscle weakness and their impaired coordination can lead to decreased levels of spirometry indices and restrictive lung disease [5]. Of interest, emerging evidence demonstrated that increased levels of cytokines like interleukin (e.g., IL6) have been associated with decreased lung functions [21]. Cytokines are soluble proteins with wide-range effects on functions of multiple organs such as the nervous system, skin, and respiratory system [22], and changes in their levels due to A-T may somewhat justify increased risk of different A-T manifestations.

9.3 Nijmegen Breakage Syndrome

9.3.1 Background

Nijmegen breakage syndrome (NBS) is a rare autosomal recessive condition first introduced in 1981 [23]. Most patients with NBS carry founder mutation c.657_661del5 in exon 6 of the *NBN* gene, called the Slavic mutation [24]. The worldwide prevalence of NBS has not been estimated, but it has been realized that eastern European populations are more prone to develop NBS [25]. The highest carrier frequencies of this condition are observed in the Czech Republic, Ukraine, and Poland, with prevalence of 1:154, 1:182, and 1:190, respectively [25].

Various systemic manifestations have been described in individuals with NBS. These include growth retardation, progressive microcephaly, intellectual disabilities, and gonadal dysfunction [26]. Subjects with this condition are at increased risk of developing cancer. A retrospective study reported that over 40% of NBS people were diagnosed with malignancies, and they were the main causes of deaths [27]. Lymphoma and leukemia are the commonest types of malignancies among this population, but other types including medulloblastoma, neuroblastoma, dysgerminoma, and thyroid cancer have also been identified [27]. Immunodeficiency is another clinical feature of NBS. Highly variable combined defects in cellular and humeral immune systems were recognized in NBS population. Low serum IgG and IgA concentrations were reported in most of the patients. Conversely, serum IgM levels were reported to be normal or even higher than normal in this population [27].

Reduced number of total B- and T-cells and significant reduction in their functions were also described [27].

9.3.2 Respiratory Manifestations

Respiratory infections are the most frequent infections reported in NBS people [26]. A retrospective cohort reported that pneumonia was the commonest clinical manifestation of NBS (46%), followed by acute bronchitis (39%) and chronic bronchitis (23%), respectively [27]. Bronchiectasis (16%), recurrent upper respiratory tract infections (12%), recurrent sinusitis (8%), chronic sinusitis with polyp (4%), fungal pneumonia (4%), lung tuberculosis (2%), pulmonary fibrosis (1%), and chronic respiratory insufficiency (1%) have also been reported as common respiratory manifestations of NBS [27]. It appears that most respiratory tract infections were caused by community-acquired pathogens. Predisposition to recurrent and/or chronic respiratory tract infections correlated with the severity of humoral immune deficiency [27]. Intravenous immunoglobulin (IVIg) therapy can be a good option for treatment of respiratory manifestations. However, this method of treatment failed to prevent the progression of infections in some patients [27].

9.4 Bloom Syndrome

9.4.1 Background

Bloom syndrome (BS) is an autosomal recessive condition caused by mutations in *BLM* gene located at 15q26. This gene codes for BLM protein, which is a DNA helicase involved in DNA replication and repair. BS was first described in dwarfs with congenital telangiectatic erythema in 1954 [28]. Only few individuals with BS have been reported, and its prevalence has not been estimated. However, it appears that this rare disease is more common among Ashkenazi Jews [29].

The involvement of multiple organs has been described in BS individuals. It is characterized by growth retardation, sparseness of subcutaneous fat tissue, and short stature. Skin lesions including erythematous, café-au-lait macules, and red, sun-sensitive skin lesions are more frequent in people with BS compared to general population. Gastroesophageal reflux (GER) is the main gastrointestinal symptom of BS patients [29]. This can cause otitis and lung infections due to the aspiration of gastric content. Men with BS are often infertile mostly caused by azoospermia and severe oligospermia. However, women are frequently fertile but with premature menopause [30]. Malignancy is the most frequent complication and the commonest cause of death among BS subjects [31]. Immunodeficiency is another main feature of BS, leading to an increased risk of different infections. One cohort study with six

BS patients demonstrated defects in maturation of B-cells. In fact, the naïve B-cell subsets were in the normal range, but the absolute numbers of natural effector B-cells and memory B-cells were significantly lower than the age-matched controls. Decreased number of CD4+ T-cells was also recognized [32].

9.4.2 Respiratory Manifestations

Pneumonia is a very common infection among people with BS, and up to 20% of these patients were reported to have pneumonia [29]. Studies indicated that pneumonia in this population did react well on antibiotics. It appears that the occurrence rate of pneumonia and other infections is higher throughout infancy and early childhood and then decreases with time [32]. Chronic obstructive pulmonary diseases including chronic bronchitis and bronchiectasis were described as serious complications in people with BS, and they were reported as the causes of deaths in few individuals [29]. A case report study described a 7-year-old child with BS and complete left lung volume loss with parenchymal destruction and areas of bronchiectatic changes indicating a destroyed lung [33]. She finally died from pulmonary complications. Upper and lower respiratory tract carcinomas are other associated pulmonary complications in patients with BS [29]. To date, no study has evaluated the efficacy of treatments may be useful for respiratory manifestations in these individuals. As immunodeficiency is the main cause of respiratory infections, IVIg may be a good option for treatment. Furthermore, management of GER may decrease the frequency of these infections.

9.5 ICF Syndrome

9.5.1 Background

The immunodeficiency, centromeric instability, and facial anomalies (ICF) syndrome is a rare autosomal recessive disorder, first described in 1978 [34]. About half of ICF subjects carry mutations of DNA methyltransferase 3B (*DNMT3B*) gene and are considered to have ICF type 1 [35]. About 30% of patients with ICF have mutations of *ZBTB24* and are considered to have ICF type 2 [36]. Recently ICF type 3 and 4 have also been described with the mutations of *CDCA7* and *HELLS* [37].

Immunodeficiency, autoimmune conditions, facial abnormalities, growth retardation, and cognitive impairment are the main reported clinical manifestations in people with ICF [38]. Immunodeficiency and recurrent infections are more frequent in individuals with ICF type 1, while mental retardation is more common in type 2 of this condition (38). Different types of facial anomalies in this population include high forehead with frontal bossing, flat nasal bridge, up-turned nose, hypertelorism, epicanthus, low-set ears, micrognathia, and macroglossia [38]. Regarding immunodeficiency, agammaglobulinemia or hypogammaglobulinemia is more common in ICF type 1 compared to type 2 of the disease [39]. Decreased numbers of memory B-cells and low levels of T-cell proliferation were also recognized in patients with ICF [38, 40].

9.5.2 *Respiratory Manifestations*

Respiratory infections are predominant clinical features in people with ICF, particularly in its type 1. One retrospective study investigating the clinical data of ICF patients indicated that bronchopneumonia was the most frequent infection among all types of ICFs [39]. Noted, respiratory infections due to opportunistic organism (*Pneumocystis jirovecii*) were also identified. Another cohort study with nine ICF subjects demonstrated that all but one of patients had respiratory infections and three of them had bronchiectasis [38]. Viral, bacterial, and fungal infections were all described. It is worth to mention that the only patient in this study, who didn't have respiratory infection, had an early diagnosis of ICF and was treated with IVIg. Overall, studies on few individuals reported the efficacy of IVIg and hematopoietic stem cell transplantation in treatment and prevention of infections like respiratory ones due to the reinforcement of immune system [38, 41], but further studies in this area need to be performed.

9.6 PMS2 Deficiency

9.6.1 *Background*

Postmeiotic segregation increased 2 (*PMS2*) gene found in clusters on chromosome 7 expresses to produce PMS2 protein. This product is involved in DNA mismatch repair (MMR) [42]. Overall, in human, seven MMR proteins have been found including MLH1, MLH3, MSH2, MSH3, MSH6, PMS1, and PMS2 [43]. Impaired production of these proteins may affect genomic stability and manifest as different malignancies at an early age, often colon and brain tumors [44]. Hereditary nonpolyposis colorectal cancer (HNPCC) or Lynch syndrome is a common condition caused by defects in MMR [45].

Among the abovementioned MMR proteins, less is known about PMS2. Isolated loss of PMS2 has been found in about 4% of tumors with microsatellite instability [46, 47]. The clinical features of Lynch syndrome due to PMS2 deficiency were reported to be unusual, and these patients had a lower lifetime risk of colorectal carcinomas compared to people with MLH1 or MSH2 deficiencies [48]. Furthermore, colorectal carcinomas associated with PMS2 variants develop less frequently and in patients of older ages [49].

Immunoglobulin class-switch recombination (CSR) deficiencies are rare primary immunodeficiencies characterized by the lack of switched isotype (IgG/IgA/IgE) production and mostly lead to increased levels of IgM (hyper IgM syndrome) [50]. Impaired CSR due to PMS2 deficiency was first described by *Péron et al.* [51]. They reported three patients with CSR deficiency and deleterious, homozygous mutations in the gene encoding the PMS2 component. Noted, studies also described this rare type of immunodeficiency in A-T and NBS too [52, 53].

9.6.2 Respiratory Manifestations

To date, no study has investigated the pulmonary manifestations of PMS2 deficiency. It appears that impaired CSR associated with PMS2 deficiency increases the risk of infections [51]. However, increased risk of pulmonary infections has not been clearly described. Future studies should focus on comorbidities of PMS2 deficiency and its respiratory manifestations.

9.7 Wolf-Hirschhorn Syndrome

9.7.1 Background

Micro-deletion of the short arm of chromosome 4 causes a rare congenital disorder first introduced by *Cooper and Hirschhorn* in 1961 [54]. They described a child with defects of midline fusion, low birth weight, poor development, and seizures at early ages. Similar features were also identified in another patient by *Wolf et al.* in 1965 [55]. Wolf-Hirschhorn syndrome (WHS) was then used to name this condition. The birth incidence of WHS was estimated to be at least 1 per 50,000 births and was reported to be more frequent in females [56, 57]. One of the main clinical findings in this population is their craniofacial features. They include wide bridge of the nose, microcephaly, high forehead, prominent glabella, poorly differentiated and low-set ears, highly arched eyebrows, widely spaced eyes, epicanthal folds, short philtrum, distinct mouth, and micrognathia [58]. Many other systemic manifestations have also been reported, such as growth retardation, skeletal anomalies, and defects in the heart, urinary tract system, and skin [58]. Epilepsy is the main neurologic finding in individuals with WHS [59].

Defects in B-cells of immune system were reported in people with WHS. A prior study on 13 infection-prone children with WHS demonstrated that 9 of them had antibody deficiencies [60]. IgA and IgG2 deficiencies, as well as impaired polysaccharide responsiveness, were recognized in these patients. However, it seems that cellular immunity remained intact due to WHS [60].

9.7.2 Respiratory Manifestations

A retrospective cross-sectional study investigating epidemiology, life expectancy, and causes of deaths in individuals with WHS indicated that among 32 subjects, lower respiratory tract infection was the leading cause of death (25%) [56]. Frequent upper respiratory tract infections have also been reported in case reports [61]. Aspiration pneumonia, otitis media, sinusitis, and chronic coughs are common respiratory manifestations in this population [62]. Although impaired humeral system in WHS people may increase the risk of respiratory features, other factors should not be discounted. High prevalence of GER and recurrent aspiration in patients with WHS and muscular hypotonia are the examples which may also justify the increased risk of respiratory manifestations [62].

9.8 Hyper-IgE Syndromes

9.8.1 Background

Hyper-IgE syndromes (HIES) were first described by *Davis et al.* [63] as Job's syndrome. They reported two patients with eczematoid dermatitis, recurrent *Staphylococcal* abscesses, and pneumonia. In 1972, *Buckley et al.* [64] identified similar clinical findings and elevated levels of IgE and brought HIES for description of this condition. Most cases are sporadic ones, but autosomal dominant (AD-HIES) and recessive (AR-HIES) forms of HIES were also recognized. Mutations in signal transducer and activator of transcription 3 (*STAT3*) were recognized to be the most frequent genetic basis in AD-HIES [65]. On the other side, mutations in dedicator of cytokinesis 8 (*DOCK8*), tyrosine kinase 2 (*TYK2*), and phosphoglucomutase 3 (*PGM3*) were reported in AR-HIES [66–68].

HIES associated with mutations in *STAT3*, *DOCK8*, *TYK2*, and *PGM3* shows some disease manifestations characteristic for each subtype. AD-HIES due to *STAT3* mutations commonly presents with facial features; dental abnormalities; skin findings including newborn rash, eczema, and recurrent abscesses; and abnormalities in connective tissue and skeletal system [69]. In patients with AR-HIES, recurrent viral infections, various allergic diseases, autoimmune conditions, and neurologic impairments like developmental delay and cognitive dysfunction mainly occur [68, 70]. Connective tissue and skeletal abnormalities were rarely reported in AR-HIES [68]. Comparing different types of AR-HIES, viral infections and allergies are more common in individuals with mutations in *DOCK8*. Cutaneous viral infections are the most distinguishing feature of *DOCK8* deficiency. The most common viruses involved in this type are herpes simplex virus, human papillomavirus, molluscum contagiosum virus, and varicella zoster virus [71]. Neurologic involvement mostly presents in people with *PGM3* mutations [68]. Unusual presentation of bacille Calmette-Guérin (BCG) infection was described in TYK2-deficient patients [67].

9.8.2 Respiratory Manifestations Due to AD-HIES

Recurrent bacterial pneumonias mainly occur in AD-HIES and typically lead to pneumatocele formation [72]. Five cohort studies investigating different features in STAT3-deficient individuals reported that recurrent pneumonia occurred in about 90–100% of their samples [69, 73–75]. Furthermore, pneumatocele was estimated to occur in up to 75% of patients [75]. *Streptococcus pneumoniae* and *Staphylococcus aureus* were the most common implicated bacteria. *Haemophilus influenzae*, *Pseudomonas aeruginosa*, *Stenotrophomonas maltophilia*, anaerobic bacteria, and *Mycoplasma pneumoniae* were other frequently reported bacteria [69]. Delayed diagnosis of pulmonary infections often occurs due to the lack of inflammatory systemic signs and symptoms. Therefore, different complications may appear. Bronchiectasis is a common respiratory manifestation and occurs more frequently in patients with STAT3 deficiency compared to patients with other mutations. Its prevalence was estimated to be about 65% [69]. Bronchopleural fistulas, hemoptysis, pneumothorax and/or pneumomediastinum, and tracheal stenosis were other reported lung complications. It was identified that almost one-fifth of STAT3-deficient patients required at least one lung lobectomy [69].

9.8.3 Respiratory Manifestations Due to AR-HIES

Different respiratory manifestations were reported in different types of AR-HIES. One retrospective study on 136 individuals with mutations in *DOCK8* demonstrated that recurrent respiratory infections occurred in approximately 90% of patients [76]. Asthma was another common respiratory manifestation with the frequency of 55%. Like STAT3-HIES, bronchiectasis and pneumatocele were also identified in these patients, but their prevalence was significantly lower than AD-HIES (bronchiectasis, 44%, and pneumatocele, 3%). Among bacterial organisms, *Staphylococcus aureus* and *Streptococcus pneumoniae* were the commonest causes of infections [76]. *Cytomegalovirus* (CMV) was the most frequent viral organism, and *Aspergillus* was the commonest fungus leading to infections. As eosinophilia is a frequent feature in DOCK8-HIES, increased risk of allergies and asthma can be justified. Furthermore, eosinophilic pneumonia was reported in case reports [77].

Two studies reporting clinical features of individuals with PGM3 deficiency showed that about 75% to 100% of patients suffered from pneumonia [78, 79]. Bronchiectasis and asthma were also reported with the frequency of 65% and 10–40%, respectively. These complications can have significant negative impacts on prognosis of patients as chronic respiratory failure was reported to be a cause of death and bilateral lung transplantation in one study [79]. Noted, only few cases with mutations in *TYK2* were identified, and its respiratory manifestations have not been recognized.

9.9 Wiskott-Aldrich Syndrome

9.9.1 Background

The characterization of Wiskott-Aldrich syndrome (WAS), a rare X-linked primary immunodeficiency syndrome, was first described by Alfred Wiskott in 1937. He described WAS in three brothers with episodic fever, microthrombocytopenia, bloody diarrhea, recurrent otitis, and eczema [80]. The incidence of WAS is estimated to be less than 1 in 100,000 live births [81].

WAS occurs as the result of mutations in *WAS* gene (position Xp11.22–p11.23) leading to functional disturbances of WAS protein (WASP) which is responsible for relaying signals from cell surface to the actin cytoskeleton [82]. The classic WAS presents with microthrombocytopenia, recurrent infections especially upper respiratory tract infections, eczema, and an elevated risk for autoimmunity and malignancies. It occurs when the gene mutations cause complete absence of WASP. Mutations with decreased protein expressions, known as X-linked thrombocytopenia, mainly present with thrombocytopenia with a milder eczema and immunodeficiency compared to the classic form [83–86]. The third type called X-linked neutropenia includes symptoms like neutropenia and myelodysplasia [87–89].

WAS affects different domains of immune system, mainly cellular immunity. Decreased numbers of T-cells and their impaired development are common in this population and continue with aging due to abnormal thymic output in addition to elevated rates of apoptosis [90, 91]. The development of B-cells, however, is not mostly affected in WAS, but severe decrease in numbers of B-cells was reported [92–94]. Of note there is an increased susceptibility for autoimmunity in WAS patients which raises the possibility of T regulatory cell defects in WAS [95]. In WAS patients, serum IgG levels mostly are normal, IgM levels are decreased, and IgA and IgE levels are increased. Antibody responses are normal to some antigens (e.g., live measles vaccine) and inadequate to some (e.g., polysaccharide antigens) [96, 97].

9.9.2 Respiratory Manifestations

Infections of upper and lower respiratory tract including otitis media (78% of WAS patients), sinusitis (24%), and pneumonia (45%) are the most frequent infectious and respiratory manifestations of WAS. *Pneumocystis carinii* pneumonia was also reported in 9% of WAS patients [84]. Furthermore, there is a significant increase in occurrence of *Pneumocystis jirovecii* pneumonia in classic form of WAS [98].

Increased risk of malignancies in respiratory tract system was also reported which are mostly associated with EBV infections (30–60%). The general risk of developing respiratory tract tumors among primary immune deficiencies varies between 1% and 25%, but it is higher in common variable immune deficiency (CVID) disorder and WAS [99].

9.10 Netherton Syndrome

9.10.1 Background

Netherton syndrome (NS) is a rare autosomal recessive condition characterized by ichthyosis, hair abnormality known as trichorrhexis invaginata (bamboo hair), and atopy-prone state [2]. It mainly occurs during mutations in the serine protease inhibitor Kazal-type 5 (SPINK5) gene, located on chromosome 5q32, resulting in a loss or reduced expression of the multi-domain serine protease inhibitor lympho-epithelial Kazal-type 5-related inhibitor (LEKTI) [100, 101]. Infections are frequent in these patients possibly due to the impairments of immune system. However, only few studies investigated the occurrence of immune system dysfunction in this population, and results were conflicting [102, 103].

9.10.2 Respiratory Manifestations

A study on nine NS individuals indicated that all but one of them had recurrent upper and lower respiratory tract infections, most frequently recurrent otitis [102]. Pneumonia and infection-related respiratory distress were also described in patients. Asthma is another frequent manifestation occurring in NS people. *Kutsal et al.* reported the youngest Netherton patient (a 6-month-old girl) with infantile asthma [104]. Respiratory distress as the result of pulmonary hypertension is another respiratory manifestation of NS and was reported in two studies [105, 106].

9.11 Dyskeratosis Congenita

9.11.1 Background

Dyskeratosis congenita (DC) is a rare inherited condition caused by premature telomere erosion at the ends of chromosomes in hematopoietic cells, immune cells, and epithelial cells. It was first characterized by the triad of abnormal skin pigmentation, nail dystrophy, and mucosal leukoplakia [107]. Three distinct patterns of inheritance have been found, including X-linked recessive, autosomal recessive, and autosomal dominant [108–110]. Most DC patients have X-linked recessive inheritance also known as Hoyeraal-Hreidarsson syndrome [111]. It appears that DC individuals with autosomal dominant form have lower severe manifestations and better prognosis compared to other types [112]. Various systemic manifestations have been reported in these individuals. Skeletal, dental, gastrointestinal, and genitourinary involvements, as well as aplastic anemia due to the bone marrow failure, were all described in this population [113]. Increased risk of occurrence of malignancies was also described [114].

Bone marrow failure and immunodeficiency are the main causes of death among DC patients. Studies have indicated different dysfunctions of immune system in this population. Both humeral- and cell-mediated immunities have been identified to be impaired. Dramatic decreased numbers of B-cells and natural killer cells were the most prominent findings, but decreased numbers of CD3, CD4, and CD8 T-cells were also recognized in minority of patients [115, 116]. Furthermore, low levels of IgM, IgG, and IgA were also reported.

9.11.2 Respiratory Manifestations

Over 20% of DC individuals have pulmonary complications. Postmortem examination revealed that pulmonary fibrosis and abnormalities in pulmonary microvasculature are the commonest pulmonary findings of these patients [117]. Case reports and small case series also detected pulmonary arteriovenous malformations in their subjects [118–120]. Dyspnea, orthopnea, platypnea, cyanosis, and digital clubbing are all the symptoms of patients with pulmonary fibrosis or arteriovenous malformations [120]. Aging and progression of DC are associated with progression of pulmonary abnormalities. Of interest, different trials indicated that hematopoietic stem cell transplant due to the treatment of aplastic anemia in DC patients increased the risk of pulmonary complications [121, 122]. This can be due to the nature of DC itself or underlying sensitivity to cytotoxic agents due to aberrant cellular DNA damage repair and dysregulated reactive oxidative species [122].

Studies on spirometry of patients showed that about one-third of cases had abnormal findings. Restrictive pattern (normal FEV1/FVC and low total lung capacity (TLC)) was more frequent, but obstruction (low FEV1/FVC and normal TLC) and mixed pattern (low FEV1/FVC and low TLC) were also noticed [123]. Individuals with abnormal spirometry were more likely to develop pulmonary complications. These abnormal findings were more detected in DC cases with bone marrow failure [123].

References

1. Gennery AR, Marodi L, Ziegler JB, Español T, Grimbacher B. Other well-defined immunodeficiencies. In: Rezaei N, Aghamohammadi A, Notarangelo L, editors. Primary immunodeficiency diseases. Berlin/Heidelberg: Springer; 2017.
2. Comel M. Ichthyosis linearis circumflexa. Dermatologica. 1949;98:133–6.
3. Boder E, Sedgwick RP. A familial syndrome of progressive cerebellar ataxia, oculocutaneous telangiectasia and frequent pulmonary infection: a preliminary report on 7 children, an autopsy, and a case history. Univ South Calif Med Bull. 1957;9:15–28.

4. Swift M, Morrell D, Cromartie E, Chamberlin AR, Skolnick MH, Bishop DT. The incidence and gene frequency of ataxia-telangiectasia in the United States. Am J Hum Genet. 1986;39:573–83.
5. Rothblum-Oviatt C, Wright J, Lefton-Greif MA, McGrath-Morrow SA, Crawford TO, Lederman HM. Ataxia telangiectasia: a review. Orphanet J Rare Dis. 2016;11:159.
6. Lin DD, Barker PB, Lederman HM, Crawford TO. Cerebral abnormalities in adults with ataxia-telangiectasia. AJNR Am J Neuroradiol. 2014;35:119–23.
7. Lefton-Greif MA, Crawford TO, Winkelstein JA, Loughlin GM, Koerner CB, Zahurak M, Lederman HM. Oropharyngeal dysphagia and aspiration in patients with ataxia-telangiectasia. J Pediatr. 2000;136:225–31.
8. Nissenkorn A, Levy-Shraga Y, Banet-Levi Y, Lahad A, Sarouk I, Modan-Moses D. Endocrine abnormalities in ataxia telangiectasia: findings from a national cohort. Pediatr Res. 2016;79:889–94.
9. Connelly PJ, Smith N, Chadwick R, Exley AR, Shneerson JM, Pearson ER. Recessive mutations in the cancer gene Ataxia Telangiectasia mutated (ATM), at a locus previously associated with metformin response, cause dysglycaemia and insulin resistance. Diabet Med. 2016;33:371–5.
10. McGrath-Morrow SA, Sterni L, McGinley B, Lefton-Greif MA, Rosquist K, Lederman H. Polysomnographic values in adolescents with ataxia telangiectasia. Pediatr Pulmonol. 2008;43:674–9.
11. Mostofsky SH, Kunze JC, Cutting LE, Lederman HM, Denckla MB. Judgment of duration in individuals with ataxia-telangiectasia. Dev Neuropsychol. 2000;17:63–74.
12. Suarez F, Mahlaoui N, Canioni D, Andriamanga C, Dubois d'Enghien C, Brousse N, Jais JP, Fischer A, Hermine O, Stoppa-Lyonnet D. Incidence, presentation, and prognosis of malignancies in ataxia-telangiectasia: a report from the French national registry of primary immune deficiencies. J Clin Oncol. 2014;33:202–8.
13. Driessen GJ, Jspeert H, Weemaes CM, Haraldsson Á, Trip M, Warris A, van der Flier M, Wulffraat N, Verhagen MM, Taylor MA, van Zelm MC. Antibody deficiency in patients with ataxia telangiectasia is caused by disturbed B- and T-cell homeostasis and reduced immune repertoire diversity. J Allergy Clin Immunol. 2013;131:1367–75.e9.
14. Kraus M, Lev A, Simon AJ, Levran I, Nissenkorn A, Levi YB, Berkun Y, Efrati O, Amariglio N, Rechavi G, Somech R. Disturbed B and T cell homeostasis and neogenesis in patients with ataxia telangiectasia. J Clin Immunol. 2014;34:561–72.
15. Pasini AM, Gagro A, Roić G, Vrdoljak O, Lujić L, Žutelija-Fattorini M. Ataxia telangiectasia and juvenile idiopathic arthritis. Pediatrics. 2017;139:e20161279.
16. Patiroglu T, Gungor H, Unal E. Autoimmune diseases detected in children with primary immunodeficiency diseases: results from a reference centre at middle anatolia. Acta Microbiol Immunol Hung. 2012;59:343–53.
17. Boder E. Ataxia–telangiectasia: some historic, clinical and pathologic observations. Birth Defects Orig Artic Ser. 1975;11:255–70.
18. Schroeder SA, Zielen S. Infections of the respiratory system in patients with ataxia–telangiectasia. Pediatr Pulmonol. 2014;49:389–99.
19. Vilozni D, Lavie M, Sarouk I, Bar-Aluma BE, Dagan A, Ashkenazi M, Ofek M, Efrati O. FVC deterioration, airway obstruction determination, and life span in Ataxia telangiectasia. Respir Med. 2015;109:890–6.
20. Berkun Y, Vilozni D, Levi Y, Borik S, Waldman D, Somech R, Nissenkorn A, Efrati O. Reversible airway obstruction in children with ataxia telangiectasia. Pediatr Pulmonol. 2010;45:230–5.
21. McGrath-Morrow SA, Collaco JM, Detrick B, Lederman HM. Serum interleukin-6 levels and pulmonary function in ataxia-telangiectasia. J Pediatr. 2016;171:256–61.
22. Amanat M, Salehi M, Rezaei N. Neurological and psychiatric disorders in psoriasis. Rev Neurosci. 2018;29:805–13. https://doi.org/10.1515/revneuro-2017-0108.

23. Weemaes CM, Hustinx TW, Scheres JM, van Munster PJ, Bakkeren JA, Taalman RD. A new chromosomal instability disorder: the Nijmegen breakage syndrome. Acta Paediatr Scand. 1981;70:557–64.
24. Varon R, Vissinga C, Platzer M, Cerosaletti KM, Chrzanowska KH, Saar K, Beckmann G, Seemanová E, Cooper PR, Nowak NJ, Stumm M. Nibrin, a novel DNA double strand break protein, is mutated in Nijmegen breakage syndrome. Cell. 1998;93:467–76.
25. Varon R, Seemanova E, Chrzanowska K, Hnateyko O, Piekutowska-Abramczuk D, Krajewska-Walasek M. Clinical ascertainment of Nijmegen breakage syndrome (NBS) and prevalence of the major mutation, 657del5, in three slav populations. Eur J Hum Genet. 2000;8:900–2.
26. Varon R, Demuth I, Digweed M. Nijmegen breakage syndrome. In: Pagon RA, Adam MP, Ardinger HH, et al., editors. GeneReviews®. Seattle: University of Washington; 1993. (updated 2017).
27. Wolska-Kuśnierz B, Gregorek H, Chrzanowska K, Piątosa B, Pietrucha B, Heropolitańska-Pliszka E, Pac M, Klaudel-Dreszler M, Kostyuchenko L, Pasic S, Marodi L. Nijmegen breakage syndrome: clinical and immunological features, long-term outcome and treatment options–a retrospective analysis. J Clin Immunol. 2015;35:538–49.
28. Bloom D. Congenital telangiectatic erythema resembling lupus erythematosus in dwarfs; probably a syndrome entity. AMA Am J Dis Child. 1954;88:754–8.
29. Sanz MM, German J. Bloom's syndrome. In: Pagon RA, Adam MP, Ardinger HH, Wallace SE, Amemiya A, Bean LJH, Bird TD, Fong CT, Mefford HC, Smith RJH, Stephens K, Ledbetter N, Hand JL, editors. GeneReviews®. Seattle: University of Washington; 2006. (updated 2016).
30. Cunniff C, Bassetti JA, Ellis NA. Bloom's syndrome: clinical spectrum, molecular pathogenesis, and cancer predisposition. Mol Syndromol. 2017;8:4–23.
31. Postema FA, Hopman SM, Hennekam RC, Merks JH. Consequences of diagnosing a tumor predisposition syndrome in children with cancer: a literature review. Pediatr Blood Cancer. 2018;65:e26718.
32. Schoenaker MH, Henriet SS, Zonderland J, van Deuren M, Pan-Hammarström Q, Posthumus-van Sluijs SJ, Pico-Knijnenburg I, Weemaes CM, IJspeert H. Immunodeficiency in Bloom's syndrome. J Clin Immunol. 2018;38:35–44.
33. Relhan V, Sinha S, Bhatnagar T, Garg VK, Kochhar A. Bloom syndrome with extensive pulmonary involvement in a child. Indian J Dermatol. 2015;60:217.
34. Tiepolo L, Maraschio P, Gimelli G, Cuoco C, Gargani GF. Romano C multibranched chromosomes 1, 9, and 16 in a patient with combined IgA and IgE deficiency. Hum Genet. 1979;51:127–37.
35. Xu GL, Bestor TH, Bourc'his D, Hsieh CL, Tommerup N, Bugge M, Hulten M, Qu X, Russo JJ, Viegas-Pequignot E. Chromosome instability and immunodeficiency syndrome caused by mutations in a DNA methyltransferase gene. Nature. 1999;402:187–91.
36. de Greef JC, Wang J, Balog J, den Dunnen JT, Frants RR, Straasheijm KR, Aytekin C, van der Burg M, Duprez L, Ferster A, et al. Mutations in ZBTB24 are associated with immunodeficiency, centromeric instability, and facial anomalies syndrome type 2. Am J Hum Genet. 2011;88:796–804.
37. Thijssen PE, Ito Y, Grillo G, Wang J, Velasco G, Nitta H, Unoki M, Yoshihara M, Suyama M, Sun Y, Lemmers RJ. Mutations in CDCA7 and HELLS cause immunodeficiency–centromeric instability–facial anomalies syndrome. Nat Commun. 2015;6:7870.
38. Sterlin D, Velasco G, Moshous D, Touzot F, Mahlaoui N, Fischer A, Suarez F, Francastel C, Picard C. Genetic, cellular and clinical features of ICF syndrome: a French national survey. J Clin Immunol. 2016;36:149–59.
39. Weemaes CM, Van Tol MJ, Wang J, Van Ostaijen-Ten Dam MM, Van Eggermond MC, Thijssen PE, Aytekin C, Brunetti-Pierri N, Van Der Burg M, Davies EG, Ferster A. Heterogeneous clinical presentation in ICF syndrome: correlation with underlying gene defects. Eur J Hum Genet. 2013;21:1219–25.

40. von Bernuth H, Ravindran E, Du H, Fröhler S, Strehl K, Krämer N, Issa-Jahns L, Amulic B, Ninnemann O, Xiao MS, Eirich K. Combined immunodeficiency develops with age in immunodeficiency-centromeric instability-facial anomalies syndrome 2 (ICF2). Orphanet J Rare Dis. 2014;9:116.
41. Gössling KL, Schipp C, Fischer U, Babor F, Koch G, Schuster FR, Dietzel-Dahmen J, Wieczorek D, Borkhardt A, Meisel R, Kuhlen M. Hematopoietic stem cell transplantation in an infant with immunodeficiency, centromeric instability, and facial anomaly syndrome. Front Immunol. 2017;8:773.
42. Nicolaides NC, Carter KC, Shell BK, Papadopoulos N, Vogelstein B, Kinzler KW. Genomic organization of the human PMS2 gene family. Genomics. 1995;30:195–206.
43. Pal T, Permuth-Wey J, Sellers TA. A review of the clinical relevance of mismatch-repair deficiency in ovarian cancer. Cancer. 2008;113:733–42.
44. Collins SL, Hervé R, Keevil CW, Blaydes JP, Webb JS. Down-regulation of DNA mismatch repair enhances initiation and growth of neuroblastoma and brain tumour multicellular spheroids. PLoS One. 2011;6:e28123.
45. Ponti G, Castellsagué E, Ruini C, Percesepe A, Tomasi A. Mismatch repair genes founder mutations and cancer susceptibility in Lynch syndrome. Clin Genet. 2015;87:507–16.
46. Dudley B, Brand RE, Thull D, Bahary N, Nikiforova MN, Pai RK. Germline *MLH1* mutations are frequently identified in Lynch syndrome patients with colorectal and endometrial carcinoma demonstrating isolated loss of PMS2 immunohistochemical expression. Am J Surg Pathol. 2015;39:1114–20.
47. Gill S, Lindor NM, Burgart LJ, Smalley R, Leontovich O, French AJ, Goldberg RM, Sargent DJ, Jass JR, Hopper JL, Jenkins MA. Isolated loss of PMS2 expression in colorectal cancers: frequency, patient age, and familial aggregation. Clin Cancer Res. 2005;11:6466–71.
48. Alpert L, Pai RK, Srivastava A, McKinnon W, Wilcox R, Yantiss RK, Arcega R, Wang HL, Robert ME, Liu X, Pai RK. Colorectal carcinomas with isolated loss of PMS2 staining by immunohistochemistry. Arch Pathol Lab Med. 2018;142:523–8.
49. Ten Broeke SW, van Bavel TC, Jansen AM, Gómez-García E, Hes FJ, van Hest LP, Letteboer TG, Olderode-Berends MJ, Ruano D, Spruijt L, Suerink M. Molecular background of colorectal tumors from patients with Lynch syndrome associated with germline variants in PMS2. Gastroenterology. 2018; https://doi.org/10.1053/j.gastro.2018.05.020.
50. Abolhassani H, Akbari F, Mirminachi B, Bazregari S, Hedayat E, Rezaei N, Aghamohammadi A. Morbidity and mortality of Iranian patients with hyper IgM syndrome: a clinical analysis. Iran J Immunol. 2014;11:123–33.
51. Péron S, Metin A, Gardès P, Alyanakian MA, Sheridan E, Kratz CP, Fischer A, Durandy A. Human PMS2 deficiency is associated with impaired immunoglobulin class switch recombination. J Exp Med. 2008;205:2465–72.
52. Krauthammer A, Lahad A, Goldberg L, Sarouk I, Weiss B, Somech R, Soudack M, Pessach IM. Elevated IgM levels as a marker for a unique phenotype in patients with Ataxia telangiectasia. BMC Pediatr. 2018;18:185.
53. Piątosa B, van der Burg M, Siewiera K, Pac M, van Dongen JJ, Langerak AW, Chrzanowska KH, Bernatowska E. The defect in humoral immunity in patients with Nijmegen breakage syndrome is explained by defects in peripheral B lymphocyte maturation. Cytometry A. 2012;81:835–42.
54. Cooper H, Hirschhorn K. Apparent deletion of short arms of one chromosome (4 or 5) in a child with defects of midline fusion. Mamm Chrom Nwsl. 1961;4:14.
55. Wolf U, Reinwein H, Porsch R, Schröter R, Baitsch H. Defizienz an den kurzen Armen eines Chromosomes Nr. 4. Humangenetik. 1965;1:397–413.
56. Shannon NL, Maltby EL, Rigby AS, Quarrell OWJ. An epidemiological study of Wolf-Hirschhorn syndrome: life expectancy and cause of mortality. J Med Genet. 2001;38:674–9.
57. Zollino M, Lecce R, Fischetto R, Murdolo M, Faravelli F, Selicorni A, Buttè C, Memo L, Capovilla G, Neri G. Mapping the Wolf-Hirschhorn syndrome phenotype outside the cur-

rently accepted WHS critical region and defining a new critical region, WHSCR-2. Am J Hum Genet. 2003;75:590–7.
58. Battaglia A, Carey JC, South ST. Wolf-Hirschhorn syndrome: a review and update. Am J Med Genet C Semin Med Genet. 2015;169:216–23.
59. Battaglia A, Filippi T, South ST, Carey JC. Spectrum of epilepsy and electroencephalogram patterns in Wolf–Hirschhorn syndrome: experience with 87 patients. Dev Med Child Neurol. 2009;51:373–80.
60. Hanley-Lopez J, Estabrooks LL, Stiehm ER. Antibody deficiency in Wolf-Hirschhorn syndrome. J Pediatr. 1998;133:141–3.
61. Rauch A, Schellmoser S, Kraus C, Dörr HG, Trautmann U, Altherr MR, Pfeiffer RA, Reis A. First known microdeletion within the Wolf-Hirschhorn syndrome critical region refines genotype–phenotype correlation. Am J Med Genet. 2001;99:338–42.
62. Paradowska-Stolarz AM. Wolf-Hirschhorn syndrome (WHS)-literature review on the features of the syndrome. Adv Clin Exp Med. 2014;23:485–9.
63. Davis SD, Schaller J, Wdegewood RJ. Job's syndrome. Recurrent, "cold", staphylococcal abscesses. Lancet. 1966;1:1013–5.
64. Buckley RH, Wray BB, Belmaker EZ. Extreme hyperimmunoglobulinemia E and undue susceptibility to infection. Pediatrics. 1972;49:59–70.
65. Minegishi Y, Saito M, Tsuchiya S, Tsuge I, Takada H, Hara T, Kawamura N, Ariga T, Pasic S, Stojkovic O, Metin A, Karasuyama H. Dominant-negative mutations in the DNA-binding domain of STAT3 cause hyper-IgE syndrome. Nature. 2007;448:1058–62.
66. Engelhardt KR, McGhee S, Winkler S, Sassi A, Woellner C, Lopez-Herrera G, Chen A, Kim HS, Lloret MG, Schulze I, Ehl S. Large deletions and point mutations involving the dedicator of cytokinesis 8 (DOCK8) in the autosomal-recessive form of hyper-IgE syndrome. J Allergy Clin Immunol. 2009;124:1289–302.
67. Woellner C, Schäffer AA, Puck JM, Renner ED, Knebel C, Holland SM, Plebani A, Grimbacher B. The hyper IgE syndrome and mutations in TYK2. Immunity. 2007;26:535.
68. Yang L, Fliegauf M, Grimbacher B. Hyper-IgE syndromes: reviewing PGM3 deficiency. Curr Opin Pediatr. 2014;26:697–703.
69. Chandesris MO, Melki I, Natividad A, Puel A, Fieschi C, Yun L, Thumerelle C, Oksenhendler E, Boutboul D, Thomas C, Hoarau C. Autosomal dominant STAT3 deficiency and hyper-IgE syndrome molecular, cellular, and clinical features from a French national survey. Medicine (Baltimore). 2012;91:e1–19.
70. Zhang Q, Davis JC, Dove CG, Su HC. Genetic, clinical, and laboratory markers for DOCK8 immunodeficiency syndrome. Dis Markers. 2010;29:131–9.
71. Renner ED, Puck JM, Holland SM, Schmitt M, Weiss M, Frosch M, Bergmann M, Davis J, Belohradsky BH, Grimbacher B. Autosomal recessive hyperimmunoglobulin E syndrome: a distinct disease entity. J Pediatr. 2004;144:93–9.
72. Mogensen TH. STAT3 and the hyper-IgE syndrome: clinical presentation, genetic origin, pathogenesis, novel findings and remaining uncertainties. JAKSTAT. 2013;2:e23435.
73. Jiao H, Toth B, Erdos M, Fransson I, Rakoczi E, Balogh I, Magyarics Z, Derfalvi B, Csorba G, Szaflarska A, Megarbane A, Akatcherian C, Dbaibo G, Rajnavolgyi E, Hammarstrom L, Kere J, Lefranc G, Marodi L. Novel and recurrent STAT3 mutations in hyper-IgE syndrome patients from different ethnic groups. Mol Immunol. 2008;46:202–6.
74. Schimke LF, Sawalle-Belohradsky J, Roesler J, Wollenberg A, Rack A, Borte M, Rieber N, Cremer R, Maass E, Dopfer R, Reichenbach J, Wahn V, Hoenig M, Jansson AF, Roesen-Wolff A, Schaub B, Seger R, Hill HR, Ochs HD, Torgerson TR, Belohradsky BH, Renner ED. Diagnostic approach to the hyper-IgE syndromes: immunologic and clinical key findings to differentiate hyper-IgE syndromes from atopic dermatitis. J Allergy Clin Immunol. 2010;126:611–617.e1.
75. Woellner C, Gertz EM, Schaffer AA, Lagos M, Perro M, Glocker EO, Pietrogrande MC, Cossu F, Franco JL, Matamoros N, Pietrucha B, Heropolitanska-Pliszka E, Yeganeh M, Moin M, Espanol T, Ehl S, Gennery AR, Abinun M, Breborowicz A, Niehues T, Kilic SS,

Junker A, Turvey SE, Plebani A, Sanchez B, Garty BZ, Pignata C, Cancrini C, Litzman J, Sanal O, Baumann U, Bacchetta R, Hsu AP, Davis JN, Hammarstrom L, Davies EG, Eren E, Arkwright PD, Moilanen JS, Viemann D, Khan S, Marodi L, Cant AJ, Freeman AF, Puck JM, Holland SM, Grimbacher B. Mutations in STAT3 and diagnostic guidelines for hyper-IgE syndrome. J Allergy Clin Immunol. 2010;125:424–432.e8.

76. Aydin SE, Kilic SS, Aytekin C, Kumar A, Porras O, Kainulainen L, Kostyuchenko L, Genel F, Kütükcüler N, Karaca N, Gonzalez-Granado L. DOCK8 deficiency: clinical and immunological phenotype and treatment options-a review of 136 patients. J Clin Immunol. 2015;35:189–98.
77. Tsuge I, Ito K, Ohye T, Kando N, Kondo Y, Nakajima Y, Inuo C, Kurahashi H, Urisu A. Acute eosinophilic pneumonia occurring in a dedicator of cytokinesis 8 (DOCK8) deficient patient. Pediatr Pulmonol. 2014;49:E52–5.
78. Sassi A, Lazaroski S, Wu G, Haslam SM, Fliegauf M, Mellouli F, Patiroglu T, Unal E, Ozdemir MA, Jouhadi Z, Khadir K. Hypomorphic homozygous mutations in & phosphoglucomutase 3 (PGM3) impair immunity and increase serum IgE levels. J Allergy Clin Immunol. 2014;133:1410–9.
79. Zhang Y, Yu X, Ichikawa M, Lyons JJ, Datta S, Lamborn IT, Jing H, Kim ES, Biancalana M, Wolfe LA, DiMaggio T. Autosomal recessive phosphoglucomutase & 3 (PGM3) mutations link glycosylation defects to atopy, immune deficiency, autoimmunity, and neurocognitive impairment. J Allergy Clin Immunol. 2014;133:1400–9.
80. Wiskott A. Familiarer, angeborener Morbus Werlhofii? Monatsschr Kinderheilkd. 1937;68:212–6.
81. Puck JM, Candotti F. Lessons from the Wiskott-Aldrich syndrome. N Engl J Med. 2006;355:1759–61.
82. Derry JM, Ochs HD, Francke U. Isolation of a novel gene mutated in Wiskott-Aldrich syndrome. Cell. 1994;78:635–44.
83. Kirchhausen T, Rosen FS. Disease mechanism: unravelling Wiskott–Aldrich syndrome. Curr Biol. 1996;6:676–8.
84. Sullivan KE, Mullen CA, Blaese RM, Winkelstein JA. A multiinstitutional survey of the Wiskott-Aldrich syndrome. J Pediatr. 1994;125:876–85.
85. Villa A, Notarangelo L, Macchi P, Mantuano E, Cavagni G, Brugnoni D, Strina D, Patrosso MC, Ramenghi U, Sacco MG, Ugazio A. X–linked thrombocytopenia and Wiskott–Aldrich syndrome are allelic diseases with mutations in the WASP gene. Nat Genet. 1995;9:414–7.
86. Zhu Q, Zhang M, Blaese RM, Derry JM, Junker A, Francke U, Chen SH, Ochs HD. The Wiskott-Aldrich syndrome and X-linked congenital thrombocytopenia are caused by mutations of the same gene. Blood. 1995;86:3797–804.
87. Ancliff PJ, Blundell MP, Cory GO, Calle Y, Worth A, Kempski H, Burns S, Jones GE, Sinclair J, Kinnon C, Hann IM. Two novel activating mutations in the Wiskott-Aldrich syndrome protein result in congenital neutropenia. Blood. 2006;108:2182–9.
88. Beel K, Cotter MM, Blatny J, Bond J, Lucas G, Green F, Vanduppen V, Leung DW, Rooney S, Smith OP, Rosen MK. A large kindred with X-linked neutropenia with an I294T mutation of the Wiskott-Aldrich syndrome gene. Br J Haematol. 2009;144:120–6.
89. Devriendt K, Kim AS, Mathijs G, Frints SG, Schwartz M, Van den Oord JJ, Verhoef GE, Boogaerts MA, Fryns JP, You D, Rosen MK. Constitutively activating mutation in WASP causes X-linked severe congenital neutropenia. Nat Genet. 2001;27:313–7.
90. Ochs HD, Slichter SJ, Harker LA, Von Behrens WE, Clark RA, Wedgwood RJ. The Wiskott-Aldrich syndrome: studies of lymphocytes, granulocytes, and. Blood. 1980;55:243–52.
91. Park JY, Kob M, Prodeus AP, Rosen FS, Shcherbina A, Remold-O'Donnell E. Early deficit of lymphocytes in Wiskott–Aldrich syndrome: possible role of WASP in human lymphocyte maturation. Clin Exp Immunol. 2004;136:104–10.
92. Westerberg L, Larsson M, Hardy SJ, Fernández C, Thrasher AJ, Severinson E. Wiskott-Aldrich syndrome protein deficiency leads to reduced B-cell adhesion, migration, and homing, and a delayed humoral immune response. Blood. 2005;105:1144–52.

93. Recher M, Burns SO, Miguel A, Volpi S, Dahlberg C, Walter JE, Moffitt K, Mathew D, Honke N, Lang PA, Patrizi L. B cell–intrinsic deficiency of the Wiskott-Aldrich syndrome protein causes severe abnormalities of the peripheral B-cell compartment in mice. Blood. 2012;119:2819–28.
94. Westerberg LS, Dahlberg C, Baptista M, Moran CJ, Detre C, Keszei M, Eston MA, Alt FW, Terhorst C, Notarangelo LD, Snapper SB. Wiskott-Aldrich syndrome protein (WASP) and N-WASP are critical for peripheral B cell development and function. Blood. 2012;119:3966–74.
95. Dupuis-Girod S, Medioni J, Haddad E, Quartier P, Cavazzana-Calvo M, Le Deist F, de Saint BG, Delaunay J, Schwarz K, Casanova JL, Blanche S. Autoimmunity in Wiskott-Aldrich syndrome: risk factors, clinical features, and outcome in a single-center cohort of 55 patients. Pediatrics. 2003;111:e622–7.
96. Blaese RM, Strober W, Brown R, Waldmann T. The Wiskott-Aldrich syndrome a disorder with a possible defect in antigen processing or recognition. Lancet. 1968;291:1056–61.
97. Cooper MD, Chase HP, Lowman JT, Krivit W, Good RA. Wiskott-Aldrich syndrome: an immunologic deficiency disease involving the afferent limb of immunity. Am J Med. 1968;44:499–513.
98. Westerberg LS, Miguel A, Wermeling F, Ochs HD, Karlsson MC, Snapper SB, Notarangelo LD. WASP confers selective advantage for specific hematopoietic cell populations and serves a unique role in marginal zone B-cell homeostasis and function. Blood. 2008;112:4139–47.
99. Jeanes AC, Owens CM. Chest imaging in the immunocompromised child. Paediatr Respir Rev. 2002;3:59–69.
100. Chavanas S, Bodemer C, Rochat A, Hamel-Teillac D, Ali M, Irvine AD, Bonafé JL, Wilkinson J, Taïeb A, Barrandon Y, Harper JI. Mutations in SPINK5, encoding a serine protease inhibitor, cause Netherton syndrome. Nat Genet. 2000;25:141–2.
101. Hachem JP, Wagberg F, Schmuth M, Crumrine D, Lissens W, Jayakumar A, Houben E, Mauro TM, Leonardsson G, Brattsand M, Egelrud T. Serine protease activity and residual LEKTI expression determine phenotype in Netherton syndrome. J Invest Dermatol. 2006;126:1609–21.
102. Renner ED, Hartl D, Rylaarsdam S, Young ML, Monaco-Shawver L, Kleiner G, Markert ML, Stiehm ER, Belohradsky BH, Upton MP, Torgerson TR. Comel-Netherton syndrome defined as primary immunodeficiency. J Allergy Clin Immunol. 2009;124:536–43.
103. Ming JE, Stiehm ER, Graham JM Jr. Syndromes associated with immunodeficiency. Adv Pediatr Infect Dis. 1999;46:271–351.
104. Kutsal E, Gücüyener K, Bakirtaş A, Eldeş N, Oztaş M, Dursun A. Youngest netherton patient with infantile asthma. Tuberk Toraks. 2008;56:104–8.
105. Okulu E, Tunc G, Erdeve O, Mumcu Y, Atasay B, Ince E, Arsan S. Netherton syndrome: a neonatal case with respiratory insufficiency. Arch Argent Pediatr. 2018;116:e609–11.
106. Macknet CA, Morkos A, Job L, Garberoglio MC, Clark RD, Macknet KD Jr, Peverini RL. An infant with Netherton syndrome and persistent pulmonary hypertension requiring extracorporeal membrane oxygenation. Pediatr Dermatol. 2008;25:368–72.
107. Engman MF. A unique case of reticular pigmentation of the skin with atrophy. Arch Bleg Dermatol Syphiligr. 1926;13:685–7.
108. Heiss NS, Knight SW, Vulliamy TJ, Klauck SM, Wiemann S, Mason PJ, Poustka A, Dokal I. X-linked dyskeratosis congenita is caused by mutations in a highly conserved gene with putative nucleolar functions. Nat Genet. 1998;19:32–8.
109. Walne AJ, Vulliamy T, Marrone A, Beswick R, Kirwan M, Masunari Y, Al-Qurashi FH, Aljurf M, Dokal I. Genetic heterogeneity in autosomal recessive dyskeratosis congenita with one subtype due to mutations in the telomerase-associated protein NOP10. Hum Mol Genet. 2007;16:1619–29.
110. Vulliamy T, Marrone A, Goldman F, Dearlove A, Bessler M, Mason PJ, Dokal I. The RNA component of telomerase is mutated in autosomal dominant dyskeratosis congenita. Nature. 2001;413:432–5.

111. Connor JM, Teague RH. Dyskeratosis congenita. Report of a large kindred. Br J Dermatol. 1981;105:321–5.
112. Drachtman RA, Alter BP. Dyskeratosis congenita: clinical and genetic heterogeneity. Report of a new case and review of the literature. Am J Pediatr Hematol Oncol. 1992;14:297–304.
113. Dokal I. Dyskeratosis congenita in all its forms. Br J Hematol. 2000;110:768–79.
114. Alter BP, Giri N, Savage SA, Rosenberg PS. Cancer in dyskeratosis congenita. Blood. 2009;113:6549–57.
115. Jyonouchi S, Forbes L, Ruchelli E, Sullivan KE. Dyskeratosis congenita: a combined immunodeficiency with broad clinical spectrum–a single-center pediatric experience. Pediatr Allergy Immunol. 2011;22:313–9.
116. Borggraefe I, Koletzko S, Arenz T, Fuehrer M, Hoffmann F, Dokal I, Vulliamy T, Weiler V, Griese M, Belohradsky BH, Lang T. Severe variant of x-linked dyskeratosis congenita (hoyeraal-hreidarsson syndrome) causes significant enterocolitis in early infancy. J Pediatr Gastroenterol Nutr. 2009;49:359–63.
117. Ballew BJ, Savage SA. Updates on the biology and management of dyskeratosis congenita and related telomere biology disorders. Expert Rev Hematol. 2013;6:327–37.
118. Gordijn SJ, Brand PL. A boy with breathlessness, digital clubbing and central cyanosis. Eur J Pediatr. 2004;163:129–30.
119. Samuel BP, Duffner UA, Abdel-Mageed AS, Vettukattil JJ. Pulmonary arteriovenous malformations in dyskeratosis congenita. Pediatr Dermatol. 2015;32:e165–6.
120. Khincha PP, Bertuch AA, Agarwal S, Townsley DM, Young NS, Keel S, Shimamura A, Boulad F, Simoneau T, Justino H, Kuo C. Pulmonary arteriovenous malformations: an uncharacterised phenotype of dyskeratosis congenita and related telomere biology disorders. Eur Respir J. 2017;49:1601640.
121. Yabe M, Yabe H, Hattori K, Morimoto T, Hinohara T, Takakura I, Shimizu T, Shimamura K, Tang X, Kato S. Fatal interstitial pulmonary disease in a patient with dyskeratosis congenita after allogeneic bone marrow transplantation. Bone Marrow Transplant. 1997;19:389–92.
122. Sorge C, Pereboeva L, Westin E, Harris WT, Kelly DR, Goldman F. Pulmonary complications post hematopoietic stem cell transplant in dyskeratosis congenita: analysis of oxidative stress in lung fibroblasts. Bone Marrow Transplant. 2017;52:765–8.
123. Giri N, Ravichandran S, Fontana J, Alter BP, Khincha P, Savage SA. Prognostic significance of pulmonary function test abnormalities in patients with dyskeratosis congenita. Blood. 2016;128:2672.

Chapter 10
Treatment of Pulmonary Manifestations of Primary Immunodeficiency Diseases

Nahal Mansouri and Davood Mansouri

10.1 Treatment of Infectious Pulmonary Manifestations of PIDs

Respiratory infections are the most frequent presentation of PIDs. Depending on the underlying immuno deficiency, these infections include a wide array of typical, atypical, and opportunistic infections. The choice and duration of antibiotics vary based on the clinical presentation, severity of symptoms, resistance patterns in the community, and prior culture data.

Here are some examples of preventive measures and antimicrobial considerations in different immunodeficiency states:

(i) In humoral immuno deficiencies, the initial empiric antibiotic choice should cover the most common encapsulated microorganisms while taking the resistance pattern into account.

In the outpatient setting, we recommend an initial antibiotic regimen with good coverage for *Streptococcus pneumoniae*, *Haemophilus influenzae*, *Klebsiella pneumoniae*, and *Moraxella catarrhalis*. Ceftriaxone or fluoroquinolones (such as levofloxacin) are an appropriate initial therapy, while the latter is not recommended in the pediatric age group due to side effects. In critically ill patients, initiation of vancomycin or linezolid plus an antibiotic such as third-generation cephalosporin with anti-Pseudomonas coverage is recommended. If an atypical infection like *Mycoplasma pneumoniae* is suspected, the addition of a macrolide or respiratory fluoroquinolone should be

N. Mansouri
Department of Medicine, Division of Pulmonary and Critical Care Medicine, Brigham and Women's Hospital, Harvard Medical School, Boston, USA

D. Mansouri (✉)
Department of Infectious Disease and Clinical Immunology, Massih Daneshvari Hospital, Shahid Beheshti University of Medical Sciences, Tehran, Iran

S. A. Mahdaviani, N. Rezaei (eds.), *Pulmonary Manifestations of Primary Immunodeficiency Diseases*, https://doi.org/10.1007/978-3-030-00880-2_10

considered as well. Immunoglobulin therapy reduces the frequency and duration of pulmonary infections and should be considered in all patients with humoral immuno deficiencies and patients with history of serious infections as soon as possible. A higher dose of immunoglobulin is indicated in individuals with bronchiectasis and gastrointestinal symptoms [1].

(ii) In cellular and combined immuno deficiencies, in addition to typical organisms, one should have a low threshold to consider coverage for opportunistic infections such as fungal pneumonias and *Pneumocystis* pneumonia (PCP). Besides, mycobacterial and viral infections such as Epstein-Barr virus (EBV) and cytomegalovirus (CMV) are commonly seen. Treatment and prophylaxis should be specific to the underlying diagnosis and history of previous infections. As soon as an innate or cellular immunodeficiency is identified, trimethoprim-sulfamethoxazole for PCP prophylaxis should be initiated. The routine use of antifungal prophylaxis in cellular immuno deficiencies with high risk of fungal infections such as severe combined immunodeficiency or congenital neutropenia has not yet been studied. In patients with STAT3 deficiency, antifungal prophylaxis is recommended in the presence of pulmonary lesions [2].

(iii) Lung abscesses and necrotizing pneumonias are commonly seen in phagocytic immuno deficiencies. In the presence of a cavitating lung lesion, catalase-positive organisms such as *Burkholderia cepacia*, *Pseudomonas aeruginosa*, *Staphylococcus aureus*, atypical mycobacteria, and molds particularly *Aspergillus* species should be considered, and antibiotic coverage must be tailored accordingly. In terms of prophylaxis, all patients with chronic granulomatous disease should receive trimethoprim-sulfamethoxazole for prophylaxis against a broad spectrum of anticipated infections; in addition, antifungal prophylaxis with itraconazole or posaconazole and immunization against *H. influenzae*, pneumococci, and influenza virus are also recommended. In addition to antimicrobial prophylaxis, chronic subcutaneous IFN-γ therapy has been shown to be well-tolerated, reduce the frequency of severe infections, and prolong infection-free survival in patients with chronic granulomatous disease (CGD) [3–6].

(iv) In complement deficiencies, the coverage of encapsulated bacteria such as *Neisseria* species or *S. pneumoniae* is imperative. Vaccination against encapsulated bacteria in addition to influenza virus is recommended in patients with complement deficiencies and asplenia [7].

(v) The presence of Mendelian susceptibility to mycobacterial diseases (MSMDs) puts patients at a high risk for mycobacterial infections, such as non-tuberculosis or environmental mycobacteria and bacillus Calmette-Guérin (BCG), as well as *Salmonella* species and viruses such as human papillomavirus, molluscum contagiosum, EBV, CMV, and invasive fungal infections including histoplasmosis, aspergillosis, and *Exophiala* species [8, 9]. In these cases, treatment should be based on the results of culture and resistance pattern [10].

Given the high prevalence of viruses such as herpes simplex virus and cytomegalovirus in combined T- and B-cell deficiencies, early clinical suspicion leads to prompt antiviral therapy.

One should note that in the presence of structural abnormalities, such as bronchiectasis or tumors, the duration and choice of treatment would be different; as in these cases, multidrug-resistant organisms are common; therefore, longer and combination antibiotic therapy with high potency and synergistic effect may be needed.

Considering the severity of infections in these individuals, it is appropriate to initiate an empiric coverage based on the PID and narrow the antimicrobial regimen once an organism is identified.

Prolonged antibiotic prophylaxis should be considered in patients with recurrent pneumonias.

10.2 Treatment of Noninfectious Respiratory Complications of Primary Immunodeficiencies

10.2.1 Obstructive Lung Diseases

10.2.1.1 Bronchiectasis

Bronchiectasis due to recurrent pyogenic lower respiratory tract infections can develop in any PID patient [11]. Early forms of bronchiectasis may be reversible; however, more advanced forms such as varicose or saccular bronchiectasis may lead to permanent lung impairment. Management of PID-associated bronchiectasis is similar to non-cystic fibrosis bronchiectasis. Once the underlying PID is identified, the focus should be on the prevention of recurrent infections, maintenance and improvement of pulmonary function, minimizing exacerbations, and finally improving the patient's quality of life by reducing daily symptoms [12, 13].

Common variable immunodeficiency (CVID) is an uncommon cause of bronchiectasis; however, the prevalence of bronchiectasis is high in patients with CVID [14–16].

Early diagnosis and prompt immunoglobulin therapy remain the mainstay for prevention of infections, and therefore, bronchiectasis in CVID, hyper-IgM syndromes, and X-linked agammaglobulinemia [1, 17]. A trial of intravenous immunoglobulin (IVIG) therapy can also be used in other forms of humoral immunodeficiencies notably IgG subclass deficiency if antibiotic prophylaxis fails [18].

The initial antibiotic therapy during an acute exacerbation of bronchiectasis should be based on prior sputum cultures and sensitivities.

In the absence of prior culture result, an antipseudomonal antibiotic such as beta-lactams or fluoroquinolones, is appropriate as the first-line empiric choice. The musculoskeletal adverse effects, especially in the pediatric age group, should be taken into account. *Pseudomonas* infection is associated with worsening of lung function and poor outcomes in patients with cystic fibrosis (CF), and the same may be true in non-CF bronchiectasis. Therefore, in hospitalized patients, intravenous antibiotic therapy with antipseudomonal coverage is recommended. Dual anti-Pseudomonas coverage may be indicated for critically ill patients and those with prior evidence of resistant *P. aeruginosa* infection [19, 20].

Inhaled antibiotics such as tobramycin, colistin, and aztreonam have been beneficial in patients with CF bronchiectasis and may also have a role in non-CF bronchiectasis as well. The British Thoracic Society guidelines recommend prolonged inhaled antibiotics if there is evidence of three or more exacerbations per year and/or *P. aeruginosa* colonization [21–23].

Mechanical airway clearance devices such as acapella and high-frequency airway chest wall oscillation can help with symptomatic relief [12, 24, 25]. The goal of such therapies is to mobilize respiratory secretions and interrupt the vicious cycle of inflammation and infection. Despite the absence of mortality reduction with the use of airway clearance devices, their consistent use is associated with improvement in hyperinflation, sputum production, and overall quality of life. Inhaled hypertonic saline plus chest physical therapy can lead to improved sputum bacteriologic clearance and may have some immune-modulating effects as well [26, 27]. On the other hand, the use of aerosolized DNase (dornase alfa) has shown deleterious effect in non-CF bronchiectasis in contrast to CF and has not been recommended in PID-associated bronchiectasis [28].

In patients with recurrent exacerbations of bronchiectasis, chronic macrolide therapy has been associated with decreased flares of bronchiectasis and improved quality of life. In the absence of contraindications, such as prolong QT, the initiation of a macrolide in any patient with three or more exacerbations per year is recommended [29].

Based on a study in 2005, inhaled corticosteroids (ICS) can reduce sputum volume and lead to decreased inflammatory markers in the sputum; however, their use has not been associated with improvement in lung function or reduction of exacerbations [30]. Further investigations are still required to assess the role of ICS in non-CF bronchiectasis.

A meta-analysis of 6 placebo-controlled trials with a total of 278 subjects did not find a significant difference in pulmonary function test results, exacerbation rates, or sputum volume between patients using inhaled glucocorticoids and those on placebo [31].

Surgery may be beneficial in advanced localized disease, but is not helpful in primary immunodeficient patients who mostly present with diffuse pulmonary involvement. Finally, it is recommended to refer all patients with symptomatic airway disease to pulmonary rehabilitation and regular chest physical therapy.

10.2.1.2 Bronchiolitis Obliterans Syndrome (BOS)

Bronchiolitis obliterans has been reported in association with severe combined immunodeficiency syndrome (SCIDS), CVID, and ataxia telangiectasia (A-T). Treatment of BOS remains poorly defined. Given the fibrotic nature of BOS, there is no approved effect for immunosuppressive therapies such as glucocorticoids.

Although cytotoxic immunosuppressive therapy (such as azathioprine, methotrexate, and cyclophosphamide) has been used in BOS associated with connective tissue diseases, they have not been investigated in PID-associated BOS. Macrolides have indicated immunomodulatory effects and may slow the progression of BOS following hematopoietic stem cell transplantation (HSCT) [32]. Despite the lack of evidence for the use of macrolides in PID-associated BOS, due to their beneficial effects in inflammatory airway diseases, a trial of chronic macrolide therapy (e.g., azithromycin 250 mg three times a week or erythromycin 200 to 600 mg/day) may be considered as well [33].

10.2.1.3 Other Uncommon Airway Involvements

Lymphocytic bronchiolitis and granulomatous involvement of the airways are reported both in CVID and CGD. Besides, steroid therapy may be indicated in patients with significant respiratory symptoms [34].

10.2.2 Interstitial Lung Disease (ILD)

ILD is one of the most common respiratory presentations of PIDs, especially humoral immunodeficiencies.

Cryptogenic organizing pneumonia (COP) followed by lymphocytic interstitial pneumonia (LIP) and granulomatous-lymphocytic ILD (GLILD) are the most common interstitial lung diseases in primary humoral immunodeficiencies; however, other forms of ILD such as nonspecific interstitial pneumonitis (NSIP) and usual interstitial pneumonitis (UIP) have been also reported [35, 36].

Importantly, decision on when and how to treat these complications should be based on multidisciplinary discussions, patient's symptoms, pulmonary function tests (PFTs), and comorbidities.

Current studies on the treatment of PID-associated ILD are limited to case reports and retrospective studies. Due to steroid responsiveness, organizing pneumonia (OP) has the best prognosis among ILDs. Treatment includes a course of high-dose steroids followed by slow tapering. Prior reports have found similar steroid responsiveness in PID-associated OP and COP as well [37].

Although investigated in a number of studies, there is still controversy regarding the use of cytotoxic and immunosuppressive therapies in granulomatous ILD or LIP [35, 38], and clinical trials investigating efficacy of GLILD treatments are required. A small retrospective study by Chase and colleagues showed improvement in PFTs and radiographic abnormalities in patients with CVID and GLILD treated with a combination of rituximab and azathioprine [39].

In a retrospective study of 59 patients with GLILD by Boursiquot et al., complete remission was achieved with the use of either prednisone, methotrexate, or cyclophosphamide in few number of patients [40]. On the other hand, few case reports support the use of anti-TNF-α agents, such as infliximab, in granulomatous CVID; however further clinical studies are needed before considering this agent as the standard of care [40–42]. Furthermore, IVIG was not effective in PID-associated ILD [43].

Similar to non-PID-related ILDs, there are limited therapeutic options for NSIP and UIP associated with immunodeficiencies as well. Multiple studies have now identified poor outcomes with the use of immunosuppressive therapy in idiopathic pulmonary fibrosis (IPF); therefore, steroids or cytotoxic therapy such as azathioprine is not recommended in UIP associated with PID. To date, no study has investigated the beneficial effect of anti-fibrotic medications such as pirfenidone or nintedanib in PID-related IPF. Although immunosuppressive therapies (such as steroids or steroid-sparing immunomodulatory drugs) have been commonly used in NSIP, nevertheless, further studies looking into the effect of these therapies in PID-related NSIP are still required.

Diffuse parenchymal lung disease and progressive pulmonary alveolar proteinosis have been described in GATA2 deficiency (MonoMAC syndrome). As expected, the treatment of pulmonary presentations in this syndrome should target the underlying immunodeficiency [44].

10.2.3 Granulomatous Lung Disease

Sterile granulomatous involvement of the lungs can be observed in CGD and as mentioned before in association with CVID.

Prior case reports have shown successful results with the use of systemic corticosteroids in inflammatory complications of CGD such as granulomatous lung disease and fulminant mulch pneumonitis (hypersensitivity-like reaction to *Aspergillus*) [45–48]. Given the high risk of infection in these patients, immunosuppressive therapy should only be considered once adequate antibacterial and antifungal therapy is initiated.

10.2.4 Structural Lung Disease

In addition to bronchiectasis, other structural changes such as cystic lung disease and bullae can be observed in individuals with PID due to recurrent infections. For instance, in STAT3 deficiency scar formation after primary necrotizing infection (e.g., *Staphylococcus pneumonia*) or de novo mutation can lead to the formation of giant pneumatoceles that can be secondarily infected with fungi such as *Aspergillus* or *Scedosporium* species. In addition to a prolonged infectious process, fungus balls can erode into the pulmonary vasculature and cause life-threatening hemoptysis or fungemia [49]. Importantly, prophylactic antimicrobial therapy with anti-staphylococcal and antifungal coverage can delay structural damage.

The management of giant bullae depends on the clinical course and development of complications. Supportive therapy with airway clearance devices, bronchodilators, and pulmonary rehabilitation is the mainstay of therapy in symptomatic patients with cystic lung disease. Bullectomy has been shown to improve symptoms in patients with giant bullae and refractory dyspnea due to emphysema; however to our knowledge, surgical approach in bullous lung disease in immunodeficiency has not been studied yet.

10.2.5 Malignancy

Treatments of malignancies in PIDs are similar to that of immunocompetent patients, but the prognosis of malignancy in PID patients is overall worse than non-immunodeficient patients. Resistance to chemotherapy is similar between immunocompetent and immunodeficient hosts. However, there is increased prevalence of chemotherapy-induced toxicity and end-organ damage in patients with PID [50].

Shorter course of chemotherapy is preferred given the high risk of systemic toxicity and infections in these individuals. Meanwhile, chemotherapy should be combined with prophylaxis against *Pneumocystis jirovecii* pneumonia (PJP) and other opportunistic infections [51].

In the case of absolute need for radiotherapy, the lowest possible dose should be considered. Increased radiosensitivity due to impaired DNA repair has been found in patients with A-T and Nijmegen breakage syndrome (NBS) [52, 53]. In addition, lymphocytes from CVID patients are more sensitive to radiation in vitro [41, 42].

Infection control remains crucial, and immunoglobulin therapy in humoral immunodeficiencies can decrease the rate of bacterial infections during chemotherapy.

In lymphoproliferative diseases (LPD), myeloablative stem cell transplantation (SCT) may increase survival. However, there are significantly higher rates of morbidity and mortality associated with transplantation in immunocompromised individuals. Cohn et al. reported 4 years of cancer-free survival in eight patients with PID- and EBV-associated LPD after the receipt of reduced intensity conditioning SCT plus pre- and posttransplant EBV treatment (including rituximab and EBV-specific cytotoxic T-lymphocyte therapy) [54].

There is paucity of data in using prophylactic antiviral therapy such as acyclovir for reduction of lymphoproliferative transformation.

In addition to LPD cure after HST, stem cell transplantation can be curative in PIDs associated with high risk of malignancy, such as severe combined immunodeficiency (SCID), Wiskott-Aldrich syndrome (WAS), X-linked hyper-IgM syndrome, and dedicator of cytokinesis 8 (DOCK8) deficiency. Unfortunately, these patients may still be at risk of developing cancer after transplantation [55].

10.3 Other Therapies

Lung transplantation has been performed in few patients with immunodeficiency and end-stage lung disease. Given the high mortality of lung transplant in already immunosuppressed individuals, this should only be considered as a source of last resort [56, 57]. One should postulate that this is logical only if the underlying immunodeficiency has been totally corrected prior or concurrent to the lung transplantation by HSCT as the high risks of lung disease recurrence in the donor lung.

Unfortunately, the diagnosis of most PID patients, particularly in adults, is delayed to the point that extensive structural lung damage has been ensued; thus lung transplantation remains the only option for the reversal of respiratory complications.

Therefore, the management of these patients requires a multidisciplinary approach consisting of a team of immunologists, infectious disease specialists, intensivists, and pulmonologists due to high rate of complications, mortality, and unpredictable outcomes which occur as a result of multifactorial underlying problems.

10.4 Prospect

HSCT and gene editing are considered as the ultimate cure for a considerable number of immunodeficiency syndromes; however, HSCT continues to carry a high mortality and morbidity risk, and therefore, newer treatment strategies are in urgent need.

Gene editing has shown promising results in the treatment of adenosine deaminase (ADA) deficiency and X-linked SCID [58].

Despite being at the early stages of stem cell manipulation and targeted gene editing, ongoing advances in these technologies may lead to the discovery of new curative therapies for PIDs in the near future with resultant considerable decline in the rate of pulmonary complications.

References

1. Lucas M, Lee M, Lortan J, Lopez-Granados E, Misbah S, Chapel H. Infection outcomes in patients with common variable immunodeficiency disorders: relationship to immunoglobulin therapy over 22 years. J Allergy Clin Immunol. 2010;125(6):1354–60. e4
2. Aguilar C, Malphettes M, Donadieu J, Chandesris O, Coignard-Biehler H, Catherinot E, et al. Prevention of infections during primary immunodeficiency. Clin Infect Dis. 2014;59(10):1462–70.
3. Gallin JI, Alling DW, Malech HL, Wesley R, Koziol D, Marciano B, et al. Itraconazole to prevent fungal infections in chronic granulomatous disease. N Engl J Med. 2003;348(24):2416–22.

4. Marciano BE, Wesley R, De Carlo ES, Anderson VL, Barnhart LA, Darnell D, et al. Long-term interferon-γ therapy for patients with chronic granulomatous disease. Clin Infect Dis. 2004;39(5):692–9.
5. Margolis DM, Melnick DA, Ailing DW, Gallin JI. Trimethoprim-sulfamethoxazole prophylaxis in the management of chronic granulomatous disease. J Infect Dis. 1990;162(3):723–6.
6. Mouy R, Fischer A, Vilmer E, Seger R, Griscelli C. Incidence, severity, and prevention of infections in chronic granulomatous disease. J Pediatr. 1989;114(4):555–60.
7. Langley JM, Dodds L, Fell D, Langley GR. Pneumococcal and influenza immunization in asplenic persons: a retrospective population-based cohort study 1990-2002. BMC Infect Dis. 2010;10(1):219.
8. Lanternier F, Barbati E, Meinzer U, Liu L, Pedergnana V, Migaud M, et al. Inherited CARD9 deficiency in 2 unrelated patients with invasive Exophiala infection. J Infect Dis. 2015;211(8):1241–50.
9. Mansouri D, Adimi P, Mirsaedi M, Mansouri N, Tabarsi P, Amiri M, et al. Primary immune deficiencies presenting in adults: seven years of experience from Iran. J Clin Immunol. 2005;25(4):385–91.
10. Mansouri D, Adimi P, Mirsaeidi M, Mansouri N, Khalilzadeh S, Masjedi MR, et al. Inherited disorders of the IL-12-IFN-γ axis in patients with disseminated BCG infection. Eur J Pediatr. 2005;164(12):753–7.
11. Obregon RG, Lynch DA, Kaske T, Newell JD, Kirkpatrick CH. Radiologic findings of adult primary immunodeficiency disorders: contribution of CT. Chest. 1994;106(2):490–5.
12. McShane PJ, Naureckas ET, Tino G, Strek ME. Non–cystic fibrosis bronchiectasis. Am J Respir Crit Care Med. 2013;188(6):647–56.
13. Pasteur MC, Bilton D, Hill AT. British Thoracic Society guideline for non-CF bronchiectasis. Thorax. 2010;65(Suppl 1):i1–i58.
14. Di Renzo M, Pasqui A, Auteri A. Common variable immunodeficiency: a review. Clin Exp Med. 2004;3(4):211–7.
15. Driessen GJ, Dalm VA, van Hagen PM, Grashoff HA, Hartwig NG, van Rossum AM, et al. Common variable immunodeficiency and idiopathic primary hypogammaglobulinemia: two different conditions within the same disease spectrum. Haematologica. 2013;98(10):1617–23.
16. Panigrahi MK. Common variable immunodeficiency disorder-An uncommon cause for bronchiectasis. Lung India. 2014;31(4):394.
17. Rose ME, Lang DM. Evaluating and managing hypogammaglobulinemia. Cleve Clin J Med. 2006;73(2):133. -7, 40, 43-4
18. Orange JS, Hossny EM, Weiler CR, Ballow M, Berger M, Bonilla FA, et al. Use of intravenous immunoglobulin in human disease: a review of evidence by members of the Primary Immunodeficiency Committee of the American Academy of Allergy. J Allergy Clin Immunol. 2006;117(4):S525–S53.
19. Neves PC, Guerra M, Ponce P, Miranda J, Vouga L. Non-cystic fibrosis bronchiectasis. Interact Cardiovasc Thorac Surg. 2011;13(6):619–25.
20. Rogers GB, van der Gast CJ, Cuthbertson L, Thomson SK, Bruce KD, Martin ML, et al. Clinical measures of disease in adult non-CF bronchiectasis correlate with airway microbiota composition. Thorax. 2013;68(8):731–7.
21. Brodt AM, Stovold E, Zhang L. Inhaled antibiotics for stable non-cystic fibrosis bronchiectasis: a systematic review. Eur Respir J. 2014;44(2):382–93.
22. Pasteur MC, Bilton D, Hill AT. British Thoracic Society guideline for non-CF bronchiectasis. Thorax. 2010;65(7):577.
23. Tay GT, Reid DW, Bell SC. Inhaled antibiotics in cystic fibrosis (CF) and non-CF bronchiectasis. Semin Respir Crit Care Med. 2015;36:267–86. Thieme Medical Publishers
24. Eaton T, Young P, Zeng I, Kolbe J. A randomized evaluation of the acute efficacy, acceptability and tolerability of flutter and active cycle of breathing with and without postural drainage in non-cystic fibrosis bronchiectasis. Chron Respir Dis. 2007;4(1):23–30.

25. Main E, Grillo L, Rand S. Airway clearance strategies in cystic fibrosis and non-cystic fibrosis bronchiectasis. Semin Respir Crit Care Med. 2015;36:251–66. Thieme Medical Publishers
26. Reeves EP, Molloy K, Pohl K, McElvaney NG. Hypertonic saline in treatment of pulmonary disease in cystic fibrosis. Sci World J. 2012;2012:465230.
27. Reeves EP, Williamson M, O'neill SJ, Greally P, McElvaney NG. Nebulized hypertonic saline decreases IL-8 in sputum of patients with cystic fibrosis. Am J Respir Crit Care Med. 2011;183(11):1517–23.
28. O'donnell AE, Barker AF, Ilowite JS, Fick RB. Treatment of idiopathic bronchiectasis with aerosolized recombinant human DNase I. Chest. 1998;113(5):1329–34.
29. Haworth CS, Bilton D, Elborn JS. Long-term macrolide maintenance therapy in non-CF bronchiectasis: evidence and questions. Respir Med. 2014;108(10):1397–408.
30. Tsang K, Tan K, Ho P, Ooi G, Ho J, Mak J, et al. Inhaled fluticasone in bronchiectasis: a 12 month study. Thorax. 2005;60(3):239–43.
31. Kapur N, Bell S, Kolbe J, Chang AB. Inhaled steroids for bronchiectasis. Cochrane Libr. 2009;1:CD000996.
32. Maimon N, Lipton J, Chan C, Marras T. Macrolides in the treatment of bronchiolitis obliterans in allograft recipients. Bone Marrow Transplant. 2009;44(2):69.
33. Feldman C. The use of antiinflammatory therapy and macrolides in bronchiectasis. Clin Chest Med. 2012;33(2):371–80.
34. Tabarsi P, Mirsaeidi M, Karimi S, Banieghbal B, Mansouri N, Masjedi MR, et al. Lymphocytic bronchiolitis as presenting disorder in an undiagnosed adult patient with chronic granulomatous disease. Send to Iran J Allergy Asthma Immunol. 2007;6(4):219–21.
35. Cha S-I, Fessler MB, Cool CD, Schwarz MI, Brown KK. Lymphoid interstitial pneumonia: clinical features, associations and prognosis. Eur Respir J. 2006;28(2):364–9.
36. Prasse A, Kayser G, Warnatz K. Common variable immunodeficiency-associated granulomatous and interstitial lung disease. Curr Opin Pulm Med. 2013;19(5):503–9.
37. Tanaka N, Kim JS, Bates CA, Brown KK, Cool CD, Newell JD, et al. Lung diseases in patients with common variable immunodeficiency: chest radiographic, and computed tomographic findings. J Comput Assist Tomogr. 2006;30(5):828–38.
38. Nicholson AG. Lymphocytic interstitial pneumonia and other lymphoproliferative disorders in the lung. Semin Respir Crit Care Med. 2001;22:409–22. Copyright© 2001 by Thieme Medical Publishers, Inc., 333 Seventh Avenue, New York, NY 10001, USA. Tel.:+ 1 (212) 584-4662.
39. Chase NM, Verbsky JW, Hintermeyer MK, Waukau JK, Tomita-Mitchell A, Casper JT, et al. Use of combination chemotherapy for treatment of granulomatous and lymphocytic interstitial lung disease (GLILD) in patients with common variable immunodeficiency (CVID). J Clin Immunol. 2013;33(1):30–9.
40. Boursiquot J-N, Gérard L, Malphettes M, Fieschi C, Galicier L, Boutboul D, et al. Granulomatous disease in CVID: retrospective analysis of clinical characteristics and treatment efficacy in a cohort of 59 patients. J Clin Immunol. 2013;33(1):84–95.
41. Franxman TJ, Howe LE, Baker JR. Infliximab for treatment of granulomatous disease in patients with common variable immunodeficiency. J Clin Immunol. 2014;34(7):820–7.
42. Thatayatikom A, Thatayatikom S, White AJ. Infliximab treatment for severe granulomatous disease in common variable immunodeficiency: a case report and review of the literature. Ann Allergy Asthma Immunol. 2005;95(3):293–300.
43. Kainulainen L, Varpula M, Liippo K, Svedström E, Nikoskelainen J, Ruuskanen O. Pulmonary abnormalities in patients with primary hypogammaglobulinemia. J Allergy Clin Immunol. 1999;104(5):1031–6.
44. Svobodova T, Mejstrikova E, Salzer U, Sukova M, Hubacek P, Matej R, et al. Diffuse parenchymal lung disease as first clinical manifestation of GATA-2 deficiency in childhood. BMC Pulm Med. 2015;15(1):8.
45. Chin TW, Stiehm ER, Falloon J, Gallin JI. Corticosteroids in treatment of obstructive lesions of chronic granulomatous disease. J Pediatr. 1987;111(3):349–52.

46. Segal BH, Leto TL, Gallin JI, Malech HL, Holland SM. Genetic, biochemical, and clinical features of chronic granulomatous disease. Medicine. 2000;79(3):170–200.
47. Siddiqui S, Anderson VL, Hilligoss DM, Abinun M, Kuijpers TW, Masur H, et al. Fulminant mulch pneumonitis: an emergency presentation of chronic granulomatous disease. Clin Infect Dis. 2007;45(6):673–81.
48. Tafti SF, Tabarsi P, Mansouri N, Mirsaeidi M, Ghajar MAM, Karimi S, et al. Chronic granulomatous disease with unusual clinical manifestation, outcome, and pattern of inheritance in an Iranian family. J Clin Immunol. 2006;26(3):291–6.
49. Freeman AF, Holland SM. The hyper-IgE syndromes. Immunol Allergy Clin North Am. 2008;28(2):277–91.
50. Shapiro RS. Malignancies in the setting of primary immunodeficiency: implications for hematologists/oncologists. Am J Hematol. 2011;86(1):48–55.
51. Salavoura K, Kolialexi A, Tsangaris G, Mavrou A. Development of cancer in patients with primary immunodeficiencies. Anticancer Res. 2008;28(2B):1263–9.
52. Gatei M, Young D, Cerosaletti KM, Desai-Mehta A, Spring K, Kozlov S, et al. ATM-dependent phosphorylation of nibrin in response to radiation exposure. Nat Genet. 2000;25(1):115.
53. Taylor A, Metcalfe J, Thick J, Mak Y. Leukemia and lymphoma in ataxia telangiectasia. Blood. 1996;87(2):423–38.
54. Cohen JM, Sebire NJ, Harvey J, Gaspar HB, Cathy C, Jones A, et al. Successful treatment of lymphoproliferative disease complicating primary immunodeficiency/immunodysregulatory disorders with reduced-intensity allogeneic stem-cell transplantation. Blood. 2007;110(6):2209–14.
55. Griffith LM, Cowan MJ, Notarangelo LD, Puck JM, Buckley RH, Candotti F, et al. Improving cellular therapy for primary immune deficiency diseases: recognition, diagnosis, and management. J Allergy Clin Immunol. 2009;124(6):1152–60. e12
56. Hill A, Thompson R, Wallwork J, Stableforth D. Heart lung transplantation in a patient with end stage lung disease due to common variable immunodeficiency. Thorax. 1998;53(7):622–3.
57. Yeatman M, McNeil K, Smith JA, Stewart S, Sharples LD, Higenbottam T, et al. Lung transplantation in patients with systemic diseases: an eleven-year experience at Papworth Hospital. J Heart Lung Transplant. 1996;15(2):144–9.
58. Kuo CY, Kohn DB. Gene therapy for the treatment of primary immune deficiencies. Curr Allergy Asthma Rep. 2016;16(5):39.

MIX
Papier aus verantwortungsvollen Quellen
Paper from responsible sources
FSC® C105338

If you have any concerns about our products,
you can contact us on
ProductSafety@springernature.com

In case Publisher is established outside the EU,
the EU authorized representative is:
Springer Nature Customer Service Center GmbH
Europaplatz 3, 69115 Heidelberg, Germany

Printed by Libri Plureos GmbH
in Hamburg, Germany